Tropical Medicine: A Guide for Medical Practitioners

Tropical Medicine: A Guide for Medical Practitioners

Editor: Reginald Thornburg

FOSTER ACADEMICS
www.fosteracademics.com

www.fosteracademics.com

FOSTER ACADEMICS

Cataloging-in-Publication Data

Tropical medicine : a guide for medical practitioners / edited by Reginald Thornburg.
p. cm.
Includes bibliographical references and index.
ISBN 978-1-63242-521-8
1. Tropical medicine. 2. Pharmacology. I. Thornburg, Reginald.
RC961 .T76 2018
616.988 3--dc23

Foster Academics,
118-35 Queens Blvd., Suite 400,
Forest Hills, NY 11375, USA

ISBN 978-1-63242-521-8 (Hardback)

Printed and bound in China.

Contents

Preface

This book was inspired by the evolution of our times; to answer the curiosity of inquisitive minds. Many developments have occurred across the globe in the recent past which has transformed the progress in the field.

Tropical medicine is a field of medicine that deals with the study of diseases and disorders that are unique and are only found in the tropical and sub-tropical regions. The main diseases in this category are ebola virus, malaria, chagas, guinea-worm disease, hookworm, etc. This book unravels the recent studies in the field of tropical medicine. It discusses in detail the various concepts and applications of the field. The topics included in this text on tropical diseases are of utmost significance and are bound to provide incredible insights to the readers. From theories to research to practical applications, case studies related to all contemporary topics of relevance to this field have been included in it. The text will serve as a reference to a broad spectrum of readers.

This book was developed from a mere concept to drafts to chapters and finally compiled together as a complete text to benefit the readers across all nations. To ensure the quality of the content we instilled two significant steps in our procedure. The first was to appoint an editorial team that would verify the data and statistics provided in the book and also select the most appropriate and valuable contributions from the plentiful contributions we received from authors worldwide. The next step was to appoint an expert of the topic as the Editor-in-Chief, who would head the project and finally make the necessary amendments and modifications to make the text reader-friendly. I was then commissioned to examine all the material to present the topics in the most comprehensible and productive format.

I would like to take this opportunity to thank all the contributing authors who were supportive enough to contribute their time and knowledge to this project. I also wish to convey my regards to my family who have been extremely supportive during the entire project.

Editor

1

Child Health in the Peruvian Amazon: Prevalence and Factors Associated with Referred Morbidity and Health Care Access in the City of Iñapari

Maria Gabriela Silva Guimarães,[1] Athos Muniz Braña,[1] Humberto Oliart-Guzmán,[1] Fernando Luiz Cunha Castelo Branco,[1] Breno Matos Delfino,[1] Thasciany Moraes Pereira,[1] Saulo Augusto Silva Mantovani,[1] Antonio Camargo Martins,[1] Ana Paula Santos,[1] José Alcântara Filgueira-Júnior,[1] Alanderson Alves Ramalho,[1] Andreia da Silva Guimarães,[1] Cristieli Sérgio de Menezes Oliveira,[1] Thiago Santos de Araújo,[1] Carlos Hermógenes Manrique de Lara Estrada,[2] Nancy Arróspide,[3] and Mônica da Silva-Nunes[1]

[1] *Centro de Ciências da Saúde e do Desporto, Universidade Federal do Acre, Campus Universitário, BR 364, km 04, Bairro Distrito Industrial, 69920-900 Rio Branco, AC, Brazil*
[2] *Dirección Regional de Salud de Madre de Dios, Avenida Ernesto Rivero N° 475, Puerto Maldonado, Peru*
[3] *Instituto Nacional de Salud, Cápac Yupanqui 1400, Jesus María, 15072 Lima 11, Peru*

Correspondence should be addressed to Mônica da Silva-Nunes; msnunes1@yahoo.com.br

Academic Editor: Marcel Tanner

Introduction. Children under 5 years of age are more susceptible to developing morbidities such as diarrhea, respiratory infections, anemia, and malnutrition. The objective of the study is to evaluate the prevalence of reported morbidities in this age group in the city of Iñapari (Peru) and the access to health services in this municipality. *Methods.* Data collection using interviews that assessed socioeconomic and demographic conditions, child morbidity, and access to health services was performed in 2011. Statistical analysis was performed using SPSS 13.0. *Results.* Regarding morbidities that occurred during lifetime, 39.8% reported previous anemia and intestinal parasite infection. About 53.7% of the children reported any type of morbidities in the last 15 days before interview, being most frequent respiratory symptoms (38.9%), diarrhea (23,4%), and fever (23,1%). Only 63.1% of those reporting recent morbidities sought health care. These morbidities were associated with precarious sanitation and lack of infrastructure, the presence of other comorbidities, and poor access to health services. *Conclusion.* The main referred morbidities in Amazonian Peruvian children were diarrhea, respiratory symptoms, anemia, and vomiting. Incentives and improvements in the health and sanitation conditions would be important measures to improve the quality of life of the Amazonian child population.

1. Introduction

Children under five years of age are an important population group in regard to their physiological and psychosocial development [1]. As a consequence, they are more susceptible to the development of various morbidities, such as diarrhea [2, 3], respiratory infections [2, 4], anemia [5], and malnutrition [4, 6].

Most cases of acute diarrhea and mortality from this disease occur in children under five years of age [2]. This increased prevalence is due to a combination of poor hygiene habits [2], poor sanitation [2, 7], and unfavorable socioeconomic conditions [2, 7].

Respiratory infections are another frequent morbidity in this group [2]. Children suffer the greatest impact from air pollutants [8], increasing the risk of respiratory illness.

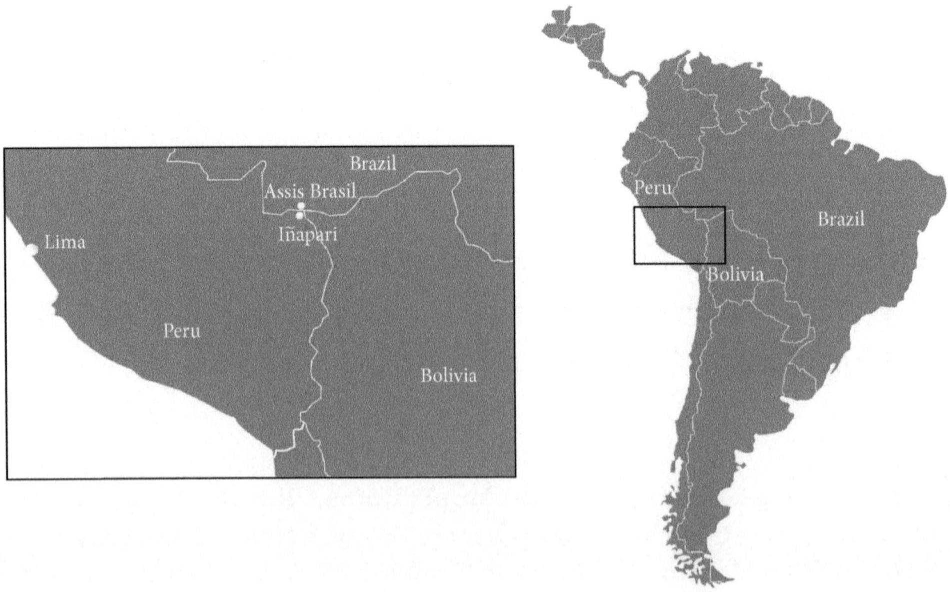

FIGURE 1: Map of Iñapari, Peru.

Additionally, contact with other children in daycare facilities promotes the acquisition of respiratory diseases due to overcrowding and exposure to possible infectious agents.

In relation to anemia, children under five years are the most vulnerable because of their increased need for iron [9], higher nutritional requirements during this period of life [10], their transition in the types of food they intake [10], and a higher susceptibility of the acquisition of intestinal parasites [11].

Malnutrition is an indicator of both health and nutrition [6]. The main causes of malnutrition are inadequate intake of nutrients [5] and infectious diseases [6], specifically respiratory and gastrointestinal diseases.

Since this age group is very susceptible to morbidity, attention must be paid to ensure that these children have access to health services. Provision of prenatal and childbirth care is effective measures in reducing infant mortality [12], as well as access to health care in both routine situations and emergencies.

Peru, located in South America and bordered to the east by Brazil, was ranked 82nd by the Human Development Index (HDI) in 2013 [10]. This is an index that considers wealth, education, and health as proxies for human development. In 2011, 36.19% of visits to Peru's health services were from children under 11 years of age [11]. According to the 2010 National Demographic and Health Census of Peru [4], 17.1% of Peruvian children under five years of age showed symptoms of acute respiratory infection and 14.9% had acute diarrheal disease.

Anemia is also one of the most prevalent nutritional problems in Peru [13]. In 2010, 50.3% of children under three years of age were anemic, with 56.6% being from rural areas [14]. Malnutrition is also a large health problem in Peru [4]. According to the National Institute of Statistics and Informatics (INEI), the prevalence of chronic malnutrition in Peruvian children under five years was 23.2% in 2010 [15].

This study aims to evaluate the prevalence of reported morbidities in children under five years of age in the municipality of Iñapari (Peru) and their access to health services in the municipality.

2. Materials and Methods

This study was conducted in the urban area of Iñapari, a municipality located in the Peruvian Amazon, in the triborder region between Brazil (Assis, Brazil), Bolivia (Bolpebra), and Peru. Iñapari is a district of the Amazon province of Tahuamanu and is located in the Madre de Dios Department (Figure 1). The estimated city population for 2010 was 1,434 people [16].

The study selected as a criterion for inclusion children under 5 years of age, because they are at greater risk of health inequalities and a greater susceptibility to the development of diseases because of that.

Children eligible for the study were identified using a census of households carried out by the health workers of Iñapari, which identified children under the age of five years living in the urban area of the city in 2011.

Data collection for the study took place between January and February 2011 using structured interviews that evaluated the socioeconomic and demographic conditions of the family (family income, maternal/guardian education level, presence of government scholarship, and maternal/guardian paid work in the last 30 or 90 days), household environmental conditions (type of housing construction, predominant material on the floor of the house, presence of electricity, presence of paved street, and type of toilet in the household), peridomestic environmental conditions (garbage collection, flooding of the peridomestic area during rain, and presence of open sewers near the house), water supply and treatment (water supply for domestic use, presence of running water inside the house, and type of water treatment), the child's demographic information (age, sex, and ethnicity), reported infant morbidity (morbidities in the last 15 days, morbidities in the last 12 months, morbidities ever in life, and hospitalization cases), and access to health services (health care, medication). Interviews were conducted by medical students who spoke Spanish, supervised by a Peruvian medical doctor and a Peruvian biologist with a M.S. degree in public health. Interviews were performed with the biological mother, and when she was not present, the biological father or the guardian of the child was interviewed. A few variables contained missing values (one or two unknown responses). The variable "is the child living with the biological father?" was a sensitive question and therefore resulted in a larger number of absences of response. Interviews were conducted by medical students who spoke Spanish, supervised by a Peruvian medical doctor and a Peruvian biologist with a M.S. degree in public health.

For statistical analysis, a database was created using SPSS Version 19.0 software (SPSS Inc., Chicago, IL). The ANOVA test was used to compare means, and Pearson's Chi-square test or Fisher's exact test was used to compare frequencies or proportions at the level of 5%.

The study was approved by the Ethics Committee for Human Research of Acre Federal University (Brazil) and of the Instituto Nacional de Salud (Lima, Peru) (processes 23107.008153/2010-92 UFAC and 2010-CI-59-INS). Informed consent was obtained from the participants in the study or from the parents or legal guardians of the minors prior to the interviews.

3. Results

The study was conducted with all children living in the urban area of the city. There were 108 children under five years of age living in the urban area of Iñapari. Of these, 46.3% were females and 53.7% were males, with a mean age of 2.11 years (standard deviation of 1.36 years and median of 2.24 years). All children were included in the study. Regarding ethnicity, 7.4% declared themselves white, 2.8% indigenous, 38.9% brown ("pardos"), and 50.9% mestizo. Almost all children (93.5%) were living with their biological mother, and 95.6% lived with their biological father. Maternal education was as follows: 68.9% of the mothers had more than eight years of schooling and 1.9% had no schooling (Table 1).

Houses were made predominantly of wood (82.4%), with latrines (67.6%) and unpaved streets or undefined streets (76.9%). Almost half (47.7%) of households reported being in flood-prone areas and 22.2% had open sewage in the peridomestic environment (Table 1).

In the study group, 39.8% of children reported having had some type of morbidity during their lifetime. The most frequently reported morbidities were anemia (23.1%) and intestinal parasites ("worms," 18.5%), and less frequent were wheezing (3.7%) and asthma (2.8%). As for the occurrence of these morbidities in the last 12 months, anemia (20.6%) and intestinal parasites (13%) were still the most frequent

TABLE 1: Epidemiological characteristics of children aged under 5 years, Iñapari, 2011.

Variables (n = 108)	N	%
Characteristics of the child		
Sex		
Male	58	53.7
Female	50	46.3
Mean and median age		
Mean	2.11 Years	—
Median	2.24 Years	—
Age		
<12 months	29	26.9
≥12 and <24 months	22	20.4
≥24 and <36 months	26	24.1
≥36 and <48 months	20	18.5
≥48 and <60 months	11	10.2
Ethnicity		
White	8	7.4
Indigenous	3	2.8
Brown ("Parda")	42	38.9
Mestizo	55	50.9
Maternal figure taking care of the child		
Biological mother	101	93.5
Grandmother	6	5.6
No maternal figure	1	0.9
Years of maternal education*		
0	2	1.9
1–4	6	5.7
5–8	25	23.6
>8	73	68.9
Living with biological father#		
Yes	87	82.9
No	18	17.1
Parental characteristics		
Paternal paid work over the past 30 days****		
No	6	6.0
Yes	94	94.0
Paternal paid work over the past 90 days****		
No	8	8.0
Yes	92	92.0
Maternal paid work over the past 30 days		
No	78	72.9
Yes	29	27.1
Maternal paid work over the past 90 days		
No	77	72.6
Yes	29	27.4

Table 1: Continued.

Variables (n = 108)	N	%
Domestic and peridomestic environment		
Type of household construction		
Predominantly made of brick	19	17.6
Predominantly made of wood	89	82.4
Presence of open sewage near house		
No	84	77.8
Yes	24	22.2
Type of street		
Soil or no street	83	76.9
Brick or asphalt	25	23.1
Type of toilet		
Flushed toilet	35	32.4
Latrine or no toilet	73	67.6
Susceptibility of household to flooding during rain***		
No	56	52.3
Yes	51	47.7
Piped water		
No	9	8.3
Yes, inside home	70	64.8
Yes, out of home	29	26.9
Domestic waste disposal		
Public garbage collection	97	89.8
Buried or burned	6	5.6
Played in the environment (open area or river)	5	4.6
House floor		
Cement, brick ceramic tile	35	32.4
Wood or land	75	67.6
Source of domestic water		
Only public system	83	76.9
Dwelling or public system	23	21.3
Other sources	2	1.9
Treatment of drinking water		
Untreated	9	8.3
Mineral untreated	28	25.9
Boiled and/or filtered and/or chlorinated	61	56.5
Only chlorinated	10	9.3
Presence of electric power		
No	7	6.5
Yes	101	93.5
Receipt of benefits		
No	43	39.8
Yes	65	60.2
Family income##		
Up to half minimum wage	2	1.9
More than half minimum wage	102	98.1

*n = 106, ***n = 107, ****n = 100, #n = 105, and ##n = 104.

Table 2: Frequency of referred morbidities in children under 5 years of age, Iñapari, 2011.

Variables (n = 108)	n	(%)
Morbidities		
Lifetime	43	39.8
Previous 12 months	36	33.3
Anemia		
Lifetime	25	23.1
Previous 12 months*	22	20.6
Intestinal parasites ("worms")		
Lifetime	20	18.5
Previous 12 months*	14	13.0
Wheezing		
Lifetime	4	3.7
Previous 12 months	4	3.7
Asthma		
Lifetime	3	2.8
Previous 12 months	2	1.9
Pneumonia		
Lifetime	7	6.5
Previous 12 months	5	4.6
Hospital admission		
Lifetime	18	16.7

*n = 107.

Table 3: Frequency of referred morbidities in the previous 30 days by children under 5 years of age, Iñapari, 2011.

Variables (n = 108)	n	%
All morbidities	61	56.5
Fever	31	28.7
Weakness	15	13.9
Headache	7	6.5
Lack of appetite	22	20.4
Stomachache*	18	16.8
Nausea*	4	3.7
Vomiting	17	15.7
Diarrhea	24	22.2
Shortness of breath	4	3.7

*n = 107.

morbidities, and less frequent were wheezing (3.7%) and asthma (1.9%) (Table 2).

The prevalence of children who had ever been consulted by a doctor or nurse was 89.8%, and the prevalence of consultation in the last 12 months was 81.5%. Only 16.7% of children were reported to have been hospitalized at least once in their life.

In relation to morbidities occurring in the last 30 days, 56.5% of the children referred to having had some morbidity. The most common were fever (28.7%) and diarrhea (22.2%), and the least common were nausea (3.7%) and shortness of breath (3.7%) (Table 3). Regarding the previous 15 days prior to the interview, 53.7% of children reported some type of morbidity. Respiratory symptoms were the most

TABLE 4: Frequency of referred morbidities in the previous 15 days by children under 5 years of age, Iñapari, 2011.

Variables (n = 108)	n	(%)
Morbidities	**58**	**53.7**
Respiratory symptoms	**42**	**38.9**
Wheezing	5	4.6
Runny nose	24	22.2
Dry cough	16	14.8
Productive cough	18	16.7
Sore throat	20	18.5
*Diarrhea**	**25**	**23.4**
Stool with blood	**1**	**0.9**
Fever	**25**	**23.1**
Vomiting	**17**	**15.7**
Dehydration	**3**	**2.8**
Lack of appetite	**22**	**20.4**
Intestinal parasites ("worm")	**2**	**1.9**
Other diseases	**9**	**8.3**

*n = 107.

TABLE 5: Search and access to health services for children under 5 years who with presented morbidities in the last 15 days, Iñapari, 2011.

Variables	n	Yes (%)
Health care seeking behavior during illness	**36/57**	**63.1**
Received health care when ill	**35/36**	**97.2**
Received drug prescription	**34/35**	**91.1**
Drug acquisition	**34/34**	**100**
Purchased from the public health care system	12/32	37.5
Purchased by the patient at the pharmacy	17/32	53.1
Purchased at the pharmacy by the health service	3/32	9.3

frequent (38.9%) and included wheezing (4.6%), runny nose (22.2%), dry cough (14.8%), productive cough (16.7%), and sore throat (18.5%). Other morbidities were diarrhea (23.4%), fever (23.1%), and vomiting (15.7%) (Table 4).

About 63.1% of children who became ill used the health service, and 97.2% of these had access to health care. A drug prescription was filled in 91.1% of cases, and in these cases the drug was purchased from the public health care system (37.5%), purchased by the patient at the pharmacy (53.1%), or in a few cases purchased at the pharmacy by the health service (9.3%) (Table 5).

For 36.8% of children who did not seek health care for their morbidities, the main reasons for such behavior were that parents did not find it necessary (68.2%), there was lack of time to seek the health service or self-medication was practiced (31.8%), or parents thought there would be no available health care (4.5%).

In Iñapari, 18.5% of the children reported the presence of worms in their lifetime and 13% reported this condition in the last 12 months. There was an association between infection and age (P = 0.006, Chi-square test), showing that, in children older than two years, the prevalence of worms was higher. There was also an association between

TABLE 6: Factors associated with respiratory symptoms in the previous 15 days in children aged under 5 years, 2011.

Variables (n = 108)	Respiratory symptoms			
	n	Yes (%)	No (%)	P value
Diarrhea in the last 15 days				
No	82	30.5	69.5	P = 0.001**
Yes	25	68.0	32.0	
Type of street				
Soil or no street	83	33.7	66.3	P = 0.04**
Brick or asphalt	25	56.0	44.0	
Type of sidewalk				
Soil or no sidewalk	68	30.9	69.1	P = 0.022**
Brick or cement	40	52.5	47.5	
Maternal smoking				
Never smoked	87	34.5	65.5	
Smoker	9	77.8	22.2	P = 0.037*
Former smoker	11	45.5	54.5	

*Chi-square test, **Fisher's exact test.

previous intestinal parasites and no piped water into the household (P = 0.038, Fisher's test) and failure to consult with and/or little follow-up by the health service, confirming the hypothesis of little access to antiparasitic drugs.

Respiratory symptoms in the last 15 days prior to the interview were associated with the presence of diarrhea in the same period of time (P = 0.001, Fisher's test), maternal smoking (P = 0.037, Chi-square test), the type of street the house was located on (brick or asphalt) (P = 0.022, Fisher's test), and the type of sidewalk (brick or cement) (P = 0.022, Fisher's test). All other variables were tested but did not show association. Variables associated with the occurrence of respiratory symptoms are shown in Table 6.

Diarrhea in the last 15 days prior to interview was also associated with the presence of fever (P = 0.018, Fisher's test), vomiting in the last 15 days (P = 0.002, Chi-square test), presence of "stomachache" in the last 30 days (P = 0.002, Chi-square test), and lack of maternal paid work over the past 90 days (P = 0.045, Fisher's test).

When analyzing the presence of diarrhea in a longer period of time (in the 30 days preceding the interview), it was possible to detect an association with other symptoms: fever (P = 0.003, Fisher's test), vomiting (P = 0.047, Chi-square test), and weakness in the last 30 days (P = 0.014, Chi-square test). Some socioeconomic variables were also associated, such as absence of maternal paid work over the past 90 days (P = 0.05, Fisher's test), lack of water piped into the household (P = 0.026, Fisher's test), not boiling water before consumption (P = 0.016, Fisher's test), and having a latrine or no toilet at home (P = 0.049, Fisher's test) (Table 7). All other variables were tested but did not show association. Variables associated with the occurrence of diarrhea in the last 30 days are shown in Table 7.

Factors associated with hospital admission anytime in life are shown in Table 8. Having been hospitalized was significantly more frequent in females, children older than two years, low maternal education, and poor prior access to

TABLE 7: Factors associated with diarrhea in the previous 30 days in children aged under 5 years, Iñapari, 2011.

Variables (n = 108)	Diarrhea			
	n	Yes (%)	No (%)	P value
Maternal paid work over the past 90 days				
No	77	27.3	72.7	$P = 0.05^{**}$
Yes	29	10.3	89.7	
Fever in previous 30 days				
No	77	14.3	85.7	$P = 0.003^{**}$
Yes	31	41.9	58.1	
Weakness in previous 30 days				
No	93	18.3	81.7	$P = 0.014^{*}$
Yes	15	46.7	53.3	
Stomachache in previous 30 days				
No	89	15.7	84.3	$P = 0.001^{*}$
Yes	18	50	50	
Vomiting in previous 30 days				
No	91	18.7	81.3	$P = 0.047^{*}$
Yes	17	41.2	58.2	
Piped water supply in household				
No	38	34.2	65.8	$P = 0.026^{**}$
Yes	70	15.7	84.3	
Source of drinking water				
Various sources	35	11.4	88.6	
Only mineral	22	45.5	54.5	$P = 0.009^{*}$
Only public system	51	19.6	80.4	
Boiling water before consumption				
No	49	32.7	67.3	$P = 0.016^{**}$
Yes	59	13.6	86.4	
Type of toilet				
Flushed toilet	35	11.4	88.6	$P = 0.049^{**}$
Latrine or no toilet	73	27.4	72.6	

*Chi-square test, **Fisher's exact test.

TABLE 8: Factors associated with hospitalization.

Variables (n = 108)	Hospitalization			
	n	Yes (%)	No (%)	P value
Sex				
Male	58	24.1	75.9	$P = 0.022^{**}$
Female	50	8.0	92.0	
Age				
<2 y.o	51	5.9	94.1	$P = 0.004^{**}$
≥2 y.o	57	26.3	73.7	
Years of maternal schooling[1]				
None	2	100.0	0.0	
1 to 4 years	6	16.7	83.3	$P = 0.016^{*}$
5 to 8 years	25	20.0	80.0	
8 years	72	13.9	86.1	
Morbidities during pregnancy[1]				
No	44	27.3	72.7	$P = 0.019^{**}$
Yes	61	9.8	90.2	
Routine health care appointment with medical doctor or nurse in 2010				
No	45	26.7	73.3	$P = 0.019^{**}$
Yes	63	9.5	90.5	
Child health care appointments				
No	13	38.5	61.5	
Yes, once in a while	26	7.7	92.3	$P = 0.011^{*}$
Yes, frequently	28	3.6	96.4	
Only when sick	41	24.4	75.6	

[1] n = 105.
*Chi-square test.
**Fisher exact test.

health care. Children whose mothers did not have morbidities during pregnancy were admitted for hospitalization more frequently than those who did.

4. Discussion

The main recently referred morbidities in this study were diarrhea, fever, vomiting, and respiratory complaints. In relation to morbidity that occurred sometime in their lives, the most frequent were anemia and intestinal parasites.

According to the World Health Organization [17], Brazil and Peru are among the Latin American countries with the highest prevalence of anemia in preschool children. According to the National Institute of Statistics and Informatics, the prevalence of anemia in children under five years of age in Peru was 37.7% in 2010 [4]. The prevalence of anemia was higher in rural areas (45.7%) [4] than in urban areas of the country (33.0%) [4]. In the Department of Madre de Dios, where Iñapari is located, the prevalence of anemia in children was 44.7%, while it was much lower (28.3%) in the Department of Lima [4].

Grantham-McGregor et al. [18] performed a review of 33 studies and found that school and preschool children were more susceptible to the development of anemia and that anemic children had lower income level in relation to nonanemic children.

Zanin et al. [19] found a prevalence rate of anemia of 35.9% in Brazilian children from Minas Gerais, which was associated with iron deficiency, parasitic infections, being at risk of or being a low length/height-for-age, and lower retinol intake. All of these are well-known risk factors for anemia in children.

A review of studies from recent, large population health surveys, carried out in 11 French-speaking African countries (Benin, Burkina Faso, Cameroon, Congo Brazzaville, Ivory Coast, Gabon, Guinea, Mali, Niger, Democratic Republic of Congo, and Senegal) identified factors associated with anemia [20]. Anemia (Hb < 11 g/dL) was found in 72.4% of the children (60.2–87.8%), with no gender difference but a slightly lower incidence in older children (62% at age of 4-5 years versus 85% at age of 9 months). In these countries, anemia was associated with location (rural areas), income (lower quintile), and low maternal education.

In Acre, Brazil, the prevalence of anemia in children under five years of age living in small communities was 57.3% in 2005, and it was primarily associated with nutritional deficiency in this age group [17]. In other municipalities of Acre, including the neighboring city of Assis, Brazil, the prevalence of anemia in children younger than five years of age was 29.2% in 2003, being higher in children under two years of age and also associated with diarrhea [21]. These are similar rates to those found in Iñapari. The prevalence of anemia during the course of life in children under five years of age was 23.1%, and the prevalence in the last 12 months was 20.6%. This is a lower frequency than appointed by National Institute of Statistics and Informatics for Madre de Dios (44.7%) [4]. This difference may be explained because our data is based on referred morbidities, and there might be undiagnosed cases among our study population since anemia is a silent disease in some cases, especially in those who do not seek health services on a regular basis. Anemia was not associated with age in this study, as it was in other studies in Acre [17, 21].

Children are most vulnerable to developing parasitic intestinal infections [22, 23], especially when in contact with other people at home or school, due to a lack of hygiene [2]. Intestinal parasites are also associated with poor socioeconomic [17, 23, 24] and sanitation conditions [23, 24]. According to the National Institute of Statistics and Information (Peru), in 2013 the proportion of people with basic sanitation in the region of Madre de Dios was only 43.8% [25], while those with access to potable water were only 93.1% [22]. These conditions are worse than those found in the Department of Lima, the capital of Peru, where basic sanitation was available to 90.3% of children from this age group and access to potable water was available to 99.3% [22, 23], thus demonstrating a higher exposure of the population of Madre de Dios to poor sanitation and related infectious diseases. In Iñapari, 67.6% of the children had a latrine at home, and 22.2% were living in houses near open sewage. Such associations are reported in children from other developing countries as well [2, 26].

Cha et al. [27] conducted a trial in rural areas of Ghana, to estimate the effects of water treatment in the incidence of diarrhea, adjusting the analysis in the presence of sanitation. The adjusted prevalence ratio of diarrhea in the intervention compared with the control communities was 0.82 (95% CI 0.71–0.96) for Krachi West, 0.95 (0.86–1.04) for Krachi East, and 0.89 (0.82–0.97) for both districts. This study provides a basis for a better approach to water quality interventions.

Data from the National Institute of Statistics and Informatics [4] show that in Peruvian children under five years of age, the prevalence of diarrhea in the last 15 days prior to the interview was 14.9% in 2010, with a higher prevalence in children living in the region of the Peruvian Amazon [4]. In Madre de Dios, the prevalence of diarrhea in the last 15 days in children was 22.4% in 2010 [4], a smaller prevalence than that found in the Department of Lima or on the Peruvian coast (13.9%) [4]. Therefore, the prevalence found in the present study in Iñapari (23.4%) in 2011 is similar to that reported for the whole Peruvian Amazon and higher than reported on the Peruvian coast. One possible cause of this discrepancy may be related to the growing urbanization of the Amazon without adequate infrastructure and sanitation [28].

Diarrhea was mainly associated with unfavorable socioeconomic conditions and poor hygiene habits, such as drinking untreated water. Children who consumed no boiled water had more diarrhea (32.7%) than those that consumed boiled water (13.6%). The same association was found in other Peruvian children [4]. Ochoa et al. [3] also found that in Peruvian children diarrhea was associated with age, breastfeeding, and natural immunity obtained by previous infections.

In Tanzania, diarrhea was associated with unfavorable socioeconomic conditions, younger age, and lack of toilet at home [24]. In Ghana, data from 3466 children showed that diarrhea was associated with household wealth quintiles, child sex and age, being the poorer, male children, and younger children more likely to have diarrhea [29].

A study with 348,706 children from 40 nations found that the prevalence of acute diarrhea was 14% [30]. The main factors associated with child diarrhea were poor household wealth and mother's lack of education. Other factors associated with diarrhea were female sex of the child, age of the child, immunization status, maternal age, and working status of the mother.

A large case-control hospital-based study conducted in Brazil [31] showed that lack of adequate excreta disposal (PAF = 12%), untreated drinking water (PAF = 11%), and a history of previous hospitalization due to acute diarrhea (PAF = 21%) were the main factors attributed to hospitalization due to diarrhea. Low socioeconomic conditions, no public water supply, crowding, and low weight-for-age were of less but still significant importance [31].

A study with 5,828 indigenous Brazilian children found an overall prevalence of recent diarrhea of 23.5%, being the highest rate in the North of the country (38.1%). Higher risk of diarrhea was observed among younger children and those who had less maternal schooling, lower household socioeconomic status, undernutrition (weight-for-age deficit), presence of another child with diarrhea in the household, and occurrence of upper respiratory infection [32].

The diarrheal process may be associated with other clinical manifestations such as fever, vomiting, and abdominal pain, as shown by other studies [33–35]. These clinical manifestations can suggest possible infectious agents involved in gastroenteritis [36], such as *Rotavirus*, *E. coli*, *Shigella*, and *Salmonella* species.

Intervention studies focusing on education about how to prevent infant diarrhea were conducted with 600 mothers in Egypt [37]. Results showed that knowledge of mothers about diarrhea (etiological factors and preventive measures) had improved significantly after the intervention and that health and nutrition education sessions were successful in improving mothers' knowledge regarding preventive measures and management of diarrhea. A meta-analysis of 22 randomized clinical trials conducted in low- and middle-income countries found that hand washing promotion probably reduces diarrhea episodes in both child daycare centers in high-income countries and among communities living in LMICs by about 30% [38]. Such measurements could be implemented by health care workers in other countries, such as Peru, in order to reduce the incidence of diarrhea in young children.

The second most prevalent morbidity in Iñapari was respiratory disease. In a study conducted in Brazilian nurseries, Pedraza et al. [2] showed that acute respiratory disease is a group of important diseases in children, as they are more vulnerable due to the immaturity of the immune system and their rapid growth. Heymann et al. [36] comment that, in the United States, hospital admission still continues to be a significant health care problem for children.

In Iñapari, the prevalence of respiratory symptoms in the last 15 days was 38.9%. In the country as a whole, the prevalence of respiratory disease in the last 15 days in children under five years of age in 2010 was 17.1%, in the Madre de Dios region it was 15.4%, and it was 18.3% in the region of Lima, suggesting a relationship between respiratory symptoms and the degree of urbanization of the area [4]. This difference in prevalence may also be the result of differences in the concept of respiratory disease among the studies. In the approach adopted by INEI [4] in Peru, the concept of respiratory disease was reported as illness associated with the presence of fast and/or troubled breathing, while, in the study in Iñapari, respiratory symptoms were defined as the occurrence of one or more symptoms such as wheezing, runny nose, cough (dry or productive), or sore throat.

Brauer et al. [39] found association of respiratory symptoms of children to environmental pollution in The Netherlands. In this study, the prevalence of respiratory symptoms was different from one region to another suggesting that regions with greater development and urbanization had higher incidence of children with respiratory symptoms, corroborating the findings in Peruvian children described above.

The association found in Iñapari between child respiratory symptoms and having tobacco users at home has been documented in previous studies [34, 36]. Gonçalves-Silva et al. [40] showed that not only can parental smoking be associated with child respiratory symptoms, but also smoking by any other resident of the household. In Iñapari, the frequency of respiratory symptoms in children whose mothers were smokers was 77.8%, while, in the study by Gonçalves-Silva et al. [40], it was 65.6%.

A review of studies from 11 French-speaking African countries also found that respiratory disease and diarrhea are common in children under 5 years of age. In the study countries, acute respiratory diseases and diarrhea affected 6.2 and 15.6% of children aged between 6 and 59 months, respectively [20].

In India, a community-based cross-sectional study found an overall prevalence of acute respiratory infections of 59.1%, which was associated with overcrowding (adjusted odds ratio (AOR) = 1.492), urban residence (AOR = 2.329), and second birth order (AOR = 0.371) [41].

Data from the Peruvian Ministry of Health [42] showed a hospitalization rate of 3.03 per 100 inhabitants in the general population in 2010. Influenza (flu) and pneumonia accounted for the largest amount of hospitalization cases in that year [43]. In Madre de Dios, in the Peruvian Amazon, intestinal infections prevailed in relation to influenza and pneumonia as a cause of hospitalization in the general population in the same year [44]. In Iñapari, hospitalization of children under five years of age was mainly due to diarrhea and other intestinal diseases, confirming the data obtained by the Ministry of Health in the region.

Shay et al. [45] estimated that 84,000 to 144,000 hospitalization cases due to lower respiratory tract disease occur annually in the USA in children under 5 years of age.

In the study of Quigley et al. [46], conducted in the UK, approximately 12% of children in the first eight months of age were hospitalized at least once. The most common causes of hospitalization were infection of the lower respiratory tract (3.2%) and diarrhea (1.1%). The study demonstrated a related protection factor to breastfeeding for hospitalization of protection related to injury.

Factors associated with child hospitalization in Iñapari were related to child age and sex, socioeconomic characteristics, and access to health care. Children whose mothers had no formal education or low education were more likely to have been hospitalized. Macedo et al. [47] also found that child hospitalization increased when maternal education was low. In Iñapari, male children had a higher frequency of hospitalization (26.3%), a finding that was reported in other studies such as Macedo et al. [47], with 53.3%, and Caetano et al. [48], with 56.9%.

Also, the frequency of hospitalization was higher in children older than 2 years (26.3%) than in those younger than 2 years (5.9%). This could be explained by the fact that as time goes by, there are more chances to get sick. The association between age and hospitalization was also described in other studies Bittencourt et al. [49] found that hospitalization was higher in children younger than six months (60.3% in public hospitals and 47.3% in private hospitals), while Caetano et al. [48] found that hospitalization was higher in children younger than 1 year (47.7%). Differences in methodology and population characteristics can explain these differences in results.

A study in rural Tanzania showed that children aged two years and older were more likely than children under one year of age to receive care at home, rather than to receive care at the health facility. Also, children aged two years and older were less likely to experience morbidity than children under one year [35].

Caetano et al. [48] describe a frequency of 56.9% of child hospitalization in children younger than 5 years, being the main causes of respiratory and parasitic diseases.

In other Latin American countries, diarrhea and respiratory diseases are also a public health problem in childhood. In Haiti, respiratory diseases accounted for 9183 (29%) hospitalization cases and 301 (17%) deaths between 2011 and 2013. Children aged 6–23 months had the highest percentage of hospitalization cases attributable to respiratory diseases (38%), whereas children aged 36–47 months had the highest proportion of deaths attributable to respiratory diseases (37%). Diarrheal diseases accounted for 8063 (26%) hospitalization cases and 224 (13%) deaths. Children aged 6–11 months had the highest percentage of diarrhea-associated hospitalization cases (39%) and deaths (29%) [50].

The occurrence of morbidity during pregnancy was inversely associated with child hospitalization. About 27.3% of children with no history of maternal morbidity during pregnancy were hospitalized at some point during life, while only 9.8% of those without maternal history of gestational morbidity had a hospitalization. This could be explained by a modified maternal behavior in child care after a gestational morbidity, leading to improved maternal care or more access to health services during pregnancy and after birth.

Children with poor health access after birth were also more likely to have a hospitalization. About 26.7% of those without a medical appointment in the previous year had hospitalization, against only 9.5% of those who attended a medical appointment in the previous year. Hospitalization cases were more frequent in children who seek health care services only when sick or who never sought health services.

Access to health care was high in Iñapari when the child was sick but lower for routine consultations. It is known that health service usage usually varies according to the degree of economic development of an area or region [51], and it can also be different in urban and in rural areas [52]. According to Pêssoa [53], consultations and physical exams are more complete in Iñapari than in the neighboring Brazilian city of Assis, but the working conditions for health care personnel and the diagnostic infrastructure are worse, with low salaries and lack of diagnostic exams. Another important difference is that in Peru access to consults and medication within the health service require payment [53], while in Brazil these are free.

This study has some strengths and weaknesses. It has the merit of being a population-based census on child health performed in the Peruvian Amazon, which is usually an understudied type of population because of the difficult physical access. Interviews were performed in Spanish by Peruvian researchers, and one of them was living in the Peruvian Amazon, so it was performed by personnel that were used to the habits and local culture, facilitating the interviews. The limitations of the study are that since it was a small community, the number of children was small and some associations may have not been identified. Also, because it was based on referred morbidities, there may be some degree of recall bias which could not be avoided.

5. Conclusion

This study showed that the main morbidities in children referred to the Iñapari municipality were related to diarrheal morbidity, respiratory symptoms, anemia, and vomiting. There was an association of these morbidities referred to as low socioeconomic conditions, precarious sanitation, and the presence of other comorbidities. Measurements to reduce morbidity and promote child health in such small Peruvian Amazonian communities would be improvements in sanitary infrastructure, water treatment, educational programs on child health for targeted families, and a more comprehensive health care with lower costs. Another important point is that free care is not always provided in Peru, which may hinder access to health care for some children. Health policies that target free universal care for infants at risk may help promote child health in this part of the Amazon.

Disclosure

The authors state that the results of the paper are not plagiarism and have not been published elsewhere.

Conflict of Interests

The authors declare they have no conflict of interests.

Acknowledgments

The authors thank the population that participated in the study for their collaboration. They also thank the local health and government authorities for their help and the health workers that helped identifying the houses included in the study. They thank staff at the Virology Laboratory at University of Sao Paulo for their help with technical issues in the serology tests. This work was supported by the Federal University of Acre (UFAC, Brazil) and Technological Foundation of Acre (FUNTAC, Brazil) through the "Research Program for SUS Announcement MS/CNPq/FDCT-FUNTAC/SESACRE nos. 01/09 and 01/10" (Statement of Grants 04/2010 and 11/2010). Research fellowships were provided by the National Research Council (CNPq, Brazil) and UFAC.

References

[1] Y. R. Gandra, "O pré-escolar de dois a seis anos de idade e o seu atendimento," *Revista de Saúde Pública*, vol. 15, supplement, pp. 3–8, 1981.

[2] D. F. Pedraza, D. Queiroz, and M. C. Sales, "Doenças infecciosas em crianças pré-escolares brasileiras assistidas em creches," *Ciência & Saúde Coletiva*, vol. 19, no. 2, pp. 511–528, 2014.

[3] T. J. Ochoa, E. H. Mercado, D. Durand et al., "Frecuencia y patotipos de *Escherichia coli* diarrogénicas en niños peruanos con y sin diarrea," *Revista Peruana de Medicina Experimental y Salud Pública*, vol. 28, no. 1, pp. 13–20, 2011.

[4] Instituto Nacional de Estadística e Informática, *Encuesta Demográfica y de Salud Familiar (ENDES)*, Instituto Nacional de Estadística e Informática (INEI), Lima, Peru, 2010, http://proyectos.inei.gob.pe/endes/endes2010/resultados/index.html.

[5] S. Fontoura, J. Coser, T. Fontoura, A. Assmann, A. Azevedo, and C. Rizzi, "Prevalência de anemia em crianças de 1 a 5 anos moradoras do bairro Passo, Vila Arneldo Matter—São Borja/RS e sua relação com estado nutricional e enteroparasitoses," *Revista Brasileira de Análises Clínicas*, vol. 41, no. 2, pp. 103–108, 2009.

[6] J. Sanchez-Abanto, "Evolución de la desnutrición crónica en menores de cinco años en el Perú," *Revista Peruana de Medicina Experimental y Salud Pública*, vol. 29, no. 3, pp. 402–405, 2015.

[7] N. V. Toscani, A. J. D. S. Santos, L. L. M. Silva et al., "Desenvolvimento e análise de jogo educativo para crianças visando à prevenção de doenças parasitológicas," *Interface*, vol. 11, no. 22, pp. 281–294, 2007.

[8] M. R. C. Farias, A. M. Rosa, S. D. S. Hacon, H. A. Castro, and E. Ignotti, "Prevalência de asma em escolares de Alta Floresta—município ao sudeste da Amazônia Brasileira," *Revista Brasileira de Epidemiologia*, vol. 13, no. 1, pp. 49–57, 2010.

[9] R. E. Jordão, J. L. D. Bernardi, and A. de Azevedo Barros Filho, "Prevalência de anemia ferropriva no Brasil: uma revisão sistemática," *Revista Paulista de Pediatria*, vol. 27, no. 1, pp. 90–98, 2009.

[10] Programa das Nações Unidas para o Desenvolvimento (PNUD), *Índice de Desenvolvimento Humano*, Programa das Nações Unidas para o Desenvolvimento (PNUD), 2013, http://www.pnud.org.br/atlas/ranking/Ranking-IDH-Global-2013.aspx.

[11] Ministerio de Salud, *Oficina General de Estadística e Informática (Base de Datos HIS)*, Ministerio de Salud, Lima, Peru, 2013, http://www.minsa.gob.pe/estadisticas/estadisticas/Servicios/Atenciones/ATENCIONESMacros.asp?00.

[12] A. Dammert, *Acceso a los Servicios de Salud y Mortalidad Infantil en el Perú*, CIES-GRADE, Lima, Peru, 2001, http://www.grade.org.pe/download/pubs/cies-ib18-ad.pdf.

[13] Perú Instituto Nacional de Estadística e Informática, *Encuesta demográfica y de salud familiar (ENDES)*, INEI, Lima, Peru, 2010, http://proyectos.inei.gob.pe/endes/images/PERU_Ind_Salud_materno_Infantil.pdf.

[14] Instituto Nacional de Estadística e Informática, *Encuesta demográfica y de salud familiar (ENDES)*, INEI, Lima, Peru, 2010, http://www.app.minsa.gob.pe/bsc/Detalle_IndBSC.asp?lcind=8&lcobj=2&lcper=1&lcfreg=8/9/2014.

[15] Instituto Nacional de Estadística e Informática, *Encuesta demográfica y de salud familiar (ENDES)*, INEI, Lima, Peru, 2010, http://www.minsa.gob.pe/estadisticas/estadisticas/indicadoresSalud/socioeconomicos/desnutricion/DESMacros.asp.

[16] Instituto Nacional de Estadística y Informática, *Censos Nacionales 2007, XI de Población y VI de Vivienda*, INEI, Lima, Peru, 2010, http://censos.inei.gob.pe/censos2007/documentos/Resultado_CPV2007.pdf.

[17] C. S. de Menezes Oliveira, M. A. Cardoso, T. S. de Araújo, and P. T. Muniz, "Anemia em crianças de 6 a 59 meses e fatores associados no Município de Jordão, Estado do Acre, Brasil," *Cadernos de Saúde Pública*, vol. 27, no. 5, pp. 1008–1020, 2011.

[18] S. Grantham-McGregor, Y. B. Cheung, S. Cueto, P. Glewwe, L. Richter, and B. Strupp, "Developmental potential in the first 5 years for children in developing countries," *The Lancet*, vol. 369, no. 9555, pp. 60–70, 2007.

[19] F. H. C. Zanin, C. A. M. da Silva, É. Bonomo et al., "Determinants of iron deficiency anemia in a cohort of children aged 6–71 months living in the Northeast of Minas Gerais, Brazil," *PLoS ONE*, vol. 10, no. 10, Article ID e0139555, 2015.

[20] S. Diouf, M. Folquet, K. Mbofung et al., "Prevalence and determinants of anemia in young children in French-speaking Africa. Role of iron deficiency," *Archives de Pédiatrie*, 2015.

[21] T. G. Castro, M. Silva-Nunes, W. L. Conde, P. T. Muniz, and M. A. Cardoso, "Anemia e deficiência de ferro em pré-escolares da Amazônia Ocidental brasileira: prevalência e fatores associados," *Cadernos de Saúde Pública*, vol. 27, no. 1, pp. 131–142, 2011.

[22] Perú Ministerio de Salud, Instituto Nacional de Estadística e Informática, INEI, Lima, Peru, 2013, http://www.app.minsa.gob.pe/bsc/detalle_indbsc.asp?lcind=79&lcobj=15&lcper=12&lcfreg=8/9/2014.

[23] L. A. Marcos Raymundo, V. Maco, A. Terashima et al., "Prevalencia de parasitosis intestinal en niños del valle del Mantaro, Jauja, Perú," *Revista Medica Herediana*, vol. 13, no. 3, pp. 85–90, 2002.

[24] J. Gascón, M. Vargas, D. Schellenberg et al., "Diarrhea in children under 5 years of age from Ifakara, tanzania: a case-control study," *Journal of Clinical Microbiology*, vol. 38, no. 12, pp. 4459–4462, 2000.

[25] Ministerio de Salud, *Instituto Nacional de Estadística e Informática*, INEI, Lima, Peru, 2013, http://www.app.minsa.gob.pe/bsc/detalle_indbsc.asp?lcind=95&lcobj=15&lcper=12&lcfreg=8/9/2014.

[26] S. H. Komagome, M. P. de Melo Romagnoli, I. T. S. Previdelli, D. L. M. Falavigna, M. L. G. G. Dias, and M. L. Gomes, "Fatores de risco para infecção parasitária intestinal em crianças e funcionários de creche," *Ciência, Cuidado e Saúde*, vol. 6, supplement 2, pp. 442–447, 2007, http://periodicos.uem.br/ojs/index.php/CiencCuidSaude/article/download/5354/3391.

[27] S. Cha, D. Kang, B. Tuffuor et al., "The effect of improved water supply on diarrhea prevalence of children under five in the Volta region of Ghana: a cluster-randomized controlled trial," *International Journal of Environmental Research and Public Health*, vol. 12, no. 10, pp. 12127–12143, 2015.

[28] F. A. Carvalho-Costa, A. Q. Gonçalves, S. L. Lassance, L. M. da Silva Neto, C. A. A. Salmazo, and M. N. Bóia, "*Giardia lamblia* and other intestinal parasitic infections and their relationships with nutritional status in children in Brazilian Amazon," *Revista do Instituto de Medicina Tropical de São Paulo*, vol. 49, no. 3, pp. 147–153, 2007.

[29] A. Kumi-Kyereme and J. Amo-Adjei, "Household wealth, residential status and the incidence of diarrhoea among children under-five years in Ghana," *Journal of Epidemiology and Global Health*, 2015.

[30] Á. M. Pinzón-Rondón, C. Zárate-Ardila, A. Hoyos-Martínez, Á. M. Ruiz-Sternberg, and A. Vélez-van-Meerbeke, "Country characteristics and acute diarrhea in children from developing nations: a multilevel study," *BMC Public Health*, vol. 15, no. 1, article 811, 2015.

[31] M. Y. Ichihara, L. C. Rodrigues, C. A. Santos, G. Teixeira Mda, and M. L. Barreto, "Risk factors for hospital admission of Brazilian children with non-rotavirus diarrhoea: a case control-study," *Transactions of the Royal Society of Tropical Medicine and Hygiene*, vol. 109, no. 7, pp. 454–461, 2015.

[32] A. L. Escobar, C. E. Coimbra Jr., J. R. Welch, B. L. Horta, R. V. Santos, and A. M. Cardoso, "Diarrhea and health inequity among indigenous children in Brazil: results from the First National Survey of Indigenous People's Health and Nutrition," *BMC Public Health*, vol. 15, no. 1, article 191, 2015.

[33] E. A. Waldman, R. d. C. B. Barata, J. C. Moraes, I. A. Guibu, and M. d. Timenetsky, "Gastroenterites e infecções respiratórias agudas em crianças menores de 5 anos, em área da região Sudeste do Brasil, 1986-1987: II—Diarréias," *Revista de Saúde Pública*, vol. 31, no. 1, pp. 62–70, 1997.

[34] E. C. Souza, M. B. Martinez, C. R. Taddei et al., "Perfil etiológico das diarréias agudas de crianças atendidas em São Paulo," *Jornal de Pediatria*, vol. 78, no. 1, pp. 31–38, 2002.

[35] A. M. Kanté, H. R. Gutierrez, A. M. Larsen et al., "Childhood illness prevalence and health seeking behavior patterns in rural Tanzania," *BMC Public Health*, vol. 15, no. 1, article 951, 2015.

[36] P. W. Heymann, H. T. Carper, D. D. Murphy et al., "Viral infections in relation to age, atopy, and season of admission among children hospitalized for wheezing," *Journal of Allergy and Clinical Immunology*, vol. 114, no. 2, pp. 239–247, 2004.

[37] S. B. Abdel-Aziz, M. A. Mowafy, and Y. S. Galal, "Assessing the impact of a community-based health and nutrition education on the management of diarrhea in an urban district, Cairo, Egypt," *Global Journal of Health Science*, vol. 8, no. 2, Article ID 46619, 2015.

[38] R. I. Ejemot-Nwadiaro, J. E. Ehiri, D. Arikpo, M. M. Meremikwu, and J. A. Critchley, "Hand washing promotion for preventing diarrhoea," *Cochrane Database of Systematic Reviews*, no. 9, Article ID CD004265, 2015.

[39] M. Brauer, G. Hoek, P. van Vliet et al., "Air pollution from traffic and the development of respiratory infections and asthmatic and allergic symptoms in children," *American Journal of Respiratory and Critical Care Medicine*, vol. 166, no. 8, pp. 1092–1098, 2002.

[40] R. M. Gonçalves-Silva, J. G. Valente, M. G. Lemos-Santos, and R. Sichieri, "Tabagismo no domicílio e doença respiratória em crianças menores de cinco anos," *Cadernos de Saúde Pública*, vol. 22, no. 3, pp. 579–586, 2006.

[41] G. S. Kumar, A. Majumdar, V. Kumar, B. N. Naik, K. Selvaraj, and K. Balajee, "Prevalence of acute respiratory infection among under-five children in urban and rural areas of puducherry, India," *Journal of Natural Science, Biology and Medicine*, vol. 6, no. 1, pp. 3–6, 2015.

[42] Ministerio de Salud, *Base de Datos Egresos Hospitalarios del Ministerio de Salud*, Ministerio de Salud, Lima, Peru, 2013, http://www.app.minsa.gob.pe/BSC/DETALLE_INDBSC.ASP?LCIND=82&LCOBJ=14&LCPER=11&LCFREG=18/7/2014.

[43] Ministerio de Salud, *Base de Datos del Ministerio de Salud*, Ministerio de Salud, Lima, Peru, 2013, http://www.minsa.gob.pe/ESTADISTICAS/ESTADISTICAS/MORBILIDAD/HSMACROS.ASP?00.

[44] Perú Ministerio de Salud, *Base de datos del Ministerio de Salud*, Perú Ministerio de Salud, Lima, Peru, 2013, http://www.minsa.gob.pe/ESTADISTICAS/ESTADISTICAS/MORBILIDAD/HSMACROS.ASP?17.

[45] D. K. Shay, R. C. Holman, R. D. Newman, L. L. Liu, J. W. Stout, and L. J. Anderson, "Bronchiolitis-associated hospitalizations among US children, 1980–1996," *Journal of the American Medical Association*, vol. 282, no. 15, pp. 1440–1446, 1999.

[46] M. A. Quigley, Y. J. Kelly, and A. Sacker, "Breastfeeding and hospitalization for diarrheal and respiratory infection in the United Kingdom millennium cohort study," *Pediatrics*, vol. 119, no. 4, pp. e837–e842, 2007.

[47] S. E. C. Macedo, A. M. B. Menezes, E. Albernaz, P. Post, and M. Knorst, "Fatores de risco para internação por doença respiratória aguda em crianças até um ano de idade," *Revista de Saúde Pública*, vol. 41, no. 3, pp. 351–358, 2007.

[48] J. R. M. Caetano, I. A. S. Bordin, R. F. Puccini, and C. D. A. Peres, "Fatores associados à internação hospitalar de crianças menores de cinco anos, São Paulo, SP," *Revista de Saúde Pública*, vol. 36, no. 3, pp. 285–291, 2002.

[49] S. A. Bittencourt, M. C. Leal, and M. O. Santos, "Hospitalizações por diarréia infecciosa no Estado do Rio de Janeiro," *Cadernos de Saúde Pública*, vol. 18, no. 3, pp. 747–775, 2002.

[50] K. Vinekar, N. Schaad, M. A. Ber Lucien et al., "Hospitalizations and deaths because of respiratory and diarrheal diseases among Haitian children under five years of age, 2011-2013," *The Pediatric Infectious Disease Journal*, vol. 34, no. 10, pp. e238–e243, 2015.

[51] C. Travassos, E. X. de Oliveira, and F. Viacava, "Desigualdades geográficas e sociais no acesso aos serviços de saúde no Brasil: 1998 e 2003," *Ciência & Saúde Coletiva*, vol. 11, no. 4, pp. 975–986, 2006.

[52] J. M. Ribeiro, S. A. Siqueira, and L. F. Pinto, "Avaliação da atenção à saúde da criança (0–5 anos) no PSF de Teresópolis (RJ) segundo a percepção dos usuários," *Ciência & Saúde Coletiva*, vol. 15, no. 2, pp. 517–527, 2010.

[53] I. N. Pêssoa, *Saúde e modos de vida em contexto amazônicos: Brasil, Peru e Bolívia [Tese de Doutorado]*, Universidade de São Paulo, São Paulo, Brazil, 2014, http://www.teses.usp.br/teses/disponiveis/6/6136/tde-02042014-114236/pt-br.php.

2

End Stage Renal Disease: Seroprevalence of Hepatitises B and C along with Associated Aetiology and Risk Factors in Children

Syed Raza Shah, Muhammad Shahzeb Khan, Muhammad Tanveer Alam, Adnan Salim, Mehwish Hussain, and Areeba Altaf

Dow University of Health Sciences (DUHS), Baba e Urdu Road, Karachi 75500, Pakistan

Correspondence should be addressed to Syed Raza Shah; syedraza91shah@live.com

Academic Editor: Aditya Prasad Dash

Background. End Stage Renal Disease (ESRD) normally requires dialysis or transplantation for survival. Since ESRD patients are on long term dialysis, infections such as Hepatitis B (HBV) and Hepatitis C (HCV) are commonly reported. *Methods.* This was a retrospective study carried out at a government hospital during a 12-month period from January 2013 to December 2013. The data was collected using a predesigned pro forma to note the etiology, gender, age, and HBsAg and anti-HCV test result of each patient. *Results.* 444 children suffering from ESRD were included in our analysis. The mean age of sample was 12.7 ± 4.1 years. Sixty percent (n = 262) of the children were boys. The most common etiology of ESRD was kidney stones (n = 44, 29.3%). HBV was positive in 11 children (2.5%) while HCV was positive in 13 (2.9%). *Conclusion.* This study asserts the need for carrying out further work to confirm these findings and expand our recommendations. It is imperative to reliably determine the burden of HBV and HCV disease and to determine the aetiology of their spread especially in children with ESRD.

1. Introduction

End Stage Renal Disease (ESRD), the stage 5 of chronic kidney disease, normally requires dialysis or transplantation for survival. The burden of ESRD in children is lesser as compared with adults; however, if ESRD occurs in children, consequences can be catastrophic. It should be pointed out that children on dialysis have 30 to 150 times higher mortality rates compared with the general children population [1]. Children with ESRD end up dying from variety of causes such as cardiovascular diseases, life threatening infections, and malignancy [2].

Since ESRD patients are on long term dialysis, infections such as Hepatitis B (HBV) and Hepatitis C (HCV) are commonly reported. HBV is a major cause of mortality in such patients [3]. Although vaccination has significantly reduced mortality rates, dialysis can shorten the duration of immunity against HBV by lowering the protective antibody levels in children who were vaccinated as infants [3, 4]. Moreover, the duration of dialysis has high predictive risk for HCV infections. This was consistent with a study in which all patients who were anti-HCV positive had been on dialysis for a mean of 105 months [5]. Furthermore, a study also reported a steady rise of the HCV antibody titres in children during the period of dialysis treatment [6]. This may be due to the number of blood transfusions at the time of haemodialysis which has been shown to be a significant risk of HCV infection [7].

Many studies have been conducted to determine the rate of HBV and HCV infections among the paediatric ESRD population. For instance a study conducted in Saudi Arabia showed that the prevalence of anti-HCV in children with ESRD was 45% compared with the prevalence of 1% among the controls [3]. Similarly, another study showed that the prevalence (11.2%) of anti-HCV was much higher in children with chronic renal disease. A study conducted back in 1985 on patients aged between 2 and 18 years with chronic renal failure showed a seroprevalence of 66.7% for HBsAg [8].

Not much data is available on this subject from our part of the world due to nonexistence of a centralized registry. While the incidence of ESRD in the United States is declining (a 5.8% decrease in 2012), it continues to be rising in Pakistan, with an estimated annual incidence of >100 new cases per million population [9, 10]. Epidemiological data on HBV and

HCV infection is therefore important for strategies to tackle the spread of the disease. Moreover, it is imperative to reliably determine the burden of HBV and HCV disease, to determine the etiology of spread especially in children with ESRD, to identify any areas with higher endemicity than the rest of the country and to understand the risk factors associated with its transmission. The primary objective of our study was to determine the frequency rate of HBsAg and anti-HCV among children with ESRD while the secondary objective was to determine the etiology, gender, and age groups that are predominantly infected.

2. Methods

This was a retrospective study carried out at a government hospital during a 12-month period from January 2013 to December 2013. All subjects' information was kept confidential and a written informed consent was obtained from each participant. All ethical responsibilities were met in accordance with Helmshki law. Since our government hospital is located in the center of the city where people come from all over the city, a good representative sample of the entire city was collected and analyzed.

The sample population included all those children under the age of 18 years who were documented cases of ESRD. ESRD was defined as individuals with a glomerular filtration rate (GFR) of $<15\,\mathrm{mL/min/1.73\,m^2}$ or with signs and symptoms of kidney failure. The latter included patients who were currently on dialysis or patients who underwent transplantation.

Blood samples were collected. HBsAg and anti-HCV were tested by in vitro immunochromatographic one step assay designed for qualitative determination. The data was collected using a predesigned pro forma to note the aetiology, gender, age, and HBsAg and anti-HCV test result of each subject. Data was collected by three investigators who were also coauthors of the study. After explaining the purpose of the study, each participant was asked to fill the consent form. Two independent authors queried the data from the database to ensure no error was made. The results were cross verified among the 2 authors to ensure integrity of data. Any discrepancy was solved through mutual consensus.

2.1. Statistical Analysis. IBM SPSS v. 21 (SPSS Inc., Illinois, US) was used to analyze the data. Mean ± standard deviation was computed to describe continuous variable. Age was classified into 3 categories, namely, 1–9 years, 10–14 years, and 15–18 years. Frequencies and percentages were calculated for presenting categorical variables such as demographic profile and clinical status of patients. Age based stratified analysis was also performed to observe pattern of clinical profile among ESRD children.

3. Results

Our sample population consisted of 444 children suffering from ESRD. The mean age of children was 12.7 ± 4.1 years. 20% (n = 91) of the children were less than 10 years of age while 39% (n = 174) were in the age group 15–18 (Table 1). 60% (n = 262) of the children were boys. The reason for ESRD was known for 33.8% (n = 150) patients only (Figure 1). The most common known aetiology of ESRD was kidney stones (n = 44, 29.3%), followed by small shrunken kidneys (n = 28, 19%) (Table 2).

HBV was positive in 11 children (2.5%) while HCV was positive in 13 (2.9%) (Table 2). The proportion of HBV positivity was found to be 1.1% (n = 1) among children less than 10 years. This proportion was higher in children with the age groups 10–14 and 15–18 years with 2.8% (n = 5) and 2.9% (n = 5), respectively. On the other hand, HCV was positive in 2.2% (n = 2), 1.7% (n = 3), and 4.6% (n = 8) of the children aged 1–9 years, 10–14 years, and 15–18 years, respectively (Table 3).

TABLE 1: Demographic profile of ESRD children.

	Frequency	Percentage
Age groups (years)		
<1	0	0%
1–9	91	20.5%
10–14	179	40.3%
15–18	174	39.2%
Gender		
Male	262	59.0%
Female	182	41.0%
Province		
Sindh	216	48.6%
Punjab	53	11.9%
KPK	9	2.0%
Baluchistan	24	5.4%
Karachi	137	30.9%
Others	5	1.1%

TABLE 2: Clinical status of ESRD children.

	Frequency	Percentage
Aetiology		
Unknown	294	66.2%
Stone	44	9.9%
Nephrotic	22	5.0%
Glomerulonephritis (nephritic)	22	5.0%
Obstructive uropathy	9	2.0%
SSK (small shrunken kidneys)	28	6.3%
Others (Wilms, BOO, gastroenteritis, etc.)	22	5.0%
VUR (vesicoureteral reflux)	3	.7%
Hepatitis B		
Positive	11	2.5%
Negative	433	97.5%
Hepatitis C		
Positive	13	2.9%
Negative	431	97.1%

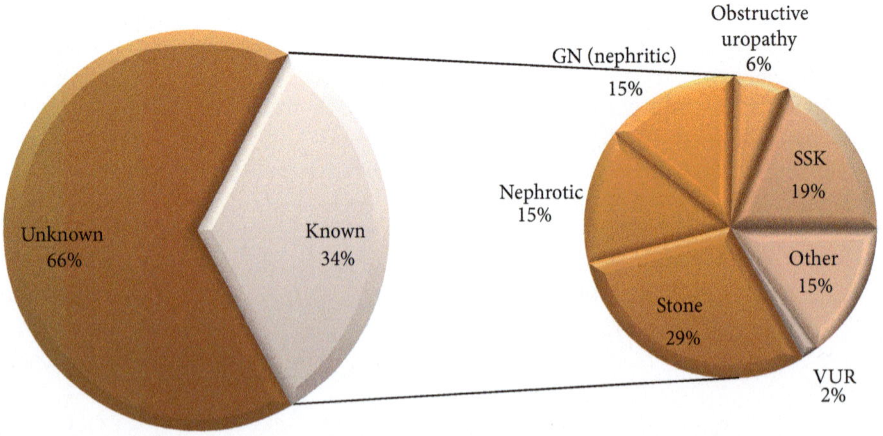

FIGURE 1: Percentage distribution of Aetiology of ESRD among children.

TABLE 3: Stratified analysis of clinical status among children with ESRD.

	Age groups (years)					
	1–9		10–14		15–19	
	Frequency	Percentage	Frequency	Percentage	Frequency	Percentage
Aetiology						
Unknown	61	67.0%	116	64.8%	117	67.2%
Stone	10	11.0%	16	8.9%	18	10.3%
Nephrotic	4	4.4%	10	5.6%	8	4.6%
GN (nephritic)	5	5.5%	7	3.9%	10	5.7%
Obstructive uropathy	1	1.1%	6	3.4%	2	1.1%
SSK	5	5.5%	15	8.4%	8	4.6%
Others (Wilms, BOO, gastroenteritis, etc.)	4	4.4%	8	4.5%	10	5.7%
VUR	1	1.1%	1	0.6%	1	0.6%
Hepatitis B						
Positive	1	1.1%	5	2.8%	5	2.9%
Negative	90	98.9%	174	97.2%	169	97.1%
Hepatitis C						
Positive	2	2.2%	3	1.7%	8	4.6%
Negative	89	97.8%	176	98.3%	166	95.4%

Table 3 shows age based stratified analysis for secondary outcome variables such as aetiology. The aetiology varied among different age groups. Kidney stones were the most common cause for ESRD among all stratified age groups. Children under the age of 10 years had the highest percentage of kidney stone being the reason for their kidney failure ($n = 10$, 11%) followed closely by the 15–18 years age group ($n = 18$, 10.3%).

4. Discussion

The prevalence of HBV and HCV in our sample population is 2.5% and 2.9%, respectively. A major hurdle in recording the prevalence of HBV and HCV in the Pakistani population is the lack of reporting to a national database. A study showed that the prevalence of HCV among the general population is 4.5% [11], while another study estimated that 17 million people in Pakistan are affected [12] compared with the global reported prevalence of less than 3%, 1.8% in Europe, and 2.3% in USA [13]. Prevalence of HBV has been shown to be 2.5% in the general population [14]. A few studies carried out in the paediatric population by Khan [15], Parker et al. [16], and Hyder et al. [17] showed that the rates of HCV are 4.09%, 1.3%, and 0.58%, respectively, while a newer study determined the prevalence to be 3.3% in the age group 9–19 years [18], while a review showed the incidence of HBV as 1.9–3.6% [19].

Keeping the route of infection in mind, some reasons for the higher prevalence of these infections in our country can be deduced. Majority of our population obtains their haircut and facial shaves from unhygienic barber shops, where the practice of using fresh blades for each individual is dubious at best. While this dangerous act used to be much more common, awareness regarding the hazards has reduced it to a great extent. There still remains a lot of work to be done, as these practices have not been completely abolished and many people do not recognize the significance of needle-stick injuries, proper disposal of used sharp objects, sharing of toothbrushes, and unsafe blood donations, apart from the pervasive presence of intravenous drug abuse. It is possible that many of the children are infected either directly through these injuries or accidents or through vertical transmission from their mothers.

Hepatitis infections in ESRD patients, especially children, represent a special subset of the population. The inflicted individuals have to undergo maintenance peritoneal dialysis, haemodialysis, or renal transplantation. All these are associated with risks of blood-borne infections being transmitted, among other complications. Being on dialysis means repetitive exposure to potentially infected instruments and hence increased risk of infections. Studies from different regions show varying trends of HBV and HCV infection in these patients. A Senegalese study showed 5.6% prevalence of HCV in ESRD patients [20], while in Libya it was shown to be 31.1%, in Germany 6.1%, in Saudi Arabia 50%, and in Turkey 20.2% [21]. On the other hand, the observed prevalence of HBV infection in ESRD patients was 2.6% in Libya, 4.1% in Europe, 2.2% in Japan, and 2.4% in USA [21]. A local study revealed frequency of HBV as 2.1% and HCV as 16.4% [22]. While these studies mostly state the frequencies among the adult populations suffering from ESRD, some researchers have worked on the paediatric ESRD patients too. From these, the prevalence in Saudi population is 45% for HCV and 15% for HBV [3], in Italian population 15% for HCV [7], and in the Egyptian paediatric ESRD population 5.9% for HBV and 94.1% for HCV [23]. All these report a much higher incidence of the investigated diseases as compared to our study. As the risk of being infected by blood-borne viruses increases with exposure, patients who are on dialysis for longer periods are at higher risk than those being started on dialysis recently. This would lead to the expectation that children with ESRD would be less likely to be infected as compared to adults with the same affliction since they have been enduring dialysis longer.

We further found that the aetiology of ESRD in our population was unknown in 66.2%. Among the known causes, the most common in our sample was urolithiasis. The main causes of ESRD in children are quite different from those in adults. Diabetes and hypertension being common culprits in the latter [24]. As far as the aetiology in children is concerned, there is a marked variety between countries and regions. While congenital anomalies and hereditary nephropathies are reported from developed nations, infections and other acquired causes make up the majority in developing countries [25, 26]. The paediatric aetiology in our population remains mostly unknown, with a high incidence of urinary tract stones which is in contrast to that reported in Western countries. Stone formation leading to renal failure has a high incidence in our region [27]. A study conducted in Karachi shows nephrolithiasis as the major factor in 16%, glomerulonephritis in 26%, and unknown in 50% [28] compared with hereditary/congenital disorders (35.9%) and glomerular disease (21.5%) in USA [9]. This is consistent with our findings which show stone formation as the leading known cause of ESRD in children.

Pakistan, among other countries of the Afro-Asian belt, has one of the highest incidences of urolithiasis in the world. This entity is observed both in adults and in children and is often neglected which leads to patients presenting with late disease; a challenge to treat [15]. Paediatric urolithiasis in Western countries occurs mainly on the backdrop of metabolic abnormalities, anatomical anomalies, and infections while the preponderant etiological basis in developing nations is not clearly defined [29]. It has been shown that there is a genetic component involved in increasing the risk of stone formation, and dietary and environmental components also contribute to the metabolic abnormalities leading to this phenomenon. Relation of physical activity and fluid intake too is well documented [30]. The importance of urolithiasis as a cause of ESRD is based on the fact that it is quite easily preventable and manageable, hence reducing the burden of patients developing renal failure.

Extrapolating on these evidences, one can make some intelligent guesses regarding the role of environment and diet on our results. In a subtropical region with the sun shining almost the whole year, high temperatures, and humidity, it is no surprise that people living in Pakistan, especially the southern coastal areas, arid Balochistan, and lower Punjab, tend to be dehydrated. Increased consumption of salt is common in our society and, with a significant portion of the population not able to afford meat, consumption of vegetables with the resultant load of oxalate provides additional risk factors. An increase in dietary calcium, associated with dairy consumption, reduces the formation of oxalate stones, which could be a possible contributory factor in those with poor feeding habits [31]. These points can help formulating advice to high-risk patients and the population in general regarding the potential prevention of stone formation, leading to decreased morbidity and mortality associated with this pathology. Prompt attention to the symptoms produced by urolithiasis is essential to achieve a reduction in incidence; clinicians should be careful not to dismiss symptoms of abdominal pain, haematuria, or dysuria. Another hurdle is neglect and delay in obtaining proper medical advice by the patients and their families; some of this is due to silent stones, but a more important cause is the practice among people, especially from rural background, to consult hakims/quacks for their ailments.

Our study has an advantage over some studies cited above in having a much larger sample size. Since this study was carried out at a dedicated center for kidney disease, the volume of patients is quite high. Not many centers operate in our country providing state-of-the-art care completely free of cost; this means that the catchment area is quite widespread in terms of geography and socioeconomic strata. It is evident from the literature review that not many studies are available regarding the epidemiology of specific diseases in special populations. Our study focuses on a subset within a subset, namely, children ailing with ESRD. While this sort of targeted researches may not be of interest to the casual investigator or practitioner, they are important for those intimately associated with these specialties as they provide important epidemiological data as well as guide important decisions on how to reduce the adverse events patients suffered from during their care.

Unarguably, our study has several limitations as well. The foremost are the facts that this was a retrospective study done in the year 2013; hence, any cases before or after that year were not accounted for. Also, the study was done at a single center. Although the center is located at the city center and would account for most of the cases reported, it still remains our limitation. Our hospital is a government based public institution. Hence, the majority of the children would represent people from a low socioeconomic background.

5. Conclusion

Our study highlights a high prevalence of HBV and HCV in paediatric ESRD patients. This unfortunate affliction represents an additional comorbidity for our patients who are already fighting a life-threatening condition. There is a need for carrying out further work to confirm these findings and expand our recommendations, particularly the sensitive issue regarding proper blood screening. NGOs and governmental institutions can play a pivotal role in bringing out the true picture as defined in earlier studies and awareness projects. Further data regarding these infections should be collected on a national level, and appropriate measures should be taken by both the government and private setups to reduce the spread of HBV and HCV as they will have a big effect on the quality of life of patients as well as playing a role in reducing mortality. Hence, focused efforts should be done to prevent the spread of HBV and HCV and thereby reduce the burden of related chronic liver disease in the country and region, as a whole, especially in a region dominated with child population.

Ethical Approval

All procedures performed in studies involving human participants were in accordance with the ethical standards of the institutional and/or national research committee and with the 1964 Helsinki declaration and its later amendments or comparable ethical standards.

Conflict of Interests

The authors declare that they have no conflict of interests.

References

[1] F. Mortazavi and M. Maleki, "Management and outcome of children with end-stage renal disease in northwest Iran," *Indian Journal of Nephrology*, vol. 22, no. 2, pp. 94–97, 2012.

[2] J. W. Groothoff, "Long-term outcomes of children with end-stage renal disease," *Pediatric Nephrology*, vol. 20, no. 7, pp. 849–853, 2005.

[3] M. Al-Mugeiren, F. Z. Al-Faleh, S. Ramia, S. Al-Rasheed, M. A. Mahmoud, and M. Al-Nasser, "Seropositivity to hepatitis C virus (HCV) in Saudi children with chronic renal failure maintained on haemodialysis," *Annals of Tropical Paediatrics*, vol. 12, no. 2, pp. 217–219, 1992.

[4] R. D. Sheth, M. F. Peskin, and X. L. Du, "The duration of hepatitis B vaccine immunity in pediatric dialysis patients," *Pediatric Nephrology*, 2014.

[5] M. M. Jonas, G. E. Zilleruelo, S. I. LaRue, C. Abitbol, J. Strauss, and Y. Lu, "Hepatitis C infection in a pediatric dialysis population," *Pediatrics*, vol. 89, no. 4, pp. 707–709, 1992.

[6] A. Peco-Antić, P. Peklar, S. Zerjev et al., "Viral hepatitis C—a problem in the treatment of children with renal insufficiency on hemodialysis," *Srpski Arhiv Za Celokupno Lekarstvo*, vol. 121, no. 3–7, pp. 81–83, 1993.

[7] M. Greco, K. Cristiano, G. Leozappa, M. Rapicetta, and G. Rizzoni, "Hepatitis C infection in children and adolescents on haemodialysis and after renal transplant," *Pediatric Nephrology*, vol. 7, no. 4, pp. 424–427, 1993.

[8] L. M. Callis, J. Clanxet, G. Fortuny, J. Caballeria, J. L. Carrasco, and R. Lardinois, "Hepatitis B virus infection and vaccination in children undergoing hemodialysis," *Acta Paediatrica Scandinavica*, vol. 74, no. 2, pp. 213–218, 1985.

[9] USRDS Annual Data Report, Volume 2—ESRD.

[10] S. A. Rizvi and K. Manzoor, "Causes of chronic renal failure in Pakistan: a single large center experience," *Saudi Journal of Kidney Diseases and Transplantation*, vol. 13, no. 3, pp. 376–379, 2002.

[11] World Health Organization, "Hepatitis-C," Fact Sheet 164, WHO, Geneva, Switzerland, 2012.

[12] M. Idrees, S. Rafique, I.-U. Rehman et al., "Hepatitis C virus genotype 3a infection and hepatocellular carcinoma: Pakistan experience," *World Journal of Gastroenterology*, vol. 15, no. 40, pp. 5080–5085, 2009.

[13] S. A. Jadoon, H. A. Jadoon, and H. S. Nazar, "Treatment of chronic hepatitis-C with standard interferon and ribavirin," *Journal of Ayub Medical College Abbottabad*, vol. 26, no. 2, pp. 212–215, 2014.

[14] C. Rodrigo and S. Rajapakse, "Current status of HIV/AIDS in South Asia," *Journal of Global Infectious Diseases*, vol. 1, no. 2, pp. 93–101, 2009.

[15] H. I. Khan, "A study of seroprevalence of hepatitis B and C in mothers and children in Lahore," *Pakistan Pediatric Journal*, vol. 20, pp. 163–166, 1996.

[16] S. P. Parker, H. I. Khan, and W. D. Cubitt, "Detection of antibodies to hepatitis C virus in dried blood spot samples from mothers and their offspring in Lahore, Pakistan," *Journal of Clinical Microbiology*, vol. 37, no. 6, pp. 2061–2063, 1999.

[17] S. N. Hyder, W. Hussain, M. Aslam, and S. Maqbool, "Seroprevalence of anti-HCV in asymptomatic children," *Pakistan Journal of Phytopathology*, vol. 12, no. 3, pp. 89–93, 2001.

[18] M. I. Anwar, M. Rahman, M. U. Hassan, and M. Iqbal, "Prevalence of active hepatitis C virus infections among general public of Lahore, Pakistan," *Virology Journal*, vol. 10, pp. 351–422, 2013.

[19] A. Bosan, H. Qureshi, K. M. Bile, I. Ahmad, and R. Hafiz, "A review of hepatitis viral infections in Pakistan," *Journal of the Pakistan Medical Association*, vol. 60, no. 12, pp. 1045–1058, 2010.

[20] S. Seck, M. Dahaba, S. Gueye, and E. Ka, "Trends in hepatitis C infection among hemodialysis patients in Senegal: results of a decade of prevention," *Saudi Journal of Kidney Diseases and Transplantation*, vol. 25, no. 6, p. 1341, 2014.

[21] W. A. Alashek, C. W. McIntyre, and M. W. Taal, "Hepatitis B and C infection in haemodialysis patients in Libya: prevalence, incidence and risk factors," *BMC Infectious Diseases*, vol. 12, article 265, 2012.

[22] M. M. Huma, D. M. Siddiqui, D. B. Bashir, D. S. Ali, D. A. Baloch, and D. M. Masroor, "Hemodialysis patients profile at Dow University of Health Sciences," *Pakistan Journal of Medical Sciences*, vol. 30, no. 6, pp. 1327–1330, 2014.

[23] A. M. Hammad and M. H. E. D. Zaghloul, "Hepatitis G virus infection in Egyptian children with chronic renal failure (single centre study)," *Annals of Clinical Microbiology and Antimicrobials*, vol. 8, article 36, 2009.

[24] B. A. Warady and V. Chadha, "Chronic kidney disease in children: the global perspective," *Pediatric Nephrology*, vol. 22, no. 12, pp. 1999–2009, 2007.

[25] J. Harambat, K. J. van Stralen, J. J. Kim, and E. J. Tizard, "Epidemiology of chronic kidney disease in children," *Pediatric Nephrology*, vol. 27, no. 3, pp. 363–373, 2012.

[26] M. Hussain, M. Lal, B. Ali, S. A. A. Naqvi, and S. A. H. Rizvi, "Urolithiasis in Sindh: a single centre experience with review of 10,000 cases," *Journal of Nephrology, Urology and Transplantation*, vol. 1, pp. 10–13, 1998.

[27] S. A. H. Rizvi, S. A. A. Naqvi, Z. Hussain et al., "Living-related pediatric renal transplants: a single-center experience from a developing country," *Pediatric Transplantation*, vol. 6, no. 2, pp. 101–110, 2002.

[28] S. A. H. Rizvi, S. Sultan, M. N. Zafar et al., "Evaluation of children with urolithiasis," *Indian Journal of Urology*, vol. 23, no. 4, pp. 420–427, 2007.

[29] D. S. Milliner and M. E. Murphy, "Urolithiasis in pediatric patients," *Mayo Clinic Proceedings*, vol. 68, no. 3, pp. 241–248, 1993.

[30] K. VanDervoort, J. Wiesen, R. Frank et al., "Urolithiasis in pediatric patients: a single center study of incidence, clinical presentation and outcome," *Journal of Urology*, vol. 177, no. 6, pp. 2300–2305, 2007.

[31] D. S. Goldfarb, "Increasing prevalence of kidney stones in the United States," *Kidney International*, vol. 63, no. 5, pp. 1951–1952, 2003.

3

Clinical Presentation, Aetiology, and Outcomes of Meningitis in a Setting of High HIV and TB Prevalence

Keneuoe Hycianth Thinyane,[1] Keanole Mofona Motsemme,[1] and Varsay Jim Lahai Cooper[2]

[1]*Department of Pharmacy, National University of Lesotho, Roma 180, Lesotho*
[2]*Department of Internal Medicine, Queen Mamohato Memorial Hospital, Maseru 100, Lesotho*

Correspondence should be addressed to Keneuoe Hycianth Thinyane; kthinyane@gmail.com

Academic Editor: Carlos E. P. Corbett

Meningitis causes significant morbidity and mortality globally. The aim of this study was to study the clinical presentation, aetiology, and outcomes of meningitis among adult patients admitted to Queen Mamohato Memorial Hospital in Maseru, Lesotho, with a diagnosis of meningitis. A cross-sectional study was conducted between February and April 2014; data collected included presenting signs and symptoms, laboratory results, and clinical outcomes. Descriptive statistics were used to summarise data; association between variables was analysed using Fisher's exact test. 56 patients were enrolled; the HIV coinfection rate was 79%. The most common presenting symptoms were altered mental status, neck stiffness, headache, and fever. TB meningitis was the most frequent diagnosis (39%), followed by bacterial (27%), viral (18%), and cryptococcal meningitis (16%). In-hospital mortality was 43% with case fatalities of 23%, 40%, 44%, and 90% for TB, bacterial, cryptococcal, and viral meningitis, respectively. Severe renal impairment was significantly associated with mortality. In conclusion, the causes of meningitis in this study reflect the high prevalence of HIV and TB in our setting. Strategies to reduce morbidity and mortality due to meningitis should include improving diagnostic services to facilitate early detection and treatment of meningitis and timely initiation of antiretroviral therapy in HIV-infected patients.

1. Introduction

Meningitis is a clinical syndrome characterized by inflammation of the meninges; it is one of the most common infectious diseases of the central nervous system (CNS) [1]. Most cases of meningitis are caused by bacteria or viruses; however fungi and parasites can also cause meningitis, especially in immunocompromised patients [2–4]. Infection with the human immunodeficiency virus (HIV) is emerging as a major risk factor for meningitis in adults [5–7]. Studies show that tuberculous meningitis (TBM) and cryptococcal meningitis (CM) are among the most common CNS opportunistic infections in patients with HIV/AIDS in sub-Saharan Africa and Asia [8–11].

Meningitis causes significant morbidity and mortality globally [3, 9, 12, 13]. Long term sequelae of bacterial meningitis in adults include hearing and visual loss, seizures, and cognitive impairment [14]. Neurological and neuropsychological deficits have also been reported in adults following cryptococcal, tuberculous, and viral meningitis [4, 15, 16]. Mortality from meningitis appears to be much higher in developing countries than in developed countries [4, 5, 17]. Factors that contribute to this high mortality include delay in diagnosis/treatment of meningitis and severe immunosuppression in HIV-infected patients [12, 13].

In Lesotho the prevalence of HIV infection is estimated at 23% of the adult population; the country also has a high incidence of tuberculosis (TB) estimated at 633 per 100 000 of the population [18, 19]. National data show that in 2009 the rate of TB-HIV coinfection among tested patients was 76.5%; 22% of all notified new TB cases during this period were extrapulmonary [19]. In Lesotho as in other countries with a high HIV burden, meningitis is a major cause of hospital admission among HIV-infected adults [8, 19]. At present there are limited data on the causes of meningitis among adults in Lesotho [20, 21]; in addition the influence of HIV infection on the pathogenesis and clinical outcomes of meningitis have not been investigated. The aim of this study was to investigate the clinical presentation, aetiology, and outcome of meningitis among patients admitted to a tertiary level hospital in Maseru, Lesotho.

2. Methods

A cross-sectional study was conducted at Queen Mamohato Memorial Hospital (QMMH), the national tertiary referral hospital in Maseru, Lesotho, over a three-month period between February and April 2014. Patients presenting with signs and symptoms suggestive of meningitis, headache, neck stiffness, fever, photophobia, and/or altered mental status, were screened on admission to the medical wards. All patients 18 years and older with an admission diagnosis of meningitis were eligible to participate in the study. Exclusion criteria were discharge or death within 24 hours of admission.

Prior to data collection, written informed consent was obtained from each patient; for patients who were too ill to communicate, permission to enroll the patients in the study was obtained from the next of kin. Data collected at admission included age, gender, and medical history (history of present illness and concurrent diseases including HIV infection). Prehospitalisation medical records were reviewed and history of antiretroviral therapy (ART), anti-TB therapy (ATT), isoniazid preventive therapy (IPT), and use of cotrimoxazole or other antimicrobial agents was noted. Clinical evaluation of patients for meningitis was carried out according to hospital protocols. All patients underwent a physical examination and neurological assessment on admission and when not contraindicated immediate lumbar puncture (LP) was performed prior to the first dose of antibiotics. Initial cerebrospinal fluid (CSF) analysis for all patients included macroscopy, white cell count (WCC) and differential, protein and glucose levels, Gram stain and culture, India ink stain, and CSF cryptococcal antigen test. Repeat LP was performed when necessary; additional investigations included bacterial antigen detection by CSF latex agglutination tests for *Streptococcus pneumoniae*, *Streptococcus* group B, *H. influenzae* B, *N. meningitidis* serogroups A, C, Y, and W-135, and *N. meningitidis* serogroup B/*E. coli* K1 and bacterial culture and antibiotic susceptibility testing. Computed tomography (CT) scanning of the head was performed in some, but not all patients with focal neurological deficits and/or altered mental status prior to lumbar puncture or within 24–48 hours of admission to exclude intracranial space occupying lesions and other causes of raised intracranial pressure. Patients with clinical suspicion of TB meningitis and/or HIV infection underwent sputum acid fast bacilli (AFB) smear and culture testing and chest radiography to screen for the presence of TB. Patients with an unknown or negative HIV status on admission were offered voluntary HIV counselling and testing; consenting patients were tested for HIV infection with a rapid test or HIV ELISA. Routine biochemical investigations for all patients included full blood count, liver function tests, and urea and electrolytes.

Clinical, radiological, microbiological, and other laboratory data were evaluated and the diagnosis of meningitis was made based on a combination of clinical and CSF findings (CSF protein and glucose levels, cell count and differential, microscopy, and culture) as explained below.

2.1. Bacterial Meningitis. Bacterial meningitis was diagnosed based on a positive CSF Gram stain and culture or a positive bacterial antigen test (BAT). In patients without a definitive microbiological diagnosis, bacterial meningitis was diagnosed when patients had a compatible clinical presentation (sudden onset of fever, headache, altered mental status, or other meningeal signs) and typical CSF findings (CSF pleocytosis with polymorphonuclear cell predominance, low glucose, and elevated protein). Patient response to antibiotic therapy was closely monitored; patients showing no clinical improvement within 7–10 days of initiation of empiric antibiotic therapy underwent further diagnostic tests.

2.2. Cryptococcal Meningitis. A diagnosis of cryptococcal meningitis was made in the presence of a positive CSF India ink stain or CSF cryptococcal antigen (CSF CRAG) test.

2.3. TB Meningitis. A diagnosis of TB meningitis was made when patients had clinical features of meningitis with negative CSF Gram stain and cultures for bacteria, negative CSF cryptococcal antigen test, and at least one of the following: (i) characteristic CSF findings (CSF pleocytosis with lymphocytic predominance, low glucose, and elevated protein); (ii) evidence of active tuberculosis at another site (e.g., the lungs); or (iii) brain CT findings suggestive of TM such as basal meningeal enhancement or hydrocephalus. Patients showing resolution of constitutional symptoms within 14–21 days of starting anti-TB treatment were continued on treatment and did not undergo further investigations before discharge. CSF acid-fast bacilli smear or culture studies were not performed.

2.4. Viral Meningitis. Viral meningitis was diagnosed when patients had clinical features of meningitis with negative CSF Gram stain and cultures for bacteria, negative CSF cryptococcal antigen test, and typical CSF findings (CSF lymphocytic predominance, normal or slightly elevated protein, and normal glucose) with exclusion of nonviral causes of aseptic meningitis. CSF polymerase chain reaction (PCR) testing for viral pathogens was not done.

All data analyses were performed using SPSS version 20.0. Descriptive statistics were represented as frequencies (%) and median and interquartile range (IQR). Fisher's exact test was conducted to examine the relationship between the dependent variable (in-hospital mortality) and other categorical variables including age, HIV status, CD4 count, and estimated glomerular filtration rate (eGFR) on admission. A p value less than 0.05 was considered statistically significant.

The study was approved by the Lesotho Ministry of Health Research and Ethics Committee.

3. Results

A total of 72 patients with clinical suspicion of meningitis were enrolled. 16 patients were subsequently excluded; of these 12 patients were diagnosed with other CNS diseases and 4 did not have a clear final diagnosis. Of the 56 patients included in the final analysis, 57% (n = 32) were female and the median age was 35 years (IQR: 28–44); 79% (n = 44) were HIV positive (Table 1). 26 of the 44 HIV-infected patients (59%) were receiving antiretroviral therapy; among these, 13 patients had been on ART for less than 3 months, 7 patients for 3–6 months, and 6 patients for more than 6 months; 5 patients were taking cotrimoxazole prophylaxis and 1 patient was on IPT. 9 patients (16%) were on antituberculosis treatment on admission. The most common clinical presentation of meningitis was altered mental status followed by neck stiffness and headache; less common symptoms included vomiting (n = 12), photophobia (n = 5), and seizures (n = 4). CD4 cell counts were measured for 66% (29/44) of the patients with HIV infection; the majority of these (24/29) had CD4 cell counts <200 cells/mm^3. More than half of all patients had one or more clinical and biochemical features consistent with critical illness including severe wasting, inability to walk/talk, serum Na^+ <130 mmol/L (n = 16), eGFR <30 mL/min (n = 10), and Hb <8.0 g/dL (n = 6).

Table 2 shows CSF findings and clinical outcomes among the 56 study participants: 22 patients (39%) were diagnosed with TB meningitis, 15 (27%) had bacterial meningitis, 10 (18%) had viral meningitis, and 9 (16%) had cryptococcal meningitis. HIV coinfection rates were greater than 70% for all types of meningitis; the proportion of patients with CD4 cell counts below 100 cells/mm^3 was 100% (9/9) for cryptococcal meningitis, 50% (5/10) for viral meningitis, 33% (5/15) for bacterial meningitis, and 0% (0/22) for TB meningitis. The majority of the patients had CSF parameters, CSF cell, protein, and glucose findings, characteristic of the various types of meningitis. Of the 15 patients diagnosed with bacterial meningitis, 9 had a CSF pleocytosis with a polymorphonuclear cell predominance reported in 7 patients; 5 patients had low CSF glucose, and 11 had elevated protein. Positive Gram stain results were obtained on initial CSF specimen for 9 patients. Six patients were diagnosed on the basis of CSF findings after repeat LP. A positive bacterial antigen test was reported in 4 patients (*S. pneumoniae*, n = 3; *H. influenzae*, n = 1) and a positive Gram stain in 3; one patient had a positive Gram stain and BAT result. Two patients with microbiologically confirmed bacterial meningitis had a normal CSF study (CSF white cell count up to 5 cells/mm^3, glucose >2.2 mmol/L, and protein <0.45 g/L). Of the 9 patients diagnosed with cryptococcal meningitis, 6 had a positive CSF India ink stain and 8 were CSF CRAG positive; 5 patients had a CSF white cell count >5 cells/mm^3 with mononuclear cell predominance in 4 patients; low CSF glucose was found in 5 and elevated protein in 8 patients. One patient had a normal CSF study at diagnosis. 22 CSF Gram stain-, bacterial antigen test-, and CSF CRAG-negative patients were diagnosed with TB meningitis. A CSF pleocytosis, median CSF WCC 217 cells/mm^3 (IQR: 58–435), was observed in all patients with TBM. 14 patients had CSF white cell counts above 100/mm^3, and 20 had a CSF lymphocytic predominance (>90% mononuclear cells). The proportion of patients with low CSF glucose and elevated CSF protein was 12/22 and 20/22, respectively. CSF analysis in patients with viral meningitis showed acellular CSF (n = 8) or a mild lymphocytic pleocytosis (CSF white cell count <30 cells/mm^3; n = 2), normal CSF glucose levels (n = 9), and elevated protein (n = 7).

Empirical antimicrobial therapy was started with intravenous ceftriaxone; 52% of the patients received adjunctive dexamethasone on admission. Patients diagnosed with TBM were started on a regimen of isoniazid, rifampicin, ethambutol, and pyrazinamide; bacterial meningitis was treated with ceftriaxone, cryptococcal meningitis with amphotericin B, and viral meningitis with acyclovir. Supportive therapy included analgesics/antipyretics and antiemetics. Patients were closely monitored and in cases of clinical deterioration, further investigations were performed and change in therapy was instituted as necessary. The median hospital stay for discharged patients was 11 days, range 6–25 days. The overall in-hospital mortality was 43% (24/56) with more than half of the deaths (14/24, 58%) occurring during the first 7 days of hospital admission. The case fatality was 90% for viral meningitis, around 40% each for bacterial and cryptococcal meningitis and 23% for TB meningitis. In-hospital mortality was higher although not statistically significant among older patients, 67% (4/6) versus 40% (20/50), patients with

TABLE 1: Demographic and baseline characteristics of the study participants.

Variable	n (%)
Female gender, N = 56	32 (57)
Age group, years, N = 56	
18–24	8 (14)
25–34	20 (36)
35–49	22 (39)
>49	6 (11)
HIV status, N = 56	
Positive	44 (79)
Negative	7 (13)
Unknown	5 (9)
% on antiretroviral therapy, N = 44	26 (59)
Clinical presentation, N = 56	
Altered mental status	42 (75)
Neck stiffness	38 (68)
Headache	30 (54)
Fever	24 (43)
Seizures	4 (7)
Baseline biochemistry, median (IQR)	
CD4 count, cells/mm^3, N = 29	100 (53–155)
Na^+, mmol/L, N = 46	131.0 (128.0–137.3)
K^+, mmol/L, N = 48	4.0 (3.4–4.9)
eGFR, mL/min, N = 46	57 (26–78)
ALT, U/L, N = 42	39 (27–77)
Hb, g/dL, N = 50	11.0 (9.0–13.0)
PLT, $\times 10^3$/L, N = 48	273 (186–336)

Data presented as n (%) unless otherwise stated; ALT: alanine transaminase; Hb: haemoglobin; n: number of patients; N: total number of patients for whom the analysis was performed; PLT: platelets.

TABLE 2: Cerebrospinal fluid analysis and clinical outcomes.

	BM ($n = 15$)	CM ($n = 9$)	TBM ($n = 22$)	VM ($n = 10$)
HIV positive, n/N (%)[a]	11/13 (85)	8/9 (89)	15/19 (79)	10/10 (100)
% on ART[b]	8/11 (73)	3/8 (38)	11/15 (73)	4/10 (40)
CD4 count, median, cells/mm^3 (IQR)	162 (91–257)	18 (12–41)	119 (100–277)	102 (75–129)
CSF analysis				
Gram stain (+)	12[c]/15 (80)	0 (0)	0 (0)	0 (0)
Bacterial antigen test (+)	4[c]/15 (27)	0 (0)	0 (0)	0 (0)
India ink (+)	0 (0)	6/9 (67)	0 (0)	0 (0)
CSF CRAG (+)	0 (0)	8/9 (89)	0 (0)	0 (0)
White blood cells				
Range, cells/mm^3	0–420	0–184	8–2393	0–18
Median, cells/mm^3 (IQR)	7 (2–147)	10 (0–86)	217 (58–435)	0 (0-0)
>5 cells/mm^3, n/N (%)	9/15 (60)	5/9 (56)	22/22 (100)	2/10 (20)
Lymphocytic pleocytosis[d]	2/9 (22)	4/5 (80)	20/22 (91)	2/2 (100)
Glucose				
Median, mmol/L (IQR)	3.0 (1.1–3.8)	2.0 (1.0–2.9)	1.1 (0.6–2.3)	3.0 (2.7–3.6)
<2.2 mmol/L, n/N (%)	5/15 (33)	5/9 (56)	14/22 (64)	1/10 (10)
Protein				
Median, g/L (IQR)	0.6 (0.4–1.5)	1.0 (0.7–1.8)	2.0 (1.7–4.4)	0.5 (0.4–0.7)
>0.45 g/L, n/N (%)	11/15 (73)	8/9 (89)	20/22 (91)	7/10 (70)
Hospital stay, median days (IQR)	11 (9–12)	17 (17–23)	11 (8–11)	23 (23-23)
Mortality rate, n/N (%)	6/24 (25)	4/24 (17)	5/24 (21)	9/24 (38)
Fatality rate, n/N (%)	6/15 (40)	4/9 (44)	5/22 (23)	9/10 (90)

[a]HIV infection rate expressed as a percentage of patients with known HIV status; [b]expressed as a percentage of patients with HIV infection; [c]positive Gram stain and bacterial antigen results reported for initial and repeat CSF specimens; [d]calculated as a percentage of patients with CSF white cells >5 cells/mm^3; BM: bacterial meningitis; CM: cryptococcal meningitis; MN: mononuclear cells; n: number of patients; N: total number of patients for whom the analysis was performed; PMN: polymorphonuclear cells; TBM: tuberculous meningitis; VM: viral meningitis.

HIV infection, 48% (21/44) versus 29% (2/7), and those with altered mental status, 50% (21/42) versus 21% (3/14) (Table 3). Severe renal impairment (eGFR < 30 mL/min) was significantly associated with in-hospital mortality, $p = 0.008$ (Fisher's exact test).

4. Discussion

We investigated the clinical presentation, aetiology, and outcomes of meningitis among adult patients admitted to a tertiary level hospital in Maseru, Lesotho. TB meningitis was the most common cause of meningitis (39%) followed by bacterial meningitis (27%), viral meningitis (18%), and cryptococcal meningitis (16%). The percentage of HIV infection was 79%, with the majority of the patients presenting with symptoms and signs of advanced HIV infection (stage III/IV events) on admission. Studies from sub-Saharan Africa show that HIV coinfection is common among adults with meningitis [7, 8, 22]. In a study conducted in South Africa, Jarvis et al. [6] found HIV coinfection rates above 90% among patients diagnosed with bacterial, cryptococcal, and tuberculous meningitis. The immunodeficiency caused by HIV predisposes individuals to opportunistic infections by pathogens such as *Cryptococcus neoformans* and *Mycobacterium tuberculosis* which typically do not cause CNS infections in immunocompetent hosts [23]. Research indicates that the spectrum of meningitis varies between countries: in parts of Africa and South East Asia, cryptococcal meningitis is the leading cause of adult meningitis, with most of the cases occurring in patients with CD4 counts <100 cells/mm^3 [10, 24, 25]. In our study, TB meningitis was the most common form of meningitis among adults, a finding which is consistent with data from other studies conducted in Southern Africa [5, 22]. Lesotho, like South Africa, has a high HIV and TB burden with HIV/TB coinfection rates above 70%. In this study, 59% of all patients ($n = 33$) were treated with anti-TB drugs during hospitalisation; of these two-thirds ($n = 22$) had been diagnosed with TB meningitis and a third had other forms of TB including pulmonary tuberculosis. Patients with HIV infection and active TB are at an increased risk of extrapulmonary tuberculosis [26]; in these patients TB meningitis is caused by the hematogenous dissemination of the tubercle bacilli from the primary site of infection such as the lungs. Research indicates that starting antiretroviral therapy early in the course of HIV infection and the use of prophylactic antimicrobial regimens might help reduce the incidence of CNS opportunistic infections in HIV-infected patients [10].

88% of the patients presented with at least two of the four signs and symptoms of fever, headache, neck stiffness,

TABLE 3: Analysis of factors associated with in-hospital mortality.

	Survived	Died	p value (Fisher's exact test)
Age, years			
>49	2	4	0.385
≤49	30	20	
Gender			
Male	14	10	1.000
Female	18	14	
HIV status			
Positive	23	21	0.436
Negative	5	2	
CD4 count, cells/mm^3			
<100	7	7	0.715
≥100	9	6	
Altered mental status			
Yes	21	21	0.072
No	11	3	
Seizures			
Yes	3	1	0.627
No	29	23	
Serum sodium, mmol/L			
<130	11	5	0.750
≥130	18	12	
eGFR, mL/min			
<30	2	8	0.008
≥30	26	10	

and altered mental status. Studies show that about 20–70% of adults with meningitis present with varying degrees of altered mental status ranging from confusion to impaired level of consciousness [27–29]. Multiple studies have shown that neurological signs at presentation are prognostic of poor clinical outcomes in patients with meningitis. In this study, mortality was higher though not statistically significant among patients with altered mental status. In a recent study, Jarvis et al. [12] found that altered mental status was an independent predictor of acute mortality in patients with cryptococcal meningitis. Similar findings have been reported for patients diagnosed with bacterial meningitis [27] and TB meningitis [22]. In general CSF cell and biochemistry findings in our study were typical of the different forms of meningitis; however CSF white cell counts were lower than those reported in adult references. More than a third of all patients with microbiologically confirmed bacterial and cryptococcal meningitis had atypical CSF findings: 6 of the 15 patients with bacterial meningitis had CSF white cell counts ≤5/mm^3 and 2 had a normal CSF study; the proportions were 4/9 and 1/9, respectively, among patients with cryptococcal meningitis. These findings are similar to those reported among populations with (predominantly) HIV-associated meningitis [6, 13, 22]. Abnormal CSF cell and biochemistry findings may cause diagnostic uncertainty especially in the presence of negative CSF microbiology results. The diagnosis of meningitis remains difficult, particularly in resource-limited settings. In diagnosing TB meningitis, CSF AFB smear has relatively low sensitivity, reported to be less than 10% in several studies [4, 13, 22], and although CSF AFB culture has greater sensitivity, it can take up to 8 weeks to obtain results, leading to a delay in diagnosis and initiation of anti-TB therapy. For these reasons ancillary investigations including neuroimaging studies and chest radiography are often necessary to confirm/rule out TB meningitis. Confirmatory diagnostic tests for viral meningitis include CSF PCR for nucleic acids and CSF viral culture; however these tests are not widely available. There is a need for sensitive, rapid laboratory tests to enable prompt diagnosis of meningitis and initiation of appropriate antimicrobial therapy.

The overall mortality was 43%; severe renal impairment (eGFR < 30 mL/min) was the only variable significantly associated with in-hospital mortality among the study participants. Some studies indicate that a positive HIV status is predictive of mortality in adults with meningitis [8, 26, 28]. In this study, the mortality rate was higher though not statistically significant among HIV-positive patients compared to those who were HIV negative. Notably, all of the patients with severe renal impairment ($n = 10$) were also HIV-infected; 6 of these patients were receiving antiretroviral therapy (tenofovir/lamivudine/efavirenz) on admission and 4 were ART naive. In the absence of other comorbidities, it is highly likely that renal impairment in these patients was HIV related; either HIV-associated nephropathy or tenofovir induced renal failure. In this study, the case fatality rate for bacterial and cryptococcal meningitis was 40% and 44%, respectively, which is similar to that reported elsewhere [5, 9, 27]. Despite advances in diagnosis and treatment, mortality from bacterial and cryptococcal meningitis remains high, especially in developing countries [12, 17]. The case fatality for TBM was 23%, which is lower than that reported in other studies [13, 22]. A possible explanation for this difference is that although the majority of the TB meningitis cases in this study were also HIV-associated, the median CD4 count among HIV-infected TBM patients (119 cells/mm^3, IQR: 100–277) was higher than that reported in the two studies above. Severe immunosuppression is significantly associated with increased in-hospital mortality in patients with TB meningitis [22]. We found a case fatality rate of 90% for patients with viral meningitis; all of the patients with viral meningitis in this study were HIV-infected. In immunocompetent adults, viral meningitis is often a benign, self-limiting condition that resolves spontaneously without any sequelae; however in immunocompromised patients, viral meningitis is frequently associated with a significant mortality [30]. Approximately 10% of HIV-infected patients develop HIV meningitis which occurs primarily at seroconversion; other aetiologic agents in HIV-associated viral meningitis include Epstein-Barr virus (EBV), herpes simplex virus (HSV) types 1 and 2, and cytomegalovirus [30, 31]. Limited data exists regarding the aetiology of viral meningitis in sub-Saharan Africa. In two recent studies conducted in Malawi [31] and Uganda [32], EBV was identified as the most common cause of viral meningitis among HIV-infected patients while HSV infection was rarely found. In our setting, viral PCR testing is not available to confirm the diagnosis of viral meningitis and guide antiviral therapy. Possible consequences of this may include misdiagnosis of patients with atypical CSF findings, inappropriate antimicrobial therapy, or a delay in starting appropriate antimicrobial therapy. In this study, all patients with suspected viral meningitis were treated with acyclovir. Acyclovir has been used successfully to treat HSV meningitis; however the treatment of viral meningitis remains challenging as there are often no definitive effective therapies for most pathogens including EBV [30].

This study has several limitations. First of all, although this was a cross-sectional study, we did not obtain a detailed medical history of the type and duration of symptoms and/or recent use of antimicrobial agents for some of the study participants; in addition some investigations such as CD4 counts were not done routinely thus limiting the use of such variables in further data analyses. Secondly, the limited range of diagnostic tests performed, low sensitivity of the available laboratory techniques, and the presence of atypical clinical and laboratory findings complicate the diagnosis of meningitis; this could have led to exclusion of some cases and misclassification of others. Finally, the study sample was small which limited statistical analysis. Despite these limitations, this study provides evidence of the association between HIV infection and meningitis and the relatively higher prevalence of TB meningitis in our setting and further highlights the difficulties in diagnosing meningitis in a resource-limited setting. In the current study, the primary outcome of interest was death or survival to hospital discharge; future research should include neuropsychological evaluation of patients to assess disability at discharge. In addition, long term follow-up studies are required to study the long term sequelae of meningitis and the incidence of meningitis recurrence especially in patients with HIV infection.

5. Conclusions

In conclusion, the majority of the meningitis cases in this study were HIV-associated. TB meningitis was the most common cause of meningitis followed by bacterial, viral, and cryptococcal meningitis. In-hospital mortality was high with case fatality rates of 23%, 40%, 44%, and 90% for TB, bacterial, cryptococcal, and viral meningitis, respectively. There is a need for sensitive, rapid, and affordable laboratory tests to enable prompt diagnosis and treatment of meningitis. Early diagnosis of HIV infection and timely initiation could reduce morbidity and mortality from HIV-associated meningitis in this setting.

Conflict of Interests

The authors declare that there is no conflict of interests regarding the publication of this paper.

Acknowledgments

The authors would like to thank the medical staff at QMMH and the study participants for their cooperation.

References

[1] R. S. Porter and J. L. Kaplan, *The Merck Manual of Diagnosis and Therapy*, Neurologic Disorders, Merck & Co, Kenilworth, NJ, USA, 19th edition, 2011.

[2] D. M. Bamberger, "Diagnosis, initial management, and prevention of meningitis," *American Family Physician*, vol. 82, no. 12, pp. 1491–1498, 2010.

[3] V. Pyrgos, A. E. Seitz, C. A. Steiner, D. R. Prevots, and P. R. Williamson, "Epidemiology of cryptococcal meningitis in the US," *PLoS ONE*, vol. 8, no. 2, Article ID e56269, 2013.

[4] A.-S. H. Christensen, Å. B. Andersen, V. T. Thomsen, P. H. Andersen, and I. S. Johansen, "Tuberculous meningitis in Denmark: a review of 50 cases," *BMC Infectious Diseases*, vol. 11, article 47, 2011.

[5] A. Bergemann and A. S. Karstaedt, "Spectrum of meningitis," *The Quarterly Journal of Medicine*, vol. 89, no. 7, pp. 499–504, 1996.

[6] J. N. Jarvis, G. Meintjes, A. Williams, Y. Brown, T. Crede, and T. S. Harrison, "Adult meningitis in a setting of high HIV and TB prevalence: findings from 4961 suspected cases," *BMC Infectious Diseases*, vol. 10, article 67, 2010.

[7] J. G. Hakim, I. T. Gangaidzo, R. S. Heyderman et al., "Impact of HIV infection on meningitis in Harare, Zimbabwe: a prospective study of 406 predominantly adult patients," *AIDS*, vol. 14, no. 10, pp. 1401–1407, 2000.

[8] C. Békondi, C. Bernede, N. Passone et al., "Primary and opportunistic pathogens associated with meningitis in adults in Bangui, Central African Republic, in relation to human immunodeficiency virus serostatus," *International Journal of Infectious Diseases*, vol. 10, no. 5, pp. 387–395, 2006.

[9] T. Berhe, Y. Melkamu, and A. Amare, "The pattern and predictors of mortality of HIV/AIDS patients with neurologic manifestation in Ethiopia: a retrospective study," *AIDS Research and Therapy*, vol. 9, article 11, 2012.

[10] I. L. Tan, B. R. Smith, G. von Geldern, F. J. Mateen, and J. C. McArthur, "HIV-associated opportunistic infections of the CNS," *The Lancet Neurology*, vol. 11, no. 7, pp. 605–617, 2012.

[11] S. K. Sharma, T. Kadhiravan, A. Banga, T. Goyal, I. Bhatia, and P. K. Saha, "Spectrum of clinical disease in a series of 135 hospitalised HIV-infected patients from north India," *BMC Infectious Diseases*, vol. 4, article 52, 2004.

[12] J. N. Jarvis, T. Bicanic, A. Loyse et al., "Determinants of mortality in a combined cohort of 501 patients with HIV-associated cryptococcal meningitis: Implications for improving outcomes," *Clinical Infectious Diseases*, vol. 58, no. 5, pp. 736–745, 2014.

[13] H. N. Luma, B. C. N. Tchaleu, B. H. M. Ngahane et al., "Tuberculous meningitis: presentation, diagnosis and outcome in HIV-infected patients at the Douala General Hospital, Cameroon: a cross sectional study," *AIDS Research and Therapy*, vol. 10, article 16, 2013.

[14] O. Hoffman and J. R. Weber, "Pathophysiology and treatment of bacterial meningitis," *Therapeutic Advances in Neurological Disorders*, vol. 2, no. 6, pp. 401–412, 2009.

[15] H. Schmidt, B. Heimann, M. Djukic et al., "Neuropsychological sequelae of bacterial and viral meningitis," *Brain*, vol. 129, no. 2, pp. 333–345, 2006.

[16] S.-H. Lan, W.-N. Chang, C.-H. Lu, C.-C. Lui, and H.-W. Chang, "Cerebral infarction in chronic meningitis: a comparison of tuberculous meningitis and cryptococcal meningitis," *QJM:*

Monthly Journal of the Association of Physicians, vol. 94, no. 5, pp. 247–253, 2001.

[17] S. B. Gordon, A. L. Walsh, M. Chaponda et al., "Bacterial meningitis in Malawian adults: pneumococcal disease is common, severe, and seasonal," *Clinical Infectious Diseases*, vol. 31, no. 1, pp. 53–57, 2000.

[18] *Lesotho Demographic and Health Survey*, Ministry of Health and Social Welfare, Bureau of Statistics, Maseru, Lesotho, 2009.

[19] Ministry of Health and Social Welfare (MOHSW), *Annual Joint Review Report 2009/10 FY*, Ministry of Health and Social Welfare (MOHSW), Maseru, Lesotho, 2010.

[20] K. H. Thinyane and V. Cooper, "Clinical profiles of HIV-infected, HAART-naive patients admitted to a tertiary level hospital in Maseru, Lesotho," *The Internet Journal of Infectious Diseases*, vol. 11, no. 1, 2013.

[21] K. H. Thinyane and V. L. J. Cooper, "Causes of hospital admission among patients receiving highly active antiretroviral therapy," *Research Journal of Medical Sciences*, vol. 7, no. 5-6, pp. 130–133, 2013.

[22] S. Marais, D. J. Pepper, C. Schutz, R. J. Wilkinson, and G. Meintjes, "Presentation and outcome of tuberculous meningitis in a high HIV prevalence setting," *PLoS ONE*, vol. 6, no. 5, Article ID e20077, 2011.

[23] J. E. Kaplan, C. Benson, K. K. Holmes, J. T. Brooks, A. Pau, and H. Masur, "Guidelines for prevention and treatment of opportunistic infections in HIV-infected adults and adolescents," *Morbidity and Mortality Weekly Report*, vol. 58, no. 4, pp. 1–198, 2009.

[24] D. J. Sloan and V. Parris, "Cryptococcal meningitis: epidemiology and therapeutic options," *Clinical Epidemiology*, vol. 6, no. 1, pp. 169–182, 2014.

[25] B. J. Park, K. A. Wannemuehler, B. J. Marston, N. Govender, P. G. Pappas, and T. M. Chiller, "Estimation of the current global burden of cryptococcal meningitis among persons living with HIV/AIDS," *AIDS*, vol. 23, no. 4, pp. 525–530, 2009.

[26] C. Vinnard and R. R. MacGregor, "Tuberculous meningitis in HIV-infected individuals," *Current HIV/AIDS Reports*, vol. 6, no. 3, pp. 139–145, 2009.

[27] E. C. Wall, K. Cartwright, M. Scarborough et al., "High mortality amongst adolescents and adults with bacterial meningitis in Sub-Saharan Africa: an analysis of 715 cases from Malawi," *PLoS ONE*, vol. 8, no. 7, Article ID e69783, 2013.

[28] J. A. Veltman, C. C. Bristow, and J. D. Klausner, "Meningitis in HIV-positive patients in sub-Saharan Africa: a review," *Journal of the International AIDS Society*, vol. 17, Article ID 19184, 2014.

[29] P. Domingo, V. Pomar, N. de Benito, and P. Coll, "The spectrum of acute bacterial meningitis in elderly patients," *BMC Infectious Diseases*, vol. 13, article 108, 2013.

[30] D. R. Chadwick, "Viral meningitis," *British Medical Bulletin*, vol. 75-76, no. 1, pp. 1–14, 2005.

[31] H. Momméja-Marin, M. Lafaurie, C. Scieux, L. Galicier, E. Oksenhendler, and J.-M. Molina, "Herpes simplex virus type 2 as a cause of severe meningitis in immunocompromised adults," *Clinical Infectious Diseases*, vol. 37, no. 11, pp. 1527–1533, 2003.

[32] L. A. Benjamin, M. Kelly, D. Cohen et al., "Detection of herpes viruses in the cerebrospinal fluid of adults with suspected viral meningitis in Malawi," *Infection*, vol. 41, no. 1, pp. 27–31, 2013.

4

Parasitic Zoonoses in Humans and Their Dogs from a Rural Community of Tropical Mexico

Antonio Ortega-Pacheco,[1] Juan F. J. Torres-Acosta,[1] Alejandro Alzina-López,[1] Eduardo Gutiérrez-Blanco,[1] Manuel E. Bolio-González,[1] Armando J. Aguilar-Caballero,[1] Roger I. Rodríguez-Vivas,[1] Edwin Gutiérrez-Ruiz,[1] Karla Y. Acosta-Viana,[2] Eugenia Guzmán-Marín,[2] Alberto Rosado-Aguilar,[1] and Matilde Jiménez-Coello[2]

[1]*Departamento Salud Animal y Medicina Preventiva, Cuerpo Académico en Salud Animal, Facultad de Medicina Veterinaria y Zootecnia, Universidad Autónoma de Yucatán, Km 15.5 Carr. Mérida-Xmatkuil, AP 4-116, Mérida, YUC, Mexico*
[2]*Laboratorio de Biología Celular, CA Biomedicina de Enfermedades Infecciosas y Parasitarias. C.I.R. "Dr. Hideyo Noguchi", Universidad Autónoma de Yucatán, Avenida Itzaes, No. 490 x C. 59, 97000 Mérida, YUC, Mexico*

Correspondence should be addressed to Antonio Ortega-Pacheco; opacheco@correo.uady.mx

Academic Editor: Marcel Tanner

A cross-sectional study was made on 89 inhabitants and their dogs from a rural community of Yucatan, Mexico, to determine the serological prevalence of some zoonotic parasitic agents. Samples were taken to monitor the presence and intensity of infection with gastrointestinal parasites in dogs. In humans, the serological prevalence of *T. canis*, *T. gondii*, and *T. spiralis* was 29.2%, 91.0%, and 6.7%, respectively. No associations were found between positive cases and studied variables. From the total of blood samples taken from dogs, 87 (97.6%) were seropositive to *T. gondii*; only 52 viable fecal samples were collected from dogs of which 46.2% had the presence of gastrointestinal parasites with low to moderate intensity; from those, 12% had the presence of *T. canis*. This study demonstrates the presence of the studied zoonotic agents in the area particularly *T. gondii* which suggest a common source of infection in dogs and humans and a high number of oocyts present in the environment. Preventive measures must be designed towards good prophylactic practices in domestic and backyard animals (*T. canis* and *T. spiralis*). Contaminated sources with *T. gondii* (food and water) should be further investigated in order to design effective control measures.

1. Introduction

Dogs are the source of several zoonotic diseases and their close contact with humans may increase the risk of zoonotic disease transmission particularly when dogs are free to roam. Dogs in urban and rural areas can be used as sentinels in humans and wildlife to evaluate the diversity and environmental contamination with parasites [1]. Backyard pigs in tropical Mexico are important for domestic consumption [2, 3]. However, their sanitary management is very poor or nonexisting [3, 4] representing a risk for the transmission of zoonotic parasitic agents. The parasites *Toxoplasma gondii* and *Toxocara* spp. are capable of producing systemic and ocular disease in dogs and humans and share soil ingestion as common mode of exposure [5]. However, the protozoa *T. gondii* are more commonly transmitted by the ingestion of contaminated food or water. Domestic dogs are the principal animal reservoir hosts for *Toxocara canis*, a common nematode throughout the world producing severe anemia and systemic disease in puppies which in humans elicits various syndromes currently characterized as generalized (visceral larva migrans and covert toxocariasis) and compartmentalized as well as ocular and neurologic [6], with more clinical manifestations on kids [7]. Diverse epidemiological studies have demonstrated that exposition to *T. canis* varies from countries and regions [8] reaching up to 83% of seropositivity in people from the Caribbean region [9]. Another important foodborne nematode *Trichinella spiralis* is transmitted to humans generally by the consumption of undercook contaminated pork meat [10].

Information related to both animal and human zoonotic parasite infections in rural communities of Mexico is scarce. To establish an effective parasite prevention and control strategies, it is necessary to understand the biology of parasites circulating in endemic regions, monitoring their presence and the risk factors associated in humans, reservoir animals, and vectors for a better planning of strategies for prevention and control of zoonotic parasitic diseases. The objective of this study was to determine the seroprevalence of humans to *T. canis*, *T. gondii*, and *T. spiralis* in a rural community of Yucatan, Mexico, together with the seroprevalence of *T. gondii* and detection of *T. canis* in their dogs.

2. Methods

2.1. Area of Study. The study was conducted in the rural community of Molas Yucatan, Mexico (20°49′ and 20°48′N and 89°37′ and 89°38′W). The community has 2014 inhabitants and 379 dwellings. A sectional, descriptive, and prospective study was conducted considering for convenience 90 dwellings reporting tenure of at least one dog. The community was divided into four sectors (north-south and east-west); 20 houses in each sector were selected.

2.2. Sampling. Each of the selected households was visited, and a directed questionnaire was applied. Samples of blood and feces of at least one dog per household were taken. In dogs, blood samples were obtained from the cephalic vein and were processed to obtain serum which was frozen at −20°C until tested. Feces were taken directly from the rectum; then, rabies vaccine was applied and dogs were dewormed. Additionally, blood samples from an adult person per household were taken. In humans, blood samples were collected by venipuncture of the brachial vein prior to written consent of the participants and according to the rules of the Bioethics Committee of the Campus of Biological and Agricultural Sciences at the Autonomous University of Yucatan (CB-CCBA-I-20014-001). Samples were processed to obtain serum and frozen at −20°C. A questionnaire was applied to all sampled persons including questions about their age, feeding habits, water sources, presence of eye lesions, and previous deworming procedures.

2.3. Laboratory Analysis. Fecal samples were processed by centrifugation-flotation technique [11]; positive samples were examined quantitatively by McMaster technique to estimate the number of eggs per gram of feces (epg) with particular attention to *T. canis*. Human sera were evaluated for the measurement of IgG *T. canis* and *T. spiralis* antigens using ELISA kit (DGR Laboratories International Inc., USA) following the manufacturer's instructions. For *T. gondii*, the presence of specific IgG antibodies was determined by indirect ELISA (International GmbH RE58241, Hamburg, Germany) containing tachyzoites of *T. gondii*. Serum samples were diluted to a ratio of 1 : 100 in PBS and secondary antibody anti-human IgG HRP-labeled anti-human IgM HRP were also marked.

Table 1: Nematode infection intensity (epg) and Eucoccidiorida (oocysts per gram of feces) in 52 dogs from a rural community of Yucatan, Mexico.

Intestinal parasites	Low	Median	High
Ancylostoma caninum	45.8%	25.0%	0.0%
Toxocara canis	12.5%	0.0%	0.0%
Trichuris vulpis	8.3%	4.2%	0.0%
Eucoccidiorida	0.0%	4.2%	0.0%
Total	66.6%	33.4%	0.0%

Low 50–100 e/g, median 101–500 e/g, and high ≥500 e/g.

2.4. Statistical Analysis. The overall prevalence of intestinal parasites in dogs was estimated. The intensity of infection (elimination of epg) was classified as low (50–100 epg), median (150–500 epg), or high (>550 epg). The overall prevalence of IgG-positive people to *T. canis*, *T. canis*, and *T. spiralis* was also estimated. A primary screening of humans seropositive to *T. canis* was assessed using 2 × 2 contingency tables of exposure variables; odds ratio and confidence interval were determined. Since very few negative cases of *T. gondii* in human and dogs and few positive cases of *T. spiralis* were found, no statistical analysis was performed. Odds ratios (OR) and 95% confidence intervals were calculated using Epi-Info software (version 6.0; CDC Atlanta, GA, USA). The level of significance was set at $P < 0.05$.

3. Results

A total of 52 viable fecal samples were collected from adult dogs of which 24 (46.2%) had at least some order/species kind of intestinal nematode. The nematode genera found in dog feces were *Ancylostoma caninum* (70.8%), *Toxocara canis* (12.5%), *Trichuris vulpis* (12.5%), and the order Eucoccidiorida (4.2%).

The intensity of infection of nematode order/species is presented in Table 1. In most cases, intensity of the infection was low followed by median intensity; no cases of high infection load were seen; from the infected dogs, all of them had only a single order/species of nematode present.

Regarding the serology from human samples, 26 (29.2%) from the 89 persons were positive to IgG anti-*T. canis* (Table 2). None of the risk factors studied were significantly associated with seropositivity in humans (Table 3). All participants owned at least one dog and none of them collected the feces from their animals. From the questionnaire, 36 persons claim vision disorders such as cloudy vision and increased tearing.

Regarding IgG anti-*T. gondii* serological results, from 89 human blood samples collected, 90.6% were positive to IgG *T. gondii* (Table 2). For dogs, 89 samples were obtained and 97.6% were seropositive to *T. gondii*. Since very few negative cases were found, no statistical inferences were feasible. From the interviews, 93% drink water from commercial carafes, 5% drink tap water, and 2% drink from both sources. Participants reported that the ingestion of meat is usually well cooked in 82% of cases and 7% claim to eat semicooked meat. 88.8% of

TABLE 2: Serological frequency of zoonotic agents identified in 89 persons from a rural community of Yucatan, Mexico.

Agent	Positive cases (*n*)	%
T. canis	26	29.2
T. gondii	81	91.0
T. spiralis	6	6.7
T. canis + *T. gondii*	26	29.2
T. spiralis + *T. gondii*	4	4.5

TABLE 3: Relationship between associated factors with *T. canis* IgG seropositivity in humans from a rural community of Yucatan, Mexico.

	n	Positive	Prevalence	OR	95% CI	*P* value
Age (years)						
20–40	29	8	27.6%	1.5	0.54–4.26	0.42 (NS)
>40–75	55	11	20.0%	—	—	—
Sex						
Male	8	1	12.5%	—	—	—
Female	76	18	23.7%	4.46	0.05–3.9	0.41 (NS)
Eyes lesions						
Yes	52	16	30.8%	1.3	0.49–3.6	0.56 (NS)
No	32	8	25.5%	—	—	—
Deworming						
Yes	32	12	37.5%	1.8	0.91–6.02	0.22 (NS)
No	52	13	25.6%	—	—	—

n: number of humans studied, OR: odds ratio, CI: confidence interval, and *P*: probability.
NS: not significant.

the interviewed persons eat sausages and from the 10 persons (11.2%) who do not eat sausages 2 were seronegative.

Only 6 (6.9%) persons were found seropositive to *T. spiralis* (Table 2).

4. Discussion

The prevalence of dogs infected with gastrointestinal parasites in this study is considered high and similar to the reported one in other regions of the world, that is, 52.4% in Argentina [12], 53% in Hungary [13], and 68% in Nigeria [14]. The high variation observed has been associated with various weather conditions, idiosyncrasies, and sanitary control of dogs. A previous study in the same community was performed four years ago and prevalence of gastrointestinal parasites in dogs was 80% with a high egg output of *A. caninum*, *T. canis*, and *T. vulpis* found; in this study, deworming of dogs was performed and talks to children, adolescents, and adults about health management of dogs were given [15]. These actions could explain the lower prevalence and intensity of infection reported at this time categorized between low and medium intensity of infection. In the specific case of *T. canis*, a higher prevalence (12.5%) was found compared to previous studies in the same area where 6.2% was found [15]. *T. canis* mainly affects puppies with frequently fatal consequences. In adult dogs, the infection is minor and usually asymptomatic. The annual variation in the number of infected puppies in the region may influence the disposal and spreading of *T. canis* eggs. The presence of infected puppies can increase the number of eggs and larvae deposited in the environment in which they can remain infective for several months infecting other dogs and with great potential to infect humans, especially children.

Human toxocariasis is worldwide distributed and occurs when embryonated eggs from the environment are ingested. This is more critical when dog overpopulation is present without the practice of preventive medicine (deworming). Children with pica are found at increased risk particularly in regions of low socioeconomic status and with proliferation of dogs and/or those who have puppies at home [7]. Adults are also at risk of infection as shown by several studies where prevalence of 26.8% in Brazil was reported [16] and 19% in Lebanon was reported [17]. In Argentina, seroprevalence of 20–38% in children and 10–39% in general population [18, 19] is reported. In Mexico, 38% of people suffering from acute nongranulomatous uveitis were seropositive for *T. canis* [20], with a prevalence of 4.6% to 17.59% reported in children less than 16 years of age [21]. Results of this study indicate a high spread of infective eggs in the rural community probably because of the high density of dogs having free access to the street and lack of health programs including a deworming program.

Although deworming has been introduced in health management of dogs in the studied community, still spreading of infected eggs and contamination of the area are present; thus, efforts to intensify the deworming of dog and cat are necessary for better control results. The ocular larva migrans syndrome is one of the major health problems associated with *T. canis* [22]. However, eye lesions were not statistically associated with seropositive persons; this syndrome is more critical in children where severe problems have been reported [7], so studies to evaluate the impact of this parasite on children should be designed and performed. *T. canis* and *T. gondii* are associated with eye lesions such as uveitis [23]. Ocular larva migrans in the case of toxocariasis may cause visual impairment as a response of granulomatous inflammatory reaction with consequences such as blindness and secondary glaucoma [7, 24]. In the present study, no association was found in patients seropositive to *T. canis* and vision disorders. However, other symptoms not evaluated in the present study may involve headache, muscle pain, influenza-like syndrome, and diarrhea in seropositive patients [25]. In a previous study conducted in Mexico, *T. canis* positive patients were highly associated with ankylosing spondylitis [26]. Young children, <5 years, are most affected with toxocariasis with clinical signs of fever, abdominal pain (probably due to hepatomegaly), and lower respiratory symptoms [7]. Further studies should be focused on children in the studied region examining the different body systems to evaluate the impact of this zoonotic agent.

The high prevalence of *T. gondii* found in dogs and their owners demonstrates a high spread of oocysts in the studied area with a probably common source of infection. The prevalence found in dogs from Brazil was 26.9% with a higher risk for dogs over five years of age [27]. However, in the present study, due to the very high prevalence found, all animals are expected to seroconvert since young ages with frequent episodes of reinfection. In Mexico, dog from shelters in Veracruz also showed a high seroprevalence reaching up to 67.3% [28]. Free roaming dogs are indicators of the high contamination of the environment with *T. gondii* oocysts as they may be sentinels of exposition. In humans, toxoplasmosis has been reported previously in the Yucatán peninsula with seroprevalence of 25% in non-cat owners [29] and also associated in patients with recent cases of spontaneous abortion [30, 31]. Seroprevalence may reach up to 87.3% in humans from rural communities from Yucatan [32]. In humans, the main route of infection of *T. gondii* is by the ingestion of tissue cysts [33]. In the present study, the oral route by consumption of undercooked meat (tissue cysts) is more likely but also the ingestion of infective oocysts from contaminated water as previously demonstrated could occur [34]. Considering the 100% *T. gondii* seroprevalence found in 50 studied cats from the same region [4], the density of cats and constant new born kittens in the village with excretion of high numbers of oocysts probably occurred, contaminating the environment and probable water sources. Even when 93% of the interviewed persons drank commercial bottled water, tap water and water from artisanal wells are also used for several other activities and may be considered as a potential source of infection with *T. gondii* oocysts. However, since dogs in the studied area are fed with human leftovers [35], contaminated meat and sausages may also be involved in the transmission cycle.

T. spiralis is a nematode capable of infecting any mammal ingesting infected raw or undercooked meat. Infection in humans with this nematode is described worldwide and outbreaks have been reported in developed countries infecting over 30% of people ingesting wild boar meat [36]. Exposition of consumers to infected meat can reach up to 65.1% of incidence, especially when meat is not tested prior to consumption when slaughter is made in households [37]. In Mexico, consumption of pork meat coming from backyard is very common in rural villages without any kind of quality test [4]. In Mexico, the Ministry of Health (NOM-194-SSA1-2014) makes the inspection of pork meat in search of *T. spiralis* compulsory. However, this is rarely done at the abattoirs or before commercialization. *T. spiralis* in Mexico has been reported since 1975 in Zacatecas state where several outbreaks have been reported in cases with mortality rates of 33% in some cases; in those outbreaks, transmission was most commonly caused by the ingestion of raw pork products or undercooked meat [38]. More recently, a prevalence of 1% using ELISA was reported in semirural county areas of Mexico [39]. In Yucatan, no proper surveys of *T. spiralis* have been performed in humans or animals. This is the first report of *T. spiralis* serological presence in humans from Yucatan. However, the *Toxocara* larval excretory antigen is normally used in serological tests that may exhibit low specificity due to cross-reaction between related helminthes, including *T. canis* [40]. Further research is needed to investigate the epidemiology of these zoonotic helminthes using more accurate techniques for diagnosis including the search of the agent in farm and backyard pigs from the region.

The main limitation of the present study was the small sample size used and consequently results may be biased or may not be representative of the rural communities from the studied area. However, this study may be a good indicator of the zoonotic situation and establish the bases for further studies including a bigger and targeted sample size from both animals and humans.

5. Conclusion

It is concluded that the dogs in a rural community of Yucatan are reservoirs of some helminthes parasites specially *T. canis*. This implies a high risk of the presence of parasites in the environment of the village and a potential risk of infection for the human community. It is important to improve the dissemination and promotion of educational programs on this important zoonosis and establish effective control measures to reduce the emission of eggs and avoid contact of human with areas contaminated with dog feces. Other important zoonotic parasites (*T. gondii* and *T. spiralis*) are also circulating.

Conflict of Interests

The authors declare that there is no conflict of interests regarding the publication of this paper.

Acknowledgments

This paper was financially supported by the Ministry of Education in Mexico through "PRODEP" (Programa para el Desarrollo Profesional Docente) as part of the project "Epidemiología de Enfermedades Zoonoticas Transmitidas por Vectores (ETV'S) de Importancia en Salud Publica."

References

[1] A. L. Salb, H. W. Barkema, B. T. Elkin et al., "Dogs as sources and sentinels of parasites in humans and wildlife, Northern Canada," *Emerging Infectious Diseases*, vol. 14, no. 1, pp. 60–63, 2008.

[2] J. G. Berdugo and C. Franco, "Ganaderia de traspatio en el Estado de Yucatan," in *Memorias de la Segunda Reunion Sobre Produccion Animal Tropical*, M. R. Godoy, J. C. Segura, and A. Arellano, Eds., pp. 114–120, Merida Yucatan, Mérida, Mexico, 1991.

[3] R. Ku-Duperón, W. Trejo-Lizama, A. J. Aguilar-Caballero et al., "Gastrointestinal parasitism in the Mexican hairless pig in backyard in the state of Yucatan, Mexico," *Revista Colombiana de Ciencia Animal*, vol. 6, pp. 17–24, 2013.

[4] M. Jimenez-Coello, K. Y. Acosta-Viana, E. Guzman-Marin et al., "The occurrence of *Toxoplasma gondii* antibodies in backyard pigs and cats from an endemic tropical area of Mexico," *Tropical and Subtropical Agroecosystems*, vol. 16, no. 1, pp. 89–92, 2013.

[5] J. L. Jones, D. Kruszon-Moran, K. Won, M. Wilson, and P. M. Schantz, "*Toxoplasma gondii* and Toxocara spp. co-infection," *American Journal of Tropical Medicine and Hygiene*, vol. 78, no. 1, pp. 35–39, 2008.

[6] L. T. Glickman and P. M. Schantz, "Epidemiology and pathogenesis of zoonotic toxocariasis," *Epidemiologic Reviews*, vol. 3, no. 1, pp. 230–250, 1981.

[7] D. Despommier, "Toxocariasis: clinical aspects, epidemiology, medical ecology, and molecular aspects," *Clinical Microbiology Reviews*, vol. 16, no. 2, pp. 265–272, 2003.

[8] H. V. Smith and R. Noordin, "Diagnostic limitations and future trends in the serodiagnosis of human toxocariasis," in *Toxocara: The Enigmatic Parasite*, C. V. Holland and H. V. Smith, Eds., chapter 7, pp. 89–112, CABI Publishing, Wallingford, UK, 2006.

[9] D. E. Thompson, D. A. P. Bundy, E. S. Cooper, and P. M. Schantz, "Edidemiological characteristics of *Toxocara canis* zoonotic infection of children in a Caribbean community," *Bulletin of the World Health Organization*, vol. 64, no. 2, pp. 283–290, 1986.

[10] J. V. Conlan, K. Vongxay, B. Khamlome et al., "Patterns and risks of *Trichinella* infection in humans and pigs in northern Laos," *PLoS Neglected Tropical Diseases*, vol. 8, no. 7, Article ID e3034, 2014.

[11] R. I. Rodríguez-Vivas and L. A. Cob-Galera, *Técnicas Diagnóstico en Parasitología Veterinaria*, Universidad Autónoma de Yucatán, Mérida, México, 2nd edition, 2005.

[12] M. F. Fontanarrosa, D. Vezzani, J. Basabe, and D. F. Eiras, "An epidemiological study of gastrointestinal parasites of dogs from Southern Greater Buenos Aires (Argentina): age, gender, breed, mixed infections, and seasonal and spatial patterns," *Veterinary Parasitology*, vol. 136, no. 3-4, pp. 283–295, 2006.

[13] E. Fok, V. Szatmári, K. Busák, and F. Rozgonyi, "Prevalence of intestinal parasites in dogs in some urban and rural areas of Hungary," *Veterinary Quarterly*, vol. 23, no. 2, pp. 96–98, 2001.

[14] B. M. Anene, T. O. Nnaji, and A. B. Chime, "Intestinal parasitic infections of dogs in the Nsukka area of Enugu State, Nigeria," *Preventive Veterinary Medicine*, vol. 27, no. 1-2, pp. 89–94, 1996.

[15] R. I. Rodríguez-Vivas, E. Gutierrez-Ruiz, M. E. Bolio-González et al., "An epidemiological study of intestinal parasites of dogs from Yucatan, Mexico, and their risk to public health," *Vector-Borne and Zoonotic Diseases*, vol. 11, no. 8, pp. 1141–1144, 2011.

[16] G. Rubinsky-Elefant, M. da Silva-Nunes, R. S. Malafronte, P. T. Muniz, and M. U. Ferreira, "Human toxocariasis in rural Brazilian Amazonia: seroprevalence, risk factors, and spatial distribution," *American Journal of Tropical Medicine and Hygiene*, vol. 79, no. 1, pp. 93–98, 2008.

[17] Z. A. Kanafani, A. Skoury, G. F. Araj et al., "Seroprevalence of toxocariasis in Lebanon: a pilot study," *Parasitology*, vol. 132, no. 5, pp. 635–639, 2006.

[18] N. E. Radman, S. M. Archelli, R. D. Fonrouge, M. D. V. Guardis, and O. R. Linzitto, "Human toxocarosis. Its seroprevalence in the City of La Plata," *Memórias do Instituto Oswaldo Cruz*, vol. 95, no. 3, pp. 281–285, 2000.

[19] J. M. Alonso, M. V. I. Bojanich, M. Chamorro, and J. O. Gorodner, "Toxocara seroprevalence in children from a subtropical city in Argentina," *Revista do Instituto de Medicina Tropical de Sao Paulo*, vol. 42, no. 4, pp. 235–237, 2000.

[20] F. Jiménez-Balderas, J. García-Jaimes, R. Ríos et al., "Isolation of IgG antibodies to *Toxocara* in ankylosing spondylitis patients with acute anterior uveítis," *Korean Journal of Ophthalmology*, vol. 28, no. 3, pp. 207–212, 2014.

[21] C. Romero Núñez, G. D. Mendoza Martínez, S. Yañez Arteaga, M. Ponce Macotela, P. Bustamante Montes, and N. Ramírez Durán, "Prevalence and risk factors associated with toxocara canis infection in children," *The Scientific World Journal*, vol. 2013, Article ID 572089, 4 pages, 2013.

[22] D. Woodhall, M. C. Starr, S. P. Montgomery et al., "Ocular toxocariasis: epidemiologic, anatomic, and therapeutic variations based on a survey of ophthalmic subspecialists," *Ophthalmology*, vol. 119, no. 6, pp. 1211–1217, 2012.

[23] S. J. Lim, S. E. Lee, S. H. Kim et al., "Prevalence of *Toxoplasma gondii* and *Toxocara canis* among patients with uveitis," *Ocular Immunology and Inflammation*, vol. 22, no. 5, pp. 360–366, 2014.

[24] S. H. Gillespie, W. J. Dinning, A. Voller, and N. S. Crowcroft, "The spectrum of ocular toxocariasis," *Eye*, vol. 7, no. 3, pp. 415–418, 1993.

[25] D. Antolavá, P. Jarcuska, M. Janicko et al., "Seroprevalence of human Toxocara infections in the Roma and non-Roma populations of Eastern Slovakia: a cross-sectional study," *Epidemiology and Infection*, vol. 143, no. 10, pp. 1–10, 2015.

[26] F. J. Jimenez-Balderas, A. Camargo-Coronel, J. Gargia-Jaimes et al., "A study on parasites in Mexican rheumatic disease patients," *Journal of the Egyptian Society of Parasitology*, vol. 42, no. 2, pp. 271–280, 2012.

[27] H. Langoni, F. Fornazari, R. C. da Silva, E. T. Monti, and F. B. Villa, "Prevalence of antibodies against *Toxoplasma gondii* and *Neospora caninum* in dogs," *Brazilian Journal of Microbiology*, vol. 44, no. 4, pp. 1327–1330, 2013.

[28] C. Alvarado-Esquivel, D. Romero-Salas, A. Cruz-Romero et al., "High prevalence of *Toxoplasma gondii* antibodies in dogs in Veracruz, Mexico," *BMC Veterinary Research*, vol. 10, article 191, 2014.

[29] M. Jiménez-Coello, E. Guzmán-Marín, A. Ortega-Pacheco, and K. Y. Acosta-Viana, "Immunological status against *Toxoplasma gondii* in non-cat owners from an endemic Region of Mexico," *Vector-Borne and Zoonotic Diseases*, vol. 11, no. 8, pp. 1057–1061, 2011.

[30] J. Zavala-Velázquez, E. Guzmán-Marín, M. Barrera-Pérez, and M. E. Rodríguez-Félix, "Toxoplasmosis and abortion in patients at the O'Horan Hospital of Merida, Yucatan," *Salud Publica de Mexico*, vol. 31, no. 5, pp. 664–668, 1989.

[31] I. A. Vado-Solís, V. Suárez-Solís, B. Jiménez-Delgadillo, J. E. Zavala-Velázquez, and J. C. Segura-Correa, "*Toxoplasma gondii* presence in women with spontaneous abortion in Yucatan, Mexico," *The Journal of Parasitology*, vol. 99, no. 2, pp. 383–385, 2013.

[32] M. Jimenez-Coello, E. Guzman-Marin, M. Rosado-Barrera M et al., "Seoprevalence of *Toxoplasma gondii* in a por rural community from Yucatan, Mexico," in *Memories from the 13th International Congress of Parasitology, August 10–15 Mexico, 2014*, 2014.

[33] A. Kijlstra and E. Jongert, "Toxoplasma-safe meat: close to reality?" *Trends in Parasitology*, vol. 25, no. 1, pp. 18–22, 2009.

[34] J. L. Jones and J. P. Dubey, "Waterborne toxoplasmosis—recent developments," *Experimental Parasitology*, vol. 124, no. 1, pp. 10–25, 2010.

[35] A. Ortega-Pacheco, J. C. Rodriguez-Buenfil, M. E. Bolio-Gonzalez, C. H. Sauri-Arceo, M. Jiménez-Coello, and C. L. Forsberg, "A survey of dog populations in Urban and rural areas of Yucatan, Mexico," *Anthrozoos*, vol. 20, no. 3, pp. 261–274, 2007.

[36] M. Faber, S. Schink, A. Mayer-Scholl et al., "Outbreak of trichinellosis due to wild boar meat and evaluation of the effectiveness of post exposure prophylaxis, Germany, 2013," *Clinical Infectious Diseases*, vol. 60, no. 2, pp. e98–e104, 2015.

[37] C. Dobrescu, H. Hriscu, M. Emandi, C. Zamfir, and C. Nemet, "Consumption of untested pork contributed to over two-thousand clinical cases of human trichinellosis in Romania," *Folia Parasitologica*, vol. 61, no. 6, pp. 558–560, 2014.

[38] J. Cabral-Soto, H. Villicaña-Fuentes, R. Fragoso-Uribe, and A. Contreras, "The epidemiological profile of trichinosis in the state of Zacatecas," *Salud Publica de Mexico*, vol. 32, no. 5, pp. 575–582, 1990.

[39] J. L. De-La-Rosa, J. G. Aranda, E. Padilla, and D. Correa, "Prevalence and risk factors associated with serum antibodies against *Trichinella spiralis*," *International Journal for Parasitology*, vol. 28, no. 2, pp. 317–321, 1998.

[40] S. Özkoç, S. Bayram Delibaş, and Ç. Akisü, "Evaluation of Trichinella cross-reactions in the serological diagnosis of toxocariasis," *Mikrobiyoloji Bulteni*, vol. 46, no. 3, pp. 456–463, 2012.

5

Leukogram Profile and Clinical Status in *vivax* and *falciparum* Malaria Patients from Colombia

Alberto Tobón-Castaño, Esteban Mesa-Echeverry, and Andrés Felipe Miranda-Arboleda

Grupo Malaria, Facultad de Medicina, Universidad de Antioquia, Calle 70, No. 52-21, Medellín, Colombia

Correspondence should be addressed to Alberto Tobón-Castaño; alberto.tobonl@udea.edu.co

Academic Editor: Ib C. Bygbjerg

Introduction. Hematological alterations are frequent in malaria patients; the relationship between alterations in white blood cell counts and clinical status in malaria is not well understood. In Colombia, with low endemicity and unstable transmission for malaria, with malaria *vivax* predominance, the hematologic profile in malaria patients is not well characterized. The aim of this study was to characterize the leukogram in malaria patients and to analyze its alterations in relation to the clinical status. *Methods.* 888 leukogram profiles of malaria patients from different Colombian regions were studied: 556 with *P. falciparum* infection (62.6%), 313 with *P. vivax* infection (35.2%), and 19 with mixed infection by these species (2.1%). *Results.* Leukocyte counts at diagnosis were within normal range in 79% of patients and 18% had leucopenia; the most frequent alteration was lymphopenia (54%) followed by monocytosis (11%); the differential granulocyte count in 298 patients revealed eosinophilia (15%) and high basophil counts (8%). Leukocytosis, eosinopenia, and neutrophilia were associated with clinical complications. The utility of changes in leukocyte counts as markers of severity should be explored in depth. A better understanding of these hematological parameters will allow their use in prompt diagnosis of malaria complications and monitoring treatment response.

1. Introduction

Malaria, a disease caused by protozoan parasites of the genus *Plasmodium*, is still considered a serious global public health problem [1]. There were approximately 198 million cases and 584,000 deaths in 2013, according to the World Health Organization (WHO) [2]; however it has been noted in recent years that there is significant underreporting of cases and deaths worldwide [3]. Fatal cases are mainly attributed to *Plasmodium falciparum*; however other plasmodia, like *P. vivax*, can cause serious illness and even death [4, 5].

Malaria can affect any organ or system, the hematological system being the most affected one. The majority of described alterations occur on the red cell line and platelets, causing anemia and thrombocytopenia [6–8]. Alterations in the white blood cell (WBC) counts are less reported and have been associated with factors such as severity, *Plasmodium* species, concurrent infections, and treatment response [9–12]. Descriptions of leukocytosis, leukopenia, neutrophilia, and neutropenia, presence of immature neutrophils, and changes in lymphocytes, monocytes, and eosinophils in these patients have been observed [13, 14], but studies have not shown a specific leukocyte profile alteration in malaria.

It has been found that WBC counts are generally lower in malaria patients compared to healthy patients and that there is a trend towards lower WBC counts in patients infected with either *P. falciparum* or *P. vivax* [15]. Additionally it has been observed that these changes are dynamic during illness, with lower lymphocyte and eosinophil counts at baseline and higher counts as the symptoms disappear [15, 16]. There have been descriptions of mortality-associated leukocytosis, presence of coinfections, and gram negative bacteremia in complicated cases of *P. falciparum* malaria [17].

Several theories attempt to explain these described hematologic disorders, including (i) bone marrow (BM) suppression secondary to immune response imbalances, (ii) lower average cell life, and (iii) leukocyte redistribution to lymphoid organs and tissues with increased inflammatory response or sequestration in microvasculature [11, 14, 18–20]. However, these findings remain poorly understood and their utility in clinical practice has not yet been established, unlike for other infectious diseases prevalent in tropical areas, such as Dengue [21].

The Complete Blood Count (CBC) assesses the cellular elements of the blood, that is, red cells, white cells, and platelets, both qualitatively and quantitatively [22] and is an essential tool in assessing hematological changes. The leukogram is part of the CBC that analyzes white blood cells; it comprises the total WBC and subpopulation counts including neutrophils, eosinophils, basophils, lymphocytes, and monocytes. Their reference values vary according to age, race, physiological condition (pregnancy), use of some drugs, and time of day [23]. The aim of this study is to characterize changes in the WBC count of patients with malaria from endemic regions in Colombia and to analyze variations according to clinical status, species of *Plasmodium*, and some sociodemographic characteristics of the patients. Our purpose is to encourage the use of easily accessible diagnostic tools, such as the CBC, allowing early identification of patients at risk for clinical complications and to implement appropriate therapeutic measures, improving patient outcome.

2. Methods and Materials

A descriptive retrospective analysis was made with clinical, laboratory, and demographic data from outpatients with *P. falciparum* or *P. vivax* malaria, from endemic regions in Colombia. The reference population consisted of patients of all ages with symptoms suggestive of malaria, with parasitological diagnosis confirmed with thick blood smear examination in first or second level of care hospitals and health care facilities in the municipalities of Turbo and Necoclí (Urabá, Antioquia), El Bagre (Bajo Cauca, Antioquia), Tumaco, Guapi, and Timbiquí (Pacific Coast), and who were enrolled in clinical and epidemiological studies conducted by the Malaria Group between 1997 and 2007 [24–26]. We also included Medellín third-level hospitals' inpatients' data from 2005 to 2010, referred from different regions. Convenience sampling was performed for this analysis; only patients with a CBC performed at hospital admission were included, obtaining a sample of 888 patients.

The thick smear examination was done according to WHO recommendations [27]. After a medical assessment, a sample of blood was taken in EDTA for cellular and biochemical studies, including a CBC within 2 hours, obtained in 3rd- and 4th-generation automated analyzers (Abbott Diagnostics Cell-Dyn3200; Beckman Coulter, Coulter HmX; and Nihon Kohden Celltac MEK, Sysmex KX-21N). Colombian population reference values for the WBC counts were applied (Table 1) [28].

The WBC count, hemoglobin values, and platelets counts were qualitatively classified as low or high if they were above or below the normal range. Complications were classified according to WHO major criteria for severity [29] and to proposed minor criteria for Colombia [26] as follows:

(1) liver failure: severe liver failure (total bilirubin >3 mg/dL; AST >120 IU/L) or mild liver failure (total bilirubin > 1.5–3 mg/dL; AST > 80–120 IU/L); (2) thrombocytopenia: profound (<25,000 platelets/μL) or severe (25–50,000 platelets/μL); (3) renal impairment: severe (BUN > 60 mg/dL or creatinine > 3 mg/dL) or mild (BUN 41–60 mg/dL or creatinine 1.5–3 mg/dL); (4) anemia: severe (hemoglobin < 5 gr/dL) or moderate (hemoglobin 5–6.9 gr/dL); (5) neurologic complication: cerebral malaria (seizures/coma) or extreme weakness; (6) pulmonary injury: acute respiratory distress syndrome (ARDS)/pulmonary edema or pleural effusion; (7) acid-base disturbance: severe acidosis (pH < 7.35 and HCO_3 < 15 mEq/L) or acidosis (pH < 7.35 and HCO_3 15–18 mEq/L); and (8) hypoglycemia: severe (<40 mg/dL) or moderate (40–49 mg/dL).

Patients were divided into five age groups for analysis. Parasitemia was classified by ranges of parasites/μL in up to 1,000; 1,001–5,000; 5,001–10,000; 10,001–50,000; 50,001–100,000; and greater than 100,000.

2.1. Statistical Analysis. The Kolmogorov-Smirnov test was used to assess normality for quantitative variables; the median values were compared with Mann-Whitney U test when variables were not normal. Associations between qualitative variables were analyzed with the χ^2 test. Spearman's rank correlation coefficient was applied to analyze some relationships between numerical data. The adopted level of statistical significance was 5% (P value <0.05). The analysis was done with IBM SPSS statistics program, 22nd version (licensed to Universidad de Antioquia).

2.2. Ethical Aspects. The patients studied prospectively were included after giving informed consent, endorsed by the Ethics Committee of the Medical Research Institute from the Medical School of the Universidad de Antioquia (Minute 31, July 2002; Minute 5, June 2005). The review of retrospectively studied patients' medical records was approved by the Hospital Ethics Committees from Hospital Pablo Tobón Uribe and Hospital San Vicente Fundación (Letter 5282, October 2009).

3. Results

Blood counts of 888 patients were analyzed. The quantitative variables showed normal distribution, except hemoglobin (KS, $P = 0.082$). The sample consisted mostly of men (62.8%) over 15 years of age, with a mean age of 26 years (median 22.8). Age ranged from 1 month to 82 years. The geographic origin of the patients is shown in Figure 1. Some demographic characteristics are described in Table 2.

The time of disease progression to first medical consultation was known for 618 patients: 30% (n = 185) consulted within the first three days of onset of symptoms, 44.9% (n = 277) between days 4 and 7, and 21.3% (n = 132) from day 8 to 15; 3.8% of the study population consulted 2 weeks after the onset of symptoms. Previous use of antimicrobials was established (not antimalarial) in 39 (4.4%) patients (particularly penicillins in 23 and cephalosporins in 7) and antimalarials in 79 (8.9%) (particularly chloroquine and primaquine in 68 and quinine in 8). Complicated malaria was diagnosed in 257 patients (29%): 110 (12%) with major criteria and 147 (16.6%) with minor criteria for severity; no deaths were reported.

Table 1: Leukogram reference values by age*.

Age	Leukocytes/μL	Neutrophils/μL	Lymphocytes/μL	Monocytes/μL	Eosinophils/μL	Basophils/μL
1–15 days	9,000–30,000	1,000–12,000	3,000–9,000	30–750	40–500	0–50
16–31 days	5,000–21,000	1,000–12,000	3,000–9,000	30–750	40–500	0–50
1–12 months	6,000–17,500	1,000–12,000	3,000–9,000	30–750	40–500	0–50
1–5 years	5,500–15,500	1,700–7,500	3,000–9,000	30–750	40–500	0–50
6–14 years	4,500–14,500	1,500–6,500	2,000–7,200	30–750	40–500	0–50
15–99 years	4,500–11,000	1,500–8,000	1,500–4,000	30–900	40–500	0–50

*Leukogram counts based on gender not shown.
Adapted from [28].

Table 2: Demographic characteristics of 888 malaria patients from Colombia.

Characteristics	n	%
Gender		
Male	558	63
Female	330	37
Age		
Less than 1 year	8	0.9
1.1 to 5 years	50	5.6
5.1 to 15 years	193	21.7
15.1 to 65 years	624	70.3
Over 65 years	13	1.5

3.1. Parasite Counts Description. *P. falciparum* infection was diagnosed in 556 patients (62.6%); *P. vivax* was in 313 (35.2%) and mixed infection by these species in 19 (2.1%). The median parasite count in 809 patients was 4,980/μL; 71.8% (n = 581) had counts lower than 10,000 parasites/μL and 1% (n = 8) had parasitemia above 100,000/μL. In parasitemia ranges, 19.9% had less than 1,000 parasites/μL, 51.8% between 1,000 and 10,000, 24.5% between 10,001 and 50,000, and 2.7% between 50,000 and 100,000.

3.2. Leukogram Findings. Leukocyte subpopulations were not normally distributed (KS, $P < 0.001$); leukocyte counts at diagnosis were within the normal range in 79% (n = 698) of patients and 18% (n = 157) had leucopenia; the median value for these cells was 6,100/μL. Figures 2 and 3 show subpopulation frequency distribution. Patients with previous use of antimicrobials had a higher frequency of leukopenia than those not taking any (35.9% versus 16.8%) (OR = 2.9; 1.4–5.7; P = 0.002); the former had lower leukocyte counts than the latter (Mann-Whitney U test; P = 0.016).

Mononuclear Cells. Lymphopenia prevailed in 54% (n = 476); the median value for these cells was 1,575/μL. Monocyte count was normal in 85% of cases (n = 749); the median count was 371 cells/μL.

Granulocytes (PMN). Some of the analyzed blood counts did not have differential granulocyte subpopulations counts and only had a total granulocyte count. Normal values were found in 91% of patients (n = 805). One-third of differential counts came from severe patients and the rest from nonsevere ones (66%)

Analyzed neutrophils in 446 patients showed normal values in 91% of cases (n = 407); the median value was 3,836 cells/μL. Only 250 patients had eosinophil counts of which 80% (n = 201) were normal and 15% (n = 37) had eosinophilia; the median value for these cells was 176/μL. Eosinopenia was present in 5% (n = 12) of patients. Only 268 patients had basophil counts, of which 92% (n = 246) were within normal values. No patient in this group had counts below normal levels.

3.2.1. Age of Patients. The median neutrophil value was lower in children; there was greater variability in their counts with the highest individual neutrophil counts. Means and medians are presented in Table 3. No significant differences between groups were observed when values were assigned into the categories of normal, low, or high ($P > 0.05$). Children were more likely to have monocytosis (RR = 2.2, 1.4–3.5; $P < 0.001$), neutrophilia (RR = 2.3, 1.0–5.2; P = 0.046), and eosinophilia (RR = 2.2, 1.1–4.5; P = 0.029) than adults (Table 4).

3.2.2. Parasitemia and Plasmodium Species. There was a negative relationship between the number of parasites and the eosinophil count (Spearman coefficient −0.2; P = 0.010); no linear correlation was found with other cell populations. There were no differences in leukocyte subpopulations medians in relation to plasmodial species ($P > 0.05$) (Table 3).

3.2.3. Severe Malaria. Neutrophilia and eosinopenia were the most common alterations in severe malaria cases. The comparison between severe malaria (overall complications, diagnosed with major or minor criteria) and nonsevere malaria shows that leukopenia and leukocytosis, lymphopenia, eosinopenia, monocytosis, and neutrophilia were linked to severity (Table 5). These associations remained when only major criteria were applied, except for leukocytosis. When only minor criteria were applied, leukopenia (OR = 1.7; 1.1–2.6; P = 0.022), leukocytosis (OR = 2.5; 1.01–2.6; P = 0.039), lymphopenia (OR = 2.2; 1.5–3.2; $P < 0.001$), and eosinopenia (OR = 10.8; 2.1–55.6; P = 0.002) were associated with severity. Leucocyte counts are compared in relation to clinical condition in Table 6.

3.2.4. Glycemia and Leukocytes. Glycemia values were obtained from 357 subjects, averaging 107.6 mg/dL (37–264) with a median of 102 mg/d. When glycemia was compared with leukocyte counts, patients with leucopenia had

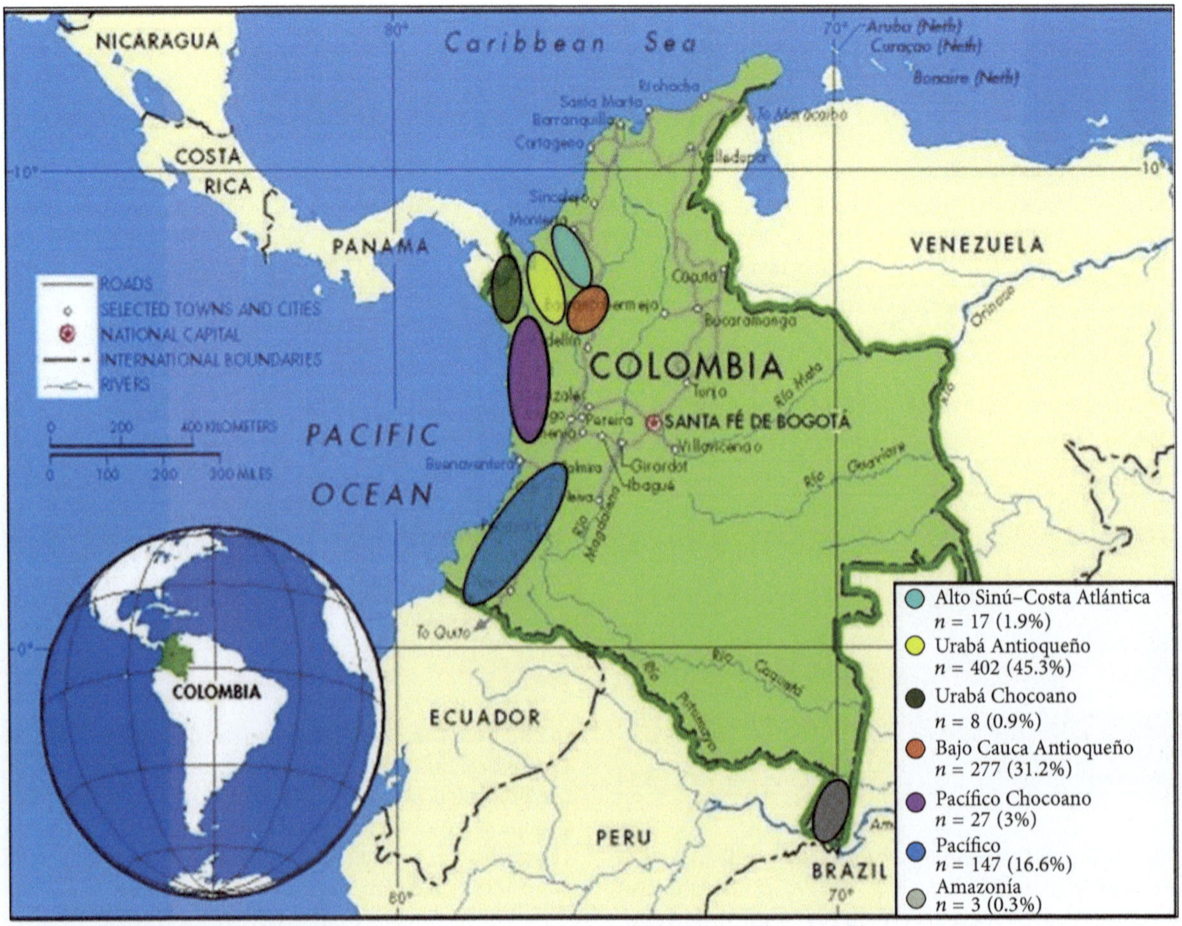

FIGURE 1: Geographical location of patients' residence by Colombian malarial endemic regions. Obtained and modified from the Cartographic Design Unit of the World Bank, 2000.

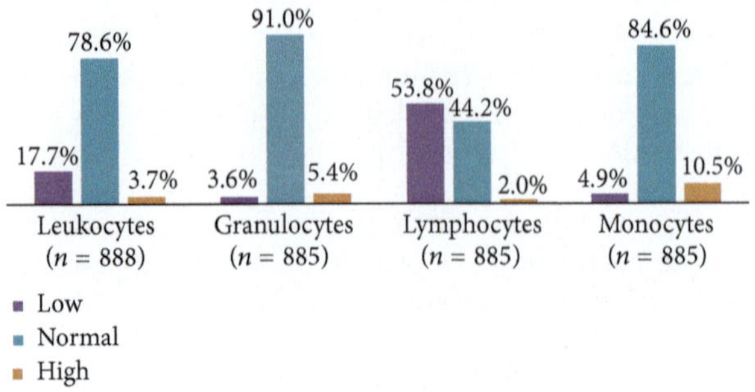

FIGURE 2: Leukocyte counts distributions.

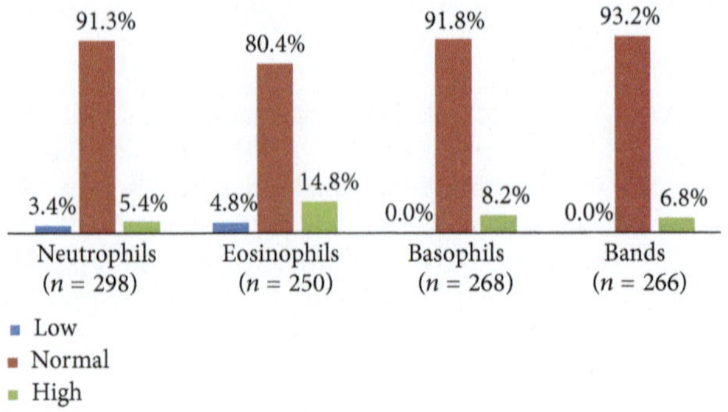

FIGURE 3: Granulocyte subpopulations counts.

significantly higher blood glucose with a median of 108 mg/dL and those with normal WBC count had a median of 101 mg/dL ($P = 0.033$, Mann-Whitney); leukopenia patients had an increased risk of elevated blood sugar levels (>140 mg/dL) (OR = 2.6; 1.4–5; $P = 0.004$) compared with patients with a normal WBC count.

Lymphopenia patients had a median blood glucose of 109 mg/dL versus 95 mg/dL in patients with normal lymphocyte counts ($P < 0.001$, Mann-Whitney); lymphopenia was associated with an increased risk of high blood glucose levels (>140 mg/dL) (OR = 2.8; 1.3–5.7; $P = 0.007$).

Low granulocyte counts were related to lower blood glucose values, with a median of 81 mg/dL versus 103 mg/dL in patients with normal granulocyte counts ($P = 0.002$, Mann-Whitney), but the values remained within normal ranges. There was no higher risk of high blood glucose ($P < 0.05$) in patients with low granulocyte counts.

Table 3: Leukocyte subpopulations (cells/μL) by age ranges and malaria etiology.

		Less than 1 year (n = 8)	1.1 to 5 years (n = 50)	5.1 to 15 years (n = 193)	15.1 to 65 years (n = 624)	Over 65 years (n = 13)	*P. falciparum*** (n = 556)	*P. vivax* (313)
Leukocytes (n = 888)	Mean	13,238	8,360	6,723	6,438	6,671	6,597	6,700
	CI*	6,592–19,883	7,480–9,240	6,289–7,158	6,250–6,627	5,676–7,667	6,385–6,810	6,414–7,086
	Median	10,050	8,200	6,200	6,000	6,000	6,000	6,200
Lymphocytes (n = 885)	Mean	5,914	3,803	2,037	1,639	1,427	1,897	1,850
	CI	3,450–8,377	3,251–4355	1,840–2,233	1,564–1,715	1,034–1,820	1,786–2,007	1,707–1,993
	Median	5,472	3,473	1,776	1,451	1,248	1,585	1,539
Monocytes (n = 885)	Mean	776	663	462	425	436	434	454
	CI	193–1,360	479–846	408–516	398–452	296	402–466	415–494
	Median	652	434	383	348	576	360	372
Granulocytes (n = 885)	Mean	6,516	3,887	4,188	4,370	4,829	4,266	4,420
	CI	1,422–11,610	3242–4533	3880–4496	4207–4532	3,772–5,885	4,098–4,435	4,164–4,675
	Median	4,502	3,590	3,768	4,128	4,210	3,950	4,015
Neutrophils (n = 446)	Mean	4,791	3,753	3,886	4,264	4,585	4,087	4,225
	CI	2,375–7,208	2,736–4,770	3,522–4,250	4,028–4,501	3,277–5,893	3,838–4,336	3,948–4,501
	Median	4,947	3,432	3,565	3,950	3,869	3,780	3,956
Eosinophils (n = 250)	Mean	662	413	405	292	68	279	469
	CI	1,595–2,919	54–773	203–606	226–358	33–101	228–330	197–741
	Median	248	224	200	179	56	168	254
Basophils (n = 268)	Mean	4	54	8	15	88	12	35
	CI	9–17	8–117	3–13	2–28	138–315	5–18	−6–77
	Median	—	—	—	—	—	—	—

*CI: 95% confidence interval. **No differences found in WBC counts when comparing between species.

Table 4: White blood cells per μL in children and adults.

Cell group	Children	Adults
Leukocytes (medians)	6.650 (n = 252) (IR* = 3,675)	6.000 (n = 636) (IR = 2,800)
Lymphocytes (medians)	2.030 (n = 251) (IR = 1,835)	1.442 (n = 634) (IR = 1,109)
Monocytes (medians)	400 (n = 251) (IR = 3,675)	348 (n = 435) (IR = 351)
Neutrophils (medians)	3.603 (n = 130) (IR = 2,154)	3,927 (n = 316) (IR = 2,371)
Eosinophils (medians)	204 (n = 79) (IR = 375)	168 (n = 171) (IR = 261)
Basophils (mean value)	17 (n = 87) (CI** = 5–30)	18 (n = 181) (CI = 4–31)
Bands (mean value)	34 (n = 87) (CI = (−3)–70)	23 (n = 179) (CI = 11–36)

*Interquartile ranges.
**95% confidence interval.

Table 5: Comparison of leukocyte alterations between complicated and noncomplicated patients.

		Normal n (%)	Low n (%)	High n (%)
	Complication (no)	516 (73.9)	96 (61.1)	19 (57.6)
Leukocytes	Complication (yes)	182 (26.1)	61 (38.9)	14 (42.4)
	OR (CI), P*		1.8 (1.3–2.6), **0.001**	2.1 (1.0–4.2), **0.038**
	Complication (no)	309 (79.0)	309 (64.9)	11 (61.1)
Lymphocytes	Complication (yes)	82 (21.0)	167 (35.1)	7 (38.9)
	OR (CI), P		2.0 (1.5–2.8), **0.000**	2.4 (0.9–6.4), 0.071
	Complication (no)	543 (72.5)	32 (74.4)	54 (58.1)
Monocytes	Complication (yes)	206 (27.5)	11 (25.6)	39 (41.9)
	OR (CI), P		0.9 (0.5–1.8), 0.783	1.9 (1.2–3.0), **0.003**
	Complication (no)	278 (68.3)	11 (73.3)	10 (41.7)
Neutrophils	Complication (yes)	129 (31.7)	4 (26.7)	14 (58.3)
	OR (CI), P		0.8 (0.3–2.5), 0.680	3.0 (1.3–6.9), **0.007**
	Complication (no)	133 (66.2)	2 (16.7)	29 (78.4)
Eosinophils	Complication (yes)	68 (33.8)	10 (83.3)	8 (21.6)
	OR (CI), P		9.8 (2.0–93.2), **0.001****	0.5 (0.2–1.2), 0.143

*Odds ratio, confidence interval, and P value; **Fisher's exact test.

3.2.5. Leukocytes and Other CBC Variables. A direct correlation between the WBC and platelet counts (Spearman coefficient 0.27, $P < 0.001$) was found. This correlation is maintained with lymphocytes (0.27; $P < 0.001$), monocytes (0.14; $P < 0.001$), granulocytes (0.18; $P < 0.001$), neutrophils (0.12; $P = 0.016$), and eosinophils (0.25; $P < 0.001$). The median platelet count differed significantly between patients with leukopenia (100,000/μL; $n = 154$) and those without leukopenia (131,000/μL; $n = 704$) ($P < 0.001$, Mann-Whitney). Thrombocytopenia defined as a platelet count <150,000/μL was a risk factor for developing leucopenia, both with (OR = 5.8; 2.7–12.4) and without anemia (OR = 3.7; 0.9–7.4). Patients with severe thrombocytopenia had significantly lower leukocyte counts if infected with *P. vivax* (median 4,850 cells/μL) compared to *P. falciparum* infections (median 6,100 cells/μL) ($P = 0.011$, Mann-Whitney), a difference that was not observed by species of *Plasmodium* among patients without thrombocytopenia.

No correlation between leukocyte and erythrocyte counts was found (Spearman = 0.032; $P = 0.364$); the median erythrocyte count did not differ ($P = 0.3133$; Mann-Whitney) between patients with leucopenia (4,365,000/mm^3; $n = 142$) and those without leukopenia (4,400,000/mm^3; $n = 620$); hemoglobin values did not differ between patients with leukopenia (11.6 mg/dL; $n = 157$) and those without leukopenia (12.1 mg/dL; $n = 698$) ($P = 0.164$, Mann-Whitney). A negative correlation between lymphocyte and erythrocyte counts (Spearman = −0.18; $P < 0.001$) and a positive one between lymphocyte and neutrophils counts (Spearman = 0.18; $P < 0.001$) were found.

A negative relationship between the number of parasites and the eosinophil count was found (Spearman coefficient −0.18; $P < 0.001$); no linear correlation was found with other cell populations.

4. Discussion

Of the studied patients, 70% consulted after three days of febrile syndrome onset and 66% of the blood counts were performed between days 4 and 15 of the disease; thus WBC counts may reflect the response to repeated erythrocytic schizogony. One of the difficulties in establishing a pattern of leukocyte alteration during malaria episodes is the presence of different infection stages when the WBC count is analyzed. This variation in hematological parameters is expected as days pass from the onset of infection and may also be the

TABLE 6: Leucocyte counts (cells/μL) in relation to clinical condition*.

Groups	Leukocytes			Lymphocytes			Monocytes			Neutrophils			Eosinophils		
	N	Median	*P*	*N*	Median	*P*	*N*	Median	*P*	*N*	Median	*P*	*N*	Median	*P*
Complicated malaria															
Yes	257	6,100	0.365	256	1,358	**0.000**	256	347	0.545	147	4,030	0.114	86	111	**0.000**
No	631	6,200		629	1,680		629	378		299	3,952		164	242	
Hepatic dysfunction															
Yes	178	6,200	0.308	178	1,295	**0.001**	178	373	0.506	105	4,040	**0.005**	55	124	0.067
No	278	5,800		277	1,526		277	392		173	3,456		69	204	
Renal dysfunction															
Yes	34	7,400	**0.014**	34	1,422	0.949	34	457	0.081	26	5,079	**0.003**	19	158	0.605
No	421	5,900		420	1,449		420	386		253	3,550		105	158	
Neurological complication															
Yes	17	7,700	0.443	17	1,716	0.319	17	418	0.578	12	3,430	0.658	10	68	**0.012**
No	871	6,100		868	1,569		868	370		434	3,836		240	186	
Pulmonary complication															
Yes	17	7,700	0.425	17	1,716	0.218	17	418	0.267	17	4,235	0.560	10	85	**0.028**
No	871	6,100		868	1,569		868	370		868	3,954		240	186	
Severe hypoglycemia (<49 gr/dL)															
Yes	4	8,300	0.318	4	807	0.246	4	191	0.209	2	8,009	**0.004**	1	N.D.	0.147
No	352	5,950		351	1,425		351	366		194	3,672		67	204	
Severe anemia															
Yes	26	8,000	0.073	26	2,346	**0.000**	26	453	**0.025**	14	3,543	0.239	10	163	0.941
No	862	6,100		859	1,540		859	368		432	3,857		240	176	
Severe Thrombocytopenia															
Yes	93	5,700	0.084	93	1,372	0.069	93	273	0.058	55	3,950	0.918	44	93	**0.003**
No	765	6,200		762	1,587		762	382		361	3,822		190	205	
Acidosis															
Yes	12	8,200	0.501	12	1,191	0.091	12	437	0.687	12	5,502	0.170	11	154	0.092
No	20	6,250		20	1,432		20	768		20	3,285		18	73	

*Major or minor criteria for severe malaria.

result of drug administration as observed with the use of antimicrobials in these patients.

The prevalent *Plasmodium* species in the cases studied was *P. falciparum*, in 63% of patients; this differs from the epidemiology of malaria in Colombia where the predominant species is *P. vivax*, a situation possibly due the fact that more *falciparum* cases require hospitalization. Parasitemia ranges were below 10,000 parasites per microliter in 72% of patients (approximately less than 0.25% of parasitized erythrocytes). This variable was not associated with leukocyte alteration, except for the negative correlation between parasitemia and eosinophil counts (Spearman, $P < 0.001$).

The leukogram profile was similar in *P. vivax* and *P. falciparum malaria*. Although a strong inflammatory response in *P. vivax* infections has been recognized [30], our study did not find a differential leukocyte response by *Plasmodium* species, except for patients with severe thrombocytopenia and *P. vivax* infection, whose leukocyte counts were significantly lower, in accordance with previous findings in the acute phase of infection [31]. Leukopenia is a common finding in *falciparum* and *vivax* malaria [15, 16, 32]. Although some studies indicate that there is a greater trend towards leukopenia in infections with *P. falciparum*, this also happens with *P. vivax* [15, 33, 34]. Therefore the presence of leukopenia or its severity does not seem to be useful for diagnosis of species.

Although *Plasmodium* sp. is a hemoparasite, it has been observed that malaria does not significantly affect WBC counts, with values that are usually normal for total leukocyte population for both granulocyte and mononuclear cell subpopulations. Publications on leukocyte alterations in patients with malaria mostly reported WBC counts within normal ranges [9, 32–36]. These findings are consistent with our results where 85% of patients had normal leukocyte counts. The leukocyte, lymphocyte, monocyte, and neutrophil counts differed significantly between children and adults, but the values were within normal limits; therefore these differences appear to be due to physiological variability between groups.

Some changes have been reported in the distribution of WBC lines during the acute phase of malaria infection as well as the return to normal values during the convalescent phase [31], and there is a clear normalizing trend of WBC counts after disease resolution [15], meaning that WBC counts could be used as an indicator for the progress of disease, providing guidance for its management.

4.1. Leukopenia. Leukopenia is an alteration present in both *falciparum* and *vivax* malaria [15, 16]. Our study found that leukopenia was more frequent (18%) than leukocytosis (4%). This is the most reported alteration in malaria with frequencies up to 22% [13, 34, 36, 37]. Leukopenia (WBC < 6,100 cells/μL) was present in 10.2% [17] of Kenyan children over 3 months of age, hospitalized with *P. falciparum* malaria. Using a cutoff value of <4,000 cells/μL to define leukopenia, this alteration was observed in 22.1% of infections by *P. vivax* and 18.4% of mixed infections [37]. In experimental infections with *P. falciparum*, counts under 3,000 cells/μL were identified in 12% ($n = 83$) and counts under 1,000 cells/μL were in 9% ($n = 79$) [38]. In the UK leukopenia was described in 7% of patients with imported *P. falciparum* malaria [39].

Leukopenia in malaria can be caused by the interaction of various events. It has been proposed that the sequestration of leukocytes causes the decline in WBC counts more than a decreased production or accelerated destruction [11]. Glycosylphosphatidylinositol (GPI), an immunogenic antigen common to all species of *Plasmodium*, stimulates the production of proinflammatory cytokines in monocytes and macrophages [15, 40]; this would increase phagocytosis generating cell debris and increasing RBC and WBC phagocytosis, thus maintaining increased proinflammatory cytokine levels, particularly TNF-α, causing altered hemopoiesis [15, 41, 42].

4.2. Leukocytosis. Leukocytosis frequency in malaria varies from one study to another [11–13, 39] and is reported predominantly in *falciparum* malaria. This alteration was identified in 4% of our patients, without statistically significant differences by *Plasmodium* species ($P > 0.05$); the presence of coinfections that may explain leukocytosis was not studied.

Leukocytosis occurs mainly by increased PMN numbers, but lymphocytosis, monocytosis, and eosinophilia can also occur [15, 17, 34]. A study of the cellular composition of BM [9] concluded that during *Plasmodium* infection there was a decrease in some core precursors and in PMN reserves, with increased circulation of immature PMN (bands) and abnormalities in their response to stimuli with drugs and endotoxin; the initial stimulus of infection on the BM reserves and increased circulating half-life of PMN lead to a transient leukocytosis. In *falciparum* malaria, leukocytosis has been explained by the stimulus of infection on the BM to release leukocytes during the paroxysms [16]; increased proinflammatory cytokines could favor the exit of leukocytes from BM [14] or by the presence of bacterial or viral coinfections [12], considering that these possible diagnoses were not excluded in some of the studies [17].

Comparative studies between severe and nonsevere malaria point out leukocytosis as a marker of severity and a predictor of death. A WBC count greater than 16,500 cells/μL was associated with a 7.14 times greater risk of death; mortality was related to the occurrence of bacteremia, polypnea, and coma [17]. When comparing severe and nonsevere patients, leukocytosis was found in 19% of severe and 12.7% of uncomplicated malaria patients; leukocytosis patients were younger and had other manifestations of severe malaria such as hypoglycemia and severe anemia and a 3.5 times greater risk of dying [12]. In our study 33 patients had leukocytosis and 42% of them had some complications (OR = 2.01; 1.1–4.2; $P = 0.040$); specifically renal dysfunction was related to this alteration.

4.3. Lymphocytes. Lymphopenia was the most common abnormality in our patients, present in 54% of cases, while only 2% had lymphocytosis; it was associated with thrombocytopenia as were lymphopenia and neutropenia ($P < 0.001$). In the acute-stage malaria infection lymphopenia (defined as an absolute lymphocyte count ≤1500 cells/μL) was common in *vivax* and *falciparum* cases [15]. This finding was similarly reported in 63% of patients with imported *falciparum* malaria; and along with thrombocytopenia it represented the most common alteration [39].

The etiology of lymphopenia is open to discussion; it has been proposed that during the onset of infection lymphocyte counts drop due to lymphocyte stimulation through inflammation and their following distribution to more active tissues [43] followed by a reorganization of cellular distribution after disease resolution with a return to normal values [44].

A study in animal models found, however, significant elevations of serum apoptotic factors such as Fas and FasL in macaques, which were more susceptible to malaria complications and developed a more pronounced lymphopenia at the expense of T cells [45]; these findings were subsequently confirmed in humans with *P. falciparum* malaria: samples from these patients showed higher values of the aforementioned apoptotic factors at diagnosis and a progressive decrease as the treatment advanced, coinciding with an increase in lymphocyte counts [46]. Despite these results, a clear correlation between elevated Fas-FasL and decreased lymphocytes counts has not been established [47] and both are believed to be the result of malaria immune hyperstimulation causing lymphocyte downregulation to maintain cellular homeostasis or a strategy of the *Plasmodium* genus parasites to decrease immune response [48]. Sequestration of lymphocytes in organs such as the spleen, presence of atypical or plasmacytoid lymphocytes, or decreased survival of these cells have been described [14, 15, 19].

Lymphopenia is a complex pathogenic phenomenon that may have important clinical effects in patients because of the transient immunodeficiency state that can occur and the increased risk of complications [44]; lymphopenia in our patients was associated, in general, with severity and specifically with moderate or severe hepatic dysfunction.

4.4. Monocytes and Granulocytes. Reported changes in other WBC like monocytes and eosinophils are less frequent; eosinopenia has been reported at malaria diagnosis [14–16], but, overall, there has been full recovery during the course of the disease, returning to normal values or even tending to mild eosinophilia at the end of treatment [16, 48]. In our patients 85% of monocyte and 91% of granulocyte counts were normal. Monocytosis presented in 11% of cases and it was associated with severe anemia, in line with the above findings for lymphocytosis. Although it has been described that PMNs are largely responsible for the elevation of leukocyte counts, a strong association of monocytosis and lymphocytosis with mortality has been highlighted [17].

Eosinophilia was the most frequent alteration in granulocytes (15% of 250 patients) while eosinopenia was identified in 5% of cases, which was associated with severe malaria and specifically with neurological, pulmonary, and renal complications and with severe thrombocytopenia. Low eosinophil levels have been reported in the early stage of acute *falciparum* and *vivax* infections (normal values $\leq$350 cells/μL), with increasing levels over the following few weeks [15]. Increased eosinophil counts have been associated with better recovery from malaria anemia secondary to allergies caused by drugs [16] and have also been proposed as an indicator of adequate response to treatment in malaria patients [14, 15].

Neutrophil counts were normal in 91% of cases, with neutrophilia prevailing over neutropenia (5% versus 3%); it was associated with severe malaria and specifically with severe hypoglycemia and moderate or severe liver and kidney dysfunction. Altered basophil counts were not associated with severity. Although differential granulocyte counts were not available for all patients, 33% came from severe cases, which ensures inclusion of complicated and noncomplicated patients in the analysis.

4.5. Leukocytes, Erythrocytes, and Platelets. Leukocyte changes were not related to the decrease in erythrocyte counts and hemoglobin, except for the relation of monocytosis and lymphocytosis with severe anemia in 26 patients. It is possible that a larger number of cases of severe anemia allow identifying other abnormalities in the WBC count. Platelet count, by contrast, positively correlated with changes in all the white lines (Spearman correlation, $P < 0.05$) and total leukocyte lymphocyte, monocyte, and eosinophil counts were lower in patients with severe thrombocytopenia though only eosinophils showed statistical significance. These findings suggest an active role of leukocytes in platelet sequestration sites, via cellular aggregation, a phenomenon described for platelets [49] and leukocytes [50].

4.6. Leukocytes and Glycemia. A trend of increasing blood glucose was observed in patients with leucopenia and the frequency of hyperglycemia was higher, with statistical significance; specifically lymphopenia was associated with higher blood sugar levels. On the contrary, neutrophilia was associated with severe hypoglycemia, a complication occurring in only 4 patients.

5. Conclusions

Malaria hematological changes are diverse and can vary according to study, *Plasmodium* species, age, gender, and other factors. Although some studies have recognized the relationship between leukocytosis and clinical complications in malaria, the general picture involving the role of leukocytes that may play a key role is not entirely clear. The few studies that analyze the leukogram profile in malaria do not delve into the relationships of the leukocyte counts and the clinical condition of patients. This is one of the largest series of leukograms published in an attempt to explain the usefulness of this information as an indicator of severity.

The leukogram profile was similar in *P. vivax* and *P. falciparum malaria.* Leukocyte counts were within normal range in 79% of patients and 18% had leucopenia; the most frequent alteration was lymphopenia (54%) followed by monocytosis (11%). In this study, alterations in leukocyte counts were related to clinical complications according to major criteria of severity; specifically lymphopenia, eosinopenia, monocytosis, and neutrophilia were indicators of serious injury. Leukopenia, lymphopenia, and eosinopenia were related to complications in patients with minor criteria, probably indicating that leukocyte changes begin early and may suggest the onset of serious injury.

Despite the limitations related to retrospective analysis, this study contributes to a better compression about the leukocyte response to plasmodial infection and its relation with the clinical status. The blood samples were processed in 3rd- and 4th-generation automated analyzers; this reflects the technological level and the devices that are available in endemic regions, used to make treatment decisions. Taking into account the limitations of the information provided by these devices, our findings' information could be used to recognize clinical deterioration and to provide adequate care and support.

This study determined changes in the WBC count of malaria patients and analyzed variations according to clinical status. Some alterations in the WBC profile were related to clinical severity and could allow early identification of patients at risk for medical complications. Their utility as markers of severity should be explored in depth, in addition to their application, to identify disease resolution. A better understanding of these hematological parameters will allow their use in early diagnosis of malaria complications and monitoring treatment response.

Conflict of Interests

The authors declare that they have no competing interests.

Authors' Contribution

Alberto Tobón-Castaño and Andrés Felipe Miranda-Arboleda participated in the study design, data collection, data analysis, and writing of the paper. Esteban Mesa-Echeverry contributed to data analysis and writing of the paper.

Acknowledgments

The authors are thankful to "Grupo Malaria, Universidad de Antioquia," "San Vicente de Paúl" and "Pablo Tobón Uribe" Hospitals, who provided data analyzed in this study, and to Ana del Mar Cortina, Ana Maria Cadavid, Lia Palacio, and Shirley Jolianiz, medical students at the School of Medicine of Universidad de Antioquia, for their support in seeking hospital medical records. This project was funded by Universidad de Antioquia, Colombia (Grupo Malaria de la Facultad de Medicina, Vicerrectoría de Investigación y CODI).

References

[1] World Health Organization, *Global Malaria Action Plan for a Malaria-Free World. Geneva, Switzerland: Roll Back Malaria Partnership; 2008*, World Health Organization, 2008.

[2] WHO, *World Malaria Report 2014*, World Health Organization, 2014.

[3] The Lancet, "New estimates of malaria deaths: concern and opportunity," *The Lancet*, vol. 379, no. 9814, p. 385, 2012.

[4] R. N. Price, N. M. Douglas, and N. M. Anstey, "New developments in *Plasmodium vivax* malaria: severe disease and the rise of chloroquine resistance," *Current Opinion in Infectious Diseases*, vol. 22, no. 5, pp. 430–435, 2009.

[5] S. Picot and A.-L. Bienvenu, "*Plasmodium vivax* infection: not so benign," *Medecine/Sciences*, vol. 25, no. 6-7, pp. 622–626, 2009.

[6] M. V. G. Lacerda, M. P. G. Mourão, H. C. Coelho, and J. B. Santos, "Thrombocytopenia in malaria: who cares?" *Memorias do Instituto Oswaldo Cruz*, vol. 106, supplement 1, pp. 52–63, 2011.

[7] J. P. Quintero, A. M. Siqueira, A. Tobón et al., "Malaria-related anaemia: a Latin American perspective," *Memorias do Instituto Oswaldo Cruz*, vol. 106, supplement 1, pp. 91–104, 2011.

[8] E. L. Martínez-Salazar and A. Tobón-Castaño, "Platelet profile is associated with clinical complications in patients with vivax and falciparum malaria in Colombia," *Revista da Sociedade Brasileira de Medicina Tropical*, vol. 47, no. 3, pp. 341–349, 2014.

[9] D. C. Dale and S. M. Wolff, "Studies of the neutropenia of acute malaria," *Blood*, vol. 41, no. 2, pp. 197–206, 1973.

[10] T. Hänscheid, M. Längin, B. Lell et al., "Full blood count and haemozoin-containing leukocytes in children with malaria: diagnostic value and association with disease severity," *Malaria Journal*, vol. 7, article 109, 2008.

[11] F. E. McKenzie, W. A. Prudhomme, A. J. Magill et al., "White blood cell counts and malaria," *Journal of Infectious Diseases*, vol. 192, no. 2, pp. 323–330, 2005.

[12] D. Modiano, B. S. Sirima, A. Konaté, I. Sanou, and A. Sawadogo, "Leucocytosis in severe malaria," *Transactions of the Royal Society of Tropical Medicine and Hygiene*, vol. 95, no. 2, pp. 175–176, 2001.

[13] W. R. J. Taylor, H. Widjaja, H. Basri et al., "Changes in the total leukocyte and platelet counts in Papuan and non Papuan adults from northeast Papua infected with acute *Plasmodium vivax* or uncomplicated *Plasmodium falciparum* malaria," *Malaria Journal*, vol. 7, article 259, 2008.

[14] S. N. Wickramasinghe and S. H. Abdalla, "Blood and bone marrow changes in malaria," *Baillieres Best Practice and Research in Clinical Haematology*, vol. 13, no. 2, pp. 277–299, 2000.

[15] N. Tangpukdee, H.-S. Yew, S. Krudsood et al., "Dynamic changes in white blood cell counts in uncomplicated *Plasmodium falciparum* and *P. vivax* malaria," *Parasitology International*, vol. 57, no. 4, pp. 490–494, 2008.

[16] B. González, H. Rodulfo, M. De Donato, M. Berrizbeitia, C. Gómez, and L. González, "Variaciones hematológicas en pacientes con malaria causada por *Plasmodium vivax* antes, durante y después del tratamiento," *Investigación Clínica*, vol. 50, no. 2, pp. 187–201, 2009.

[17] S. Ladhani, B. Lowe, A. O. Cole, K. Kowuondo, and C. R. J. C. Newton, "Changes in white blood cells and platelets in children with falciparum malaria: relationship to disease outcome," *British Journal of Haematology*, vol. 119, no. 3, pp. 839–847, 2002.

[18] Q. De Mast, F. C. G. J. Sweep, M. McCall et al., "A decrease of plasma macrophage migration inhibitory factor concentration is associated with lower numbers of circulating lymphocytes in experimental *Plasmodium falciparum* malaria," *Parasite Immunology*, vol. 30, no. 3, pp. 133–138, 2008.

[19] H. Helmby, G. Jönsson, and M. Troye-Blomberg, "Cellular changes and apoptosis in the spleens and peripheral blood of mice infected with blood-stage Plasmodium chabaudi chabaudi AS," *Infection and Immunity*, vol. 68, no. 3, pp. 1485–1490, 2000.

[20] K. Mohan and M. M. Stevenson, "Dyserythropoiesis and severe anaemia associated with malaria correlate with deficient interleukin-12 production," *British Journal of Haematology*, vol. 103, no. 4, pp. 942–949, 1998.

[21] C. J. Gregory, O. D. Lorenzi, L. Colón et al., "Utility of the tourniquet test and the white blood cell count to differentiate dengue among acute febrile illnesses in the emergency room," *PLoS Neglected Tropical Diseases*, vol. 5, no. 12, Article ID e1400, 2011.

[22] G. Campuzano, "Del hemograma manual al hemograma de cuarta generación," *Medicina & Laboratorio*, vol. 13, pp. 511–550, 2007.

[23] G. Campuzano, *Utilidad del Extendido de Sangre Periférica: Los Leucocitos*, vol. 14, Medicina & Laboratorio, 2008.

[24] A. Tobón, C. Giraldo, J. G. Piñeros, M. Arboleda, S. Blair, and J. Carmona-Fonseca, "The epidemiology of complicated falciparum malaria: case and controls study in Tumaco and Turbo, Colombia, 2003," *Revista Brasileira de Epidemiologia*, vol. 9, no. 3, pp. 283–296, 2006.

[25] S. Blair, G. Álvarez, and G. Campuzano, "Relación entre anemia y malaria en una población rural de Colombia," *Boletín de Malariología y Salud Ambiental (Venezuela)*, no. 37, pp. 7–13, 1997.

[26] A. Tobón-Castaño, C. Giraldo-Castro, and S. Blair, "Prognostic value of clinical and parasitological signs for severe malaria in patients from Colombia," *Biomédica*, vol. 32, supplement 1, pp. 79–94, 2012.

[27] F. J. Lopez Antuñano and G. Schmunis, *Diagnóstico de Malaria*, Publicación Científica no. 512, OMS, Washington, DC, USA, 1988.

[28] G. Campuzano, "Interpretación del hemograma automatizado: claves para una mejor utilización de la prueba," *Medicina & Laboratorio*, vol. 19, no. 1-2, pp. 11–68, 2013.

[29] WHO, "Severe falciparum malaria. World Health Organization, Communicable Diseases Cluster," *Transactions of the Royal Society of Tropical Medicine and Hygiene*, vol. 94, supplement 1, pp. S1–S90, 2000.

[30] B. E. Barber, T. William, M. J. Grigg et al., "Parasite biomass-related inflammation, endothelial activation, microvascular dysfunction and disease severity in vivax malaria," *PLoS Pathogens*, vol. 11, no. 1, Article ID e1004558, 2015.

[31] R. N. Rodrigues-da-Silva, J. D. C. Lima-Junior, B. D. P. F. e Fonseca et al., "Alterations in cytokines and haematological parameters during the acute and convalescent phases of *Plasmodium falciparum* and *Plasmodium vivax* infections," *Memórias do Instituto Oswaldo Cruz*, vol. 109, no. 2, pp. 154–162, 2014.

[32] C. G. Reiley and O. Barrett Jr., "Leukocyte response in acute malaria," *The American Journal of the Medical Sciences*, vol. 262, no. 3, pp. 153–158, 1971.

[33] B. Eriksson, U. Hellgren, and L. Rombo, "Changes in erythrocyte sedimentation rate, C-reactive protein and hematological parameters in patients with acute malaria," *Scandinavian Journal of Infectious Diseases*, vol. 21, no. 4, pp. 435–441, 1989.

[34] U. M. Jadhav, R. Singhvi, and R. Shah, "Prognostic implications of white cell differential count and white cell morphology in Malaria," *Journal of Postgraduate Medicine*, vol. 49, no. 3, pp. 218–220, 2003.

[35] L. H. Camacho, P. Wilairatana, G. Weiss et al., "The eosinophilic response and haematological recovery after treatment for *Plasmodium falciparum* malaria," *Tropical Medicine and International Health*, vol. 4, no. 7, pp. 471–475, 1999.

[36] E. Goldstein, "A clinical study of falciparum and vivax malaria in Vietnam servicemen," *Military Medicine*, vol. 133, no. 12, pp. 991–996, 1968.

[37] A. Rasheed, S. Saeed, and S. A. Khan, "Clinical and laboratory findings in acute malaria caused by various plasmodium species," *Journal of the Pakistan Medical Association*, vol. 59, no. 4, pp. 220–223, 2009.

[38] L. W. P. Church, T. P. Le, J. P. Bryan et al., "Clinical manifestations of *Plasmodium falciparum* malaria experimentally induced by mosquito challenge," *Journal of Infectious Diseases*, vol. 175, no. 4, pp. 915–920, 1997.

[39] M. W. Richards, R. H. Behrens, and J. F. Doherty, "Short report: hematologic changes in acute, imported *Plasmodium falciparum* malaria," *The American Journal of Tropical Medicine and Hygiene*, vol. 59, no. 6, p. 859, 1998.

[40] L. Schofield, L. Vivas, F. Hackett, P. Gerold, R. T. Schwartz, and S. Tachado, "Neutralizing monoclonal antibodies to glycosylphosphatidylinositol, the dominant TNF-α-inducing toxin of *Plasmodium falciparum*: prospects for the immunotherapy of severe malaria," *Annals of Tropical Medicine and Parasitology*, vol. 87, no. 6, pp. 617–626, 1993.

[41] A. R. Miller, J. Suttles, and R. D. Stout, "Cytokine priming reduces dependence on TNF-R2 for TNF-α-mediated induction of macrophage nitric oxide generation," *Journal of Interferon and Cytokine Research*, vol. 16, no. 12, pp. 1055–1063, 1996.

[42] H. H. Simms, T. A. Gaither, L. F. Fries, and M. M. Frank, "Monokines released during short-term FCγ receptor phagocytosis up-regulate polymorphonuclear leukocytes and monocyte-phagocytic function," *Journal of Immunology*, vol. 147, no. 1, pp. 265–272, 1991.

[43] I. M. Elhassan, L. Hviid, G. Satti et al., "Evidence of endothelial inflammation, T cell activation, and T cell reallocation in uncomplicated *Plasmodium falciparum* malaria," *The American Journal of Tropical Medicine and Hygiene*, vol. 51, no. 3, pp. 372–379, 1994.

[44] L. Hviid, J. A. L. Kurtzhals, B. Q. Goka, J. O. Oliver-Commey, F. K. Nkrumah, and T. G. Theander, "Rapid reemergence of T cells into peripheral circulation following treatment of severe and uncomplicated *Plasmodium falciparum* malaria," *Infection and Immunity*, vol. 65, no. 10, pp. 4090–4093, 1997.

[45] J. Matsumoto, S. Kawai, K. Terao et al., "Malaria infection induces rapid elevation of the soluble Fas ligand level in serum and subsequent T lymphocytopenia: possible factors responsible for the differences in susceptibility of two species of *Macaca* monkeys to *Plasmodium coatneyi* infection," *Infection and Immunity*, vol. 68, no. 3, pp. 1183–1188, 2000.

[46] P. Kern, M. Dietrich, C. Hemmer, and N. Wellinghausen, "Increased levels of soluble Fas ligand in serum in *Plasmodium falciparum* malaria," *Infection and Immunity*, vol. 68, no. 5, pp. 3061–3063, 2000.

[47] L. Hviid, K. Kemp, P. Kern et al., "What is the cause of lymphopenia in malaria?" *Infection and Immunity*, vol. 68, no. 10, pp. 6087–6089, 2000.

[48] J. A. L. Kurtzhals, C. M. Reimert, E. Tette et al., "Increased eosinophil activity in acute *Plasmodium falciparum* infection—association with cerebral malaria," *Clinical & Experimental Immunology*, vol. 112, no. 2, pp. 303–307, 1998.

[49] Q. de Mast, E. Groot, P. J. Lenting et al., "Thrombocytopenia and release of activated von Willebrand factor during early *Plasmodium falciparum* malaria," *Journal of Infectious Diseases*, vol. 196, no. 4, pp. 622–628, 2007.

[50] N. Karunaweera, D. Wanasekara, V. Chandrasekharan, K. Mendis, and R. Carter, "Plasmodium vivax: paroxysm-associated lipids mediate leukocyte aggregation," *Malaria Journal*, vol. 6, article 62, 2007.

6

A Prospective Study of Tuberculosis Drug Susceptibility in Sabah, Malaysia, and an Algorithm for Management of Isoniazid Resistance

Muhammad Redzwan S. Rashid Ali,[1] Uma Parameswaran,[2,3] Timothy William,[2,3,4] Elspeth Bird,[3] Christopher S. Wilkes,[3] Wai Khew Lee,[5] Tsin Wen Yeo,[3,6] Nicholas M. Anstey,[3,6,7] and Anna P. Ralph[3,6,7]

[1] *Department of Respiratory Medicine, Queen Elizabeth Hospital, 88000 Kota Kinabalu, Sabah, Malaysia*
[2] *Infectious Diseases Unit, Clinical Research Centre, Queen Elizabeth Hospital, 88000 Kota Kinabalu, Sabah, Malaysia*
[3] *Infectious Diseases Society Sabah-Menzies School of Health Research Clinical Research Unit, 88000 Kota Kinabalu, Sabah, Malaysia*
[4] *Sabah Department of Health, 88000 Kota Kinabalu, Sabah, Malaysia*
[5] *Luyang Outpatient Clinic, 88000 Kota Kinabalu, Sabah, Malaysia*
[6] *Global and Tropical Health Division, Menzies School of Health Research, Darwin, NT 0811, Australia*
[7] *Department of Medicine, Royal Darwin Hospital, Darwin, NT 0811, Australia*

Correspondence should be addressed to Anna P. Ralph; anna.ralph@menzies.edu.au

Academic Editor: Hans Peter Beck

Introduction. The burden of tuberculosis is high in eastern Malaysia, and rates of *Mycobacterium tuberculosis* drug resistance are poorly defined. Our objectives were to determine *M. tuberculosis* susceptibility and document management after receipt of susceptibility results. *Methods.* Prospective study of adult outpatients with smear-positive pulmonary tuberculosis (PTB) in Sabah, Malaysia. Additionally, hospital clinicians accessed the reference laboratory for clinical purposes during the study. *Results.* 176 outpatients were enrolled; 173 provided sputum samples. Mycobacterial culture yielded *M. tuberculosis* in 159 (91.9%) and nontuberculous Mycobacterium (NTM) in three (1.7%). Among outpatients there were no instances of multidrug resistant *M. tuberculosis* (MDR-TB). Seven people (4.5%) had isoniazid resistance (INH-R); all were switched to an appropriate second-line regimen for varying durations (4.5–9 months). Median delay to commencement of the second-line regimen was 13 weeks. Among 15 inpatients with suspected TB, 2 had multidrug resistant TB (one extensively drug resistant), 2 had INH-R, and 4 had NTM. *Conclusions.* Current community rates of MDR-TB in Sabah are low. However, INH-resistance poses challenges, and NTM is an important differential diagnosis in this setting, where smear microscopy is the usual diagnostic modality. To address INH-R management issues in our setting, we propose an algorithm for the treatment of isoniazid-resistant PTB.

1. Introduction

Tuberculosis (TB) is a disease of major significance in eastern Malaysia (Malaysian Borneo), especially in Sabah state. Eastern Malaysia has a disproportionally high burden of the country's TB cases [1], and Sabah's estimated TB incidence rate (131/100,000) [2] far exceeds national rates (80/100,000) [3]. Rates of *Mycobacterium tuberculosis* drug resistance are not well defined in Sabah. Where testing has occurred, it has often been reserved for treatment failure cases, limiting the generalizability of such findings. Malaysian rates of multidrug resistant- (MDR-) TB have been estimated at 0.3% in 2005 and 1.3% in 2011 [4]. In unpublished data from the Sabah state reference laboratory, 16 MDR-TB cases occurred in 2011, representing 2.1% of isolates submitted that year [5]. Isoniazid resistance (INH-R) is reported in approximately 4% of

Table 1: Treatment of isoniazid-resistant pulmonary tuberculosis: recommendations from selected references and level of evidence.

Treatment element	Reference	Study type	Level of evidence*
Drugs			
R throughout	[11]	Meta-analysis of trials and cohort studies	III
	[21]	Nonrandomised trial	IIa
REZ	[22]	Observational study	III
	[17, 23]	Expert opinion	IV
HREZ	[16]	Retrospective review	III
Add a fluoroquinolone in all instances (moxifloxacin 400 mg or levofloxacin 750–100 mg substituted for isoniazid)	[20]	Expert opinion	IV
Add a fluoroquinolone if pyrazinamide is not tolerated	[23]	Expert opinion	IV
Add a fluoroquinolone if disease is extensive	[18]	Expert opinion	IV
High-dose H is not recommended	[23]	Expert opinion	IV
Duration			
6 months (REZ)	[21]	Nonrandomised trial	IIa
6 months (REZ) if disease is not extensive	[23]	Expert opinion	IV
6 to 9 months (REZ)	[17]	Expert opinion	IV
6 to 12 months (variety of regimens)	[22]	Observational study	III
9 months (REZ) if culture-positive at 2 months	[23]	Expert opinion	IV
*Dosing frequency***			
	[11]	Meta-analysis of trials and cohort studies	III
Dosing should be daily during the intensive phase	[24]	Systematic review	
	[23]	Expert opinion	IV
Dosing can be given intermittently (thrice weekly) during the continuation phase	[25]	Expert opinion	IV
Twice or thrice weekly RZE for 6 months in HIV negative disease	[21]	Nonrandomised trial	IIa

*Ia: evidence from meta-analysis of randomized controlled trials, Ib: evidence from at least one randomized controlled trial, IIa: evidence from at least one well designed controlled trial which is not randomized, IIb: evidence from at least one well designed experimental trial, III: evidence from case, correlation, and comparative studies, IV: evidence from a panel of experts [26].
**Where dosing is self-administered rather than directly observed (as in Malaysia), there may be no advantage in an intermittent regimen.

M. tuberculosis in western Malaysia [6, 7], but rates have not been published from eastern Malaysia.

Isoniazid resistance (INH-R) is now generally acknowledged to be associated with poorer outcomes than INH-susceptible disease [8–11]. Despite INH-R TB being so common (4–10% globally [12–14]), the level of evidence to guide management is mostly level III-IV (Table 1), resulting in practices being nonuniform regarding drug choice, duration, and dosing frequency. The standard short-course regimen (isoniazid (H), rifampicin (R), ethambutol (E), and pyrazinamide (Z)) has traditionally been considered adequate [15, 16]. However 9 months of REZ (9REZ) or variations on this theme [10, 17–19] are increasingly used, and some advocate for the addition of a fluoroquinolone routinely [20], or in extensive INH-R pulmonary disease [18]. A new trial from the Tuberculosis Trials Consortium [21] provides much-needed evidence in this field; although the study was single-arm and nonrandomised, it provides evidence that twice or thrice weekly REZ for 6 months in HIV negative patients is mostly effective (3.5% failed or relapsed) but poorly tolerated [21]. Poor tolerability, especially of pyrazinamide, is a key challenge in the treatment of INH-R pulmonary TB (PTB) and a reason to require third-line options such as 12 months of a 2-drug regimen [22] or substitution with a fluoroquinolone [18].

The time taken to obtain *M. tuberculosis* susceptibility results is long if solid culture medium only is used, or where results are batched for dispatch to a reference laboratory; both these factors apply in our setting. If susceptibility results are delayed and the patient has already been switched to HR continuation phase treatment, the question of what to do after a period of effective monotherapy with rifampicin arises. Tailoring of regimens for pulmonary INH-R TB depending on factors, such as patient age, HIV status, and cavitary disease, can be difficult in high TB-burden settings accustomed to standardized regimens.

Knowledge of local susceptibility not only allows tailoring of treatment in individuals but provides local antibiogram data to aid clinicians in constructing regimens to use empirically and in culture-negative suspected tuberculosis (e.g., paediatric and extrapulmonary TB) and latent TB. Our first objective was to determine TB drug susceptibility profiles among patients with new or retreatment pulmonary TB presenting to a large community TB clinic in Kota Kinabalu, Sabah, Malaysia. Our second objective was to document clinical practice on receipt of susceptibility results.

2. Methods

This is a prospective observational study of smear-positive PTB outpatients, enrolled at Luyang Tuberculosis Outpatient Clinic, Kota Kinabalu, Malaysia. This is the main referral TB clinic in Kota Kinabalu, diagnosing and treating almost 200 patients annually. Kota Kinabalu district has a population of approximately 600,000. Participants were enrolled over 2 years, 4 July 2012–3 July 2014. Additionally, during the study period, clinicians at the Kota Kinabalu tertiary adult referral hospital, Queen Elizabeth Hospital (QEH), were able to access the services of the reference laboratory for clinical purposes, for patients in whom mycobacterial infection, particularly drug resistance, was suspected. QEH manages approximately 200 smear-positive PTB inpatients annually.

2.1. Informed Consent. Potentially eligible participants were provided with information about the study using written and pictorial materials and explanations from research staff and were required to provide written, informed consent. Consent was obtained from a parent/guardian for participants aged between 15 and 17, who additionally provided their assent.

2.2. Participants. Outpatient participants were eligible if they had sputum smear-positive pulmonary TB, were aged ≥15 years, and had received <7 days' TB treatment. They were referred for enrolment by the TB clinic doctor after being diagnosed with TB on the basis of clinical and X-ray assessment, and at least one sputum positive for acid fast bacilli (AFB) on Ziehl-Neelsen stain performed at the clinic's smear microscopy laboratory.

2.3. Procedures. A new sputum sample was provided on the day of enrolment. Samples were batched in a domestic refrigerator and transported to an international reference laboratory (Singapore General Hospital Laboratory, Singapore) as described elsewhere [27]. The BACTEC *Mycobacterium* Growth Indicator Tube (MGIT) 960 tube system was employed for culture. Drug susceptibility testing was performed for *M. tuberculosis* isolates using the nonradiometric MGIT system for isoniazid, rifampicin, ethambutol, streptomycin, and, in the instance of any first-line resistance, also for ofloxacin, kanamycin, and ethionamide. Nontuberculous mycobacteria (NTM) were identified using a DNA probe (ProbeTec, Becton-Dickinson). Further speciation, if done, was achieved using a second DNA probe (INNO-LiPA MYCOBACTERIA, Innogenetics, Ghent, Belgium) and high-performance liquid chromatography (HPLC) of mycolic acids.

HIV was tested using two rapid tests (Abbott Determine HIV-1/2 and a second locally supplied point-of-care test, as described elsewhere [28]). Positive results were confirmed by enzyme immunoassay, particle agglutination, and line immunoassay.

Table 2: Characteristics of outpatients enrolled at Luyang Clinic.

Baseline characteristic	Number
Number	176
Age in years: median (range)	30.0 (16–73)
Male: number (%)	104 (59.0%)
Nationality	
Malaysian: number (%)	117 (66.5%)
Non-Malaysian: number (%)	59 (33.5%)
HIV positive: number (%)	3 (1.7%)
Current smoker	40 (22.7%)
Past TB	13 (7.4%)

2.4. Ethical Approval. Ethical approval was obtained from the Medical Research Ethics Committee, Malaysian Ministry of Health, and the Health Research Ethics Committee of Human Research Ethics Committee of the Northern Territory Department of Health and Menzies School of Health Research, Australia.

2.5. Clinical Specimens from Hospital Patients. During the study period, clinicians at Queen Elizabeth Hospital were also able to utilise the arrangement established with the reference laboratory. Clinicians could send sputum specimens or extrapulmonary samples, with the batched research specimens, to obtain mycobacterial culture and susceptibility testing to guide clinical management. No specific inclusion criteria were applied apart from the suspicion of mycobacterial infection and difficulty obtaining results locally.

2.6. Statistics. Data were analysed using Stata 13.1. (Stata Corp., College Station, Texas, USA). Continuous variables were compared using Student's t-test or Wilcoxon Rank Sum test. Categorical variables were compared using Chi-squared or Fisher's Exact test, as appropriate.

3. Results

3.1. Outpatients. During the 2-year study period, 176 outpatients consented and were enrolled (Figure 1, Table 2). Details relating to patient demographics and HIV status are described elsewhere [28]. A sputum sample was received by the laboratory for 173 individuals. Thirteen participants reported having received TB treatment in the past (median 12.5 years ago according to patients' recollection, range 1–39 years).

3.2. Outpatient Culture and Susceptibility Results. Mycobacterial culture was positive in 162 of 173 (93.6%) samples received. One hundred and fifty-nine (91.9%) yielded *M. tuberculosis*, and three (1.7%) yielded NTM; one was *M. fortuitum*; the others were not speciated. Of patients in whom NTM was isolated, two had underlying bronchiectasis.

Susceptibility results were unavailable in 3 *M. tuberculosis* isolates due to overgrowth of the culture by contaminating organisms. In the 156 isolates from outpatients with

Table 3: Isoniazid resistance among outpatients with pulmonary tuberculosis.

	Previous TB	Change in therapy after INH-R result	Time elapsed between treatment start & change of regimen	Second line regimen	Recommended duration of second line regimen	Outcome
Patient 1	No	Yes	28 weeks	RZE	6	Cured
Patient 2	No	Yes	15 weeks	RZE	9	Defaulted but already smear negative and received 6 months' treatment in total
Patient 3	No	Yes	8 weeks	RZE	4.5	Transferred
Patient 4	No	Yes	12 weeks	RZE	9	Cured
Patient 5	No	Yes	11 weeks	RZE	6	Cured
Patient 6	No	Yes	16 weeks	RZE	6	Cured
Patient 7	No	Yes	8 weeks	RZE	6	Cured
Median			**12 Weeks**			

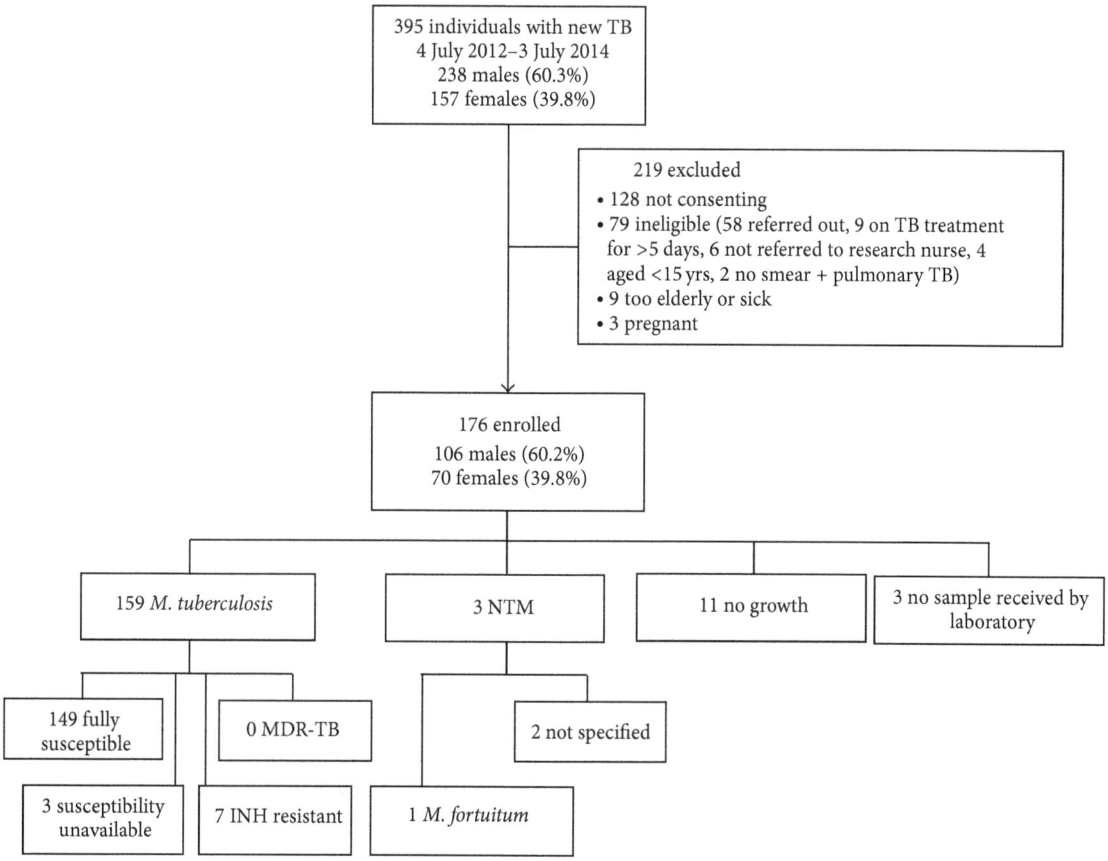

Figure 1: Outpatient study diagram showing enrolment and microbiological results.

susceptibility data, none had MDR-TB or rifampicin monoresistance. Seven people (4.5%) had infection with INH-R *M. tuberculosis*, none of whom recalled having previously received TB treatment. INH-R disease was more common in people of non-Malaysian ethnicity: 6 of the 7 (86%) were Filipino or Indonesian, compared with 50/159 (33.6%) with INH-S disease ($P = 0.009$).

One *M. tuberculosis* isolate with isoniazid resistance had additional streptomycin and ethionamide resistance. One instance of streptomycin monoresistance was also identified.

3.3. Management of Drug Resistant Cases. Among people identified as having INH-R, there were substantial delays between commencement of the first-line tuberculosis treatment regimen and change to a second-line regimen. The median delay was 13 weeks (range 8 to 28 weeks); see Table 3. Opportunities for delay included the time taken to dispatch sputum samples to the laboratory, receive the resistance report, inform the treating doctor, and recall the patient and for nursing staff to implement the doctor's new treatment regimen. The usual regimen prescribed after notification of

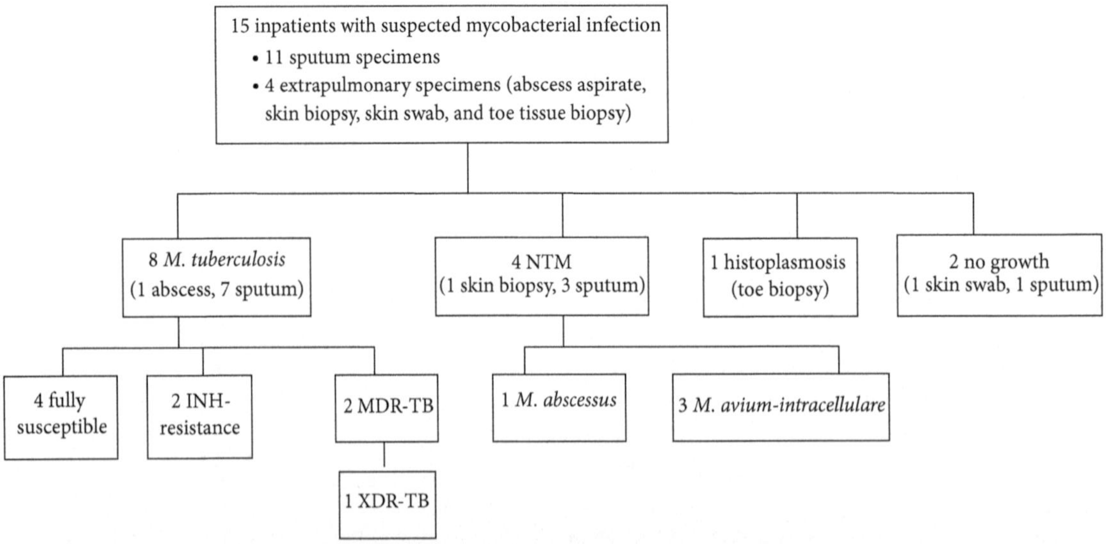

FIGURE 2: Hospital inpatients with suspected mycobacterial infection.

INH-R results was rifampicin, pyrazinamide, and ethambutol (Table 3). Three patients with INH-R disease had follow-up sputum cultures performed at two months; all three had converted their culture to negative.

3.4. Hospital Patients. Fifteen additional samples were submitted for culture from hospital inpatients with suspected pulmonary TB (10 patients), or suspected extrapulmonary TB (five patients). Of those with suspected pulmonary TB, three had prior TB treatment failure, one had defaulted, three had unknown past treatment history, and three had underlying lung disease.

Findings from hospital inpatients are shown in Figure 2. Two cases of pulmonary MDR-TB, including one case of XDR-TB, were identified, both in heavily pretreated people. The XDR-TB case is the subject of a separate case report [29]. Two instances of INH-R were also identified, one monoresistant (in a pretreated patient) and one combined with streptomycin resistance (in a TB treatment-naïve health care worker). Regarding NTM, these were isolated in specimens obtained from four of the hospitalised individuals and identified by DNA probe and HPLC as *M. abscessus* or *M. avium-intracellulare* complex (from sputum) and *M. avium-intracellulare* complex (from a skin biopsy).

4. Discussion

We have found low rates of drug resistance among outpatient cases of tuberculosis in Sabah, Borneo, but occasional cases of MDR-TB in pretreated patients in the inpatient setting. The rate of isoniazid resistance (4.5%) is, reassuringly, at the lower end of what is reported globally [12–14]. Thus, while the TB burden is high in eastern Malaysia, our study illustrates that this appears to be predominantly drug-susceptible disease. While the uncommon finding of MDR-TB reflects well on the local TB control program, high ongoing rates of drug-susceptible disease in relatively young people (median age 30 years) suggest that community transmission of TB is an important area requiring targeted intervention.

The MDR-TB rates we have found are low compared with Malaysia's immediate neighbours, where rates have been estimated as follows in new and retreatment cases, respectively: Singapore 0.1% new and 2.9% retreatment, Thailand 1.7% and 34.5%, Indonesia 2% and 14.7%, and Philippines 4.0% and 20.9% [30]. There were few retreatment cases in our series (13 outpatients and 3 hospitalised patients) to provide an accurate assessment among these patients, but the two cases of MDR-TB both occurred in pretreated individuals. These low rates also compare favourably with other member states of the WHO Western Pacific Region; MDR-TB rates in Papua New Guinea, for instance, have been estimated to be at least 26% of cases [31].

We identified substantial challenges in managing INH-resistance, particularly in the transition from protocol-based standardised care to tailored care. Despite Malaysian guidelines now recommending baseline cultures in all cases of suspected TB, routine susceptibility results are generally unavailable; usual practice in our setting is to undertake sputum mycobacterial cultures only for persistent smear-positivity after two to three months of treatment. Multifactorial delays occurred in implementing regimen changes, comprising the delay in specimens reaching the reference laboratory, the time taken to notify of the treating doctor, patient recall, and dispensing of the new regimen. A specific challenge in this context was that susceptibility results were frequently reported after completion of intensive phase treatment, when the routine switch to HR had already been made. Arising from these findings, we therefore developed an algorithm for managing this situation (Figure 3), based on the evidence summarised in Table 1. Such an algorithm does not replace clinical judgement guided by individual patient needs but provides

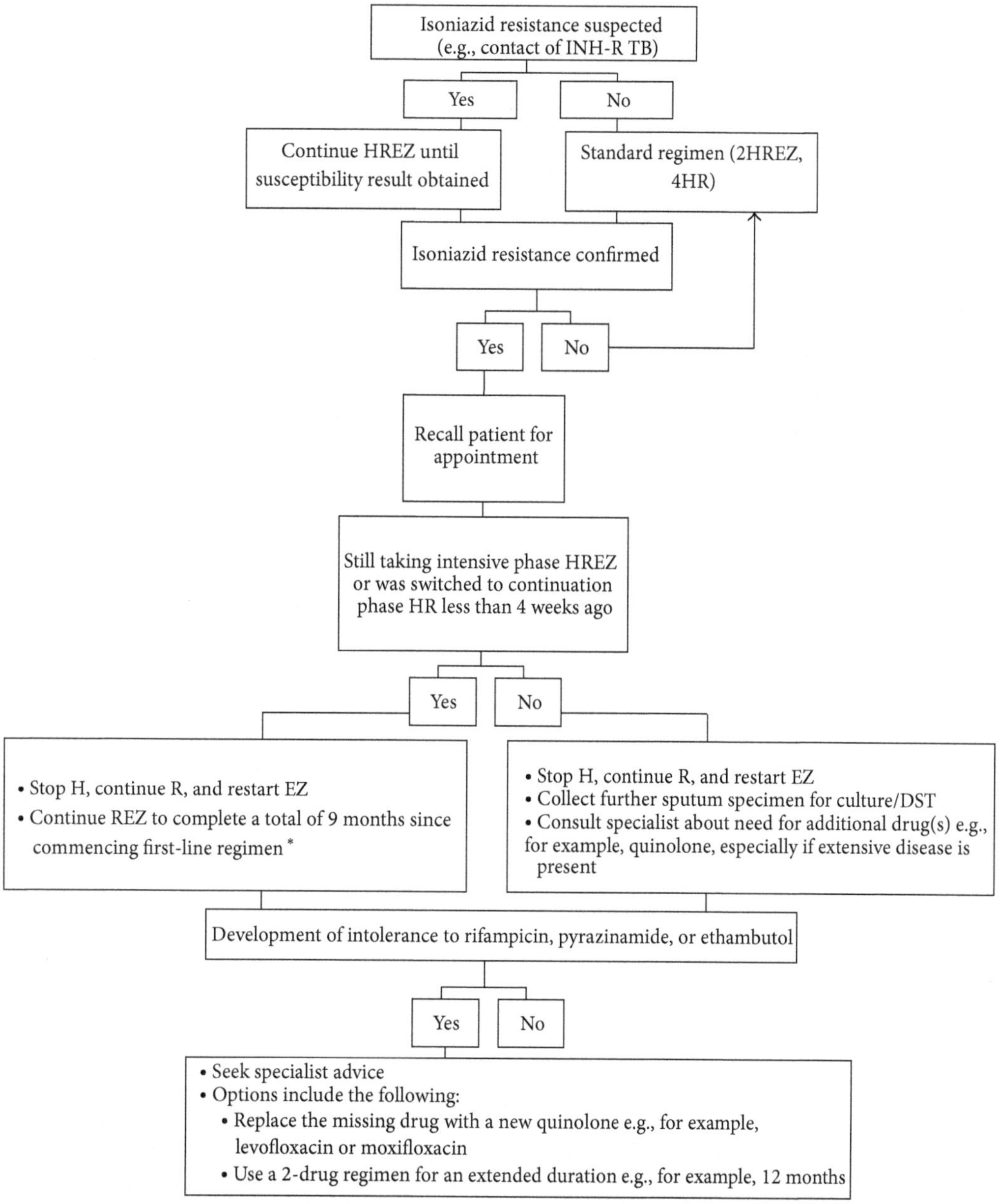

H = isoniazid, R = rifampicin, E = ethambutol, Z = pyrazinamide, DST = drug susceptibility testing

* If risk factors for drug adverse events are present (e.g., elderly, viral hepatitis) and disease is not extensive, noncavitary, and the patient is improving, 6REZ can be used instead of 9REZ. Monthly eye reviews (acuity and colour vision) are required when ethambutol is continued beyond 2 months

FIGURE 3: Algorithm for managing isoniazid resistance.

guidance for nonspecialists in the local health centre settings where most outpatient TB is managed.

NTM was detected in 7 of 191 people (outpatients and inpatients) with suspected TB. This finding illustrates the problem of NTM colonisation or infection being mistaken for TB, especially where smear microscopy is the diagnostic mainstay. NTM infections have been noted to cause a substantial burden of disease in our clinical practice and elsewhere in Malaysia [32]. Rising rates have also been reported elsewhere in Asia [33, 34]. This disease has been relatively neglected compared with TB due to lower incidence and lack of associated public health risk, yet diagnosis and management can be far more challenging than TB and outcomes poor. More research is required in Sabah to better understand and optimise management of local NTM infections. Greater local access to mycobacterial culture is needed to aid clinicians in distinguishing NTM from TB, especially in patients in whom NTM is more likely, that is, those with underlying chronic lung disease.

A limitation of the study is that findings from the outpatient setting cannot be extrapolated to all TB cases in Sabah and are not representative of the inpatient setting; we have presented results from the selected group of hospital patients to illustrate this, but more data are required on inpatient drug resistance rates, as well as treatment outcomes.

In conclusion, current rates of MDR-TB in the community in Sabah are low, reflecting well on local TB case management, but INH-resistance poses challenges. This must be addressed to avoid additional stepwise acquired resistance. Improvement in local resourcing to ensure that diagnostics such as liquid mycobacterial culture or molecular tests are available in a timely, clinically useful fashion would be a major advance in TB management in Sabah, which has Malaysia's highest TB burden. In the current scenario of delayed access to susceptibility results, our proposed management algorithm can provide guidance here and in settings facing similar issues globally.

Conflict of Interests

The authors declare that there is no conflict of interests regarding the publication of this paper.

Acknowledgments

The authors are very grateful to Kelly Nestor, Ann Wee, Thecla Tasius, Florena Maidik, and Sharon Nestor for enrolling the participants; all the staff at Luyang Outpatient Clinic particularly Dr. Eman Farhad, Dr. Maryam Amaleena, Suzie Taylor, Jenny Omar, and Dr. Elissa Soh; also Justine Peh Woei Ling at the Singapore General Hospital Mycobacteriology Laboratory; Ms. Dawn Carmel Paul for supporting the project; and Dr. Abdul Razak Mutalif (Institute of Respiratory Medicine and Head of Respiratory Services, Ministry of Health, Malaysia) for reviewing and endorsing the paper. This study was funded by the National Health and Medical Research Council (NHMRC) of Australia (Grant 605806). Anna Ralph is supported by NHMRC fellowship 1016567.

References

[1] C. Rundi, "Understanding tuberculosis: perspectives and experiences of the people of Sabah, East Malaysia," *Journal of Health, Population and Nutrition*, vol. 28, no. 2, pp. 114–123, 2010.

[2] J. F. Dony, J. Ahmad, and Y. K. Tiong, "Epidemiology of tuberculosis and leprosy, Sabah, Malaysia," *Tuberculosis*, vol. 84, no. 1-2, pp. 8–18, 2004.

[3] World Health Organization, *Global Tuberculosis Report 2014*, WHO Library Cataloguing-in-Publication Data, WHO/HTM/TB/2014.08, 2014.

[4] Ministry of Health Malaysia, Academy of Medicine M, and Malaysian Thoracic Society, *Management of Tuberculosis. Clinical Practice Guidelines*, MOH/P/PAK/258.12(GU), 3rd edition, 2012.

[5] D. C. Paul, A. Chew, N. L. Yau et al., "Multidrug resistant Mycobacterium tuberculosis complex: a laboratory perspective," in *Proceedings of the 7th Public Health Colloquium*, Sabah State Health Department, Kota Kinabalu, Malaysia, November 2012.

[6] R. D. Jalleh, I. Kuppusamy, R. Soshila, A. M. Aziah, and M. Y. Faridza, "A study of primary drug resistance in pulmonary tuberculosis in West Malaysia 1984–1987," *Medical Journal of Malaysia*, vol. 48, no. 2, pp. 113–116, 1993.

[7] Z. Hamzah, L. J. Min, I. A. Ali et al., "Drug resistance pattern of *Mycobacterium tuberculosis* complex isolated for Perak State (2006–2008)," in *Proceedings of the 1st AMDI International Biohealth Science Conference: Infectious Diseases—Current Challenges (IBSC '10)*, Poster Presentation: Conference Abstracts, p. 172, Ipoh Public Health Laboratory Data, Ministry of Health, Penang, Malaysia, November-December 2010.

[8] M. A. Espinal, S. J. Kim, P. G. Suarez et al., "Standard short-course chemotherapy drug-resistant tuberculosis: treatment outcomes in 6 countries," *The Journal of the American Medical Association*, vol. 283, no. 19, pp. 2537–2545, 2000.

[9] M. G. Farah, A. Tverdal, T. W. Steen, E. Heldal, A. B. Brantsaeter, and G. Bjune, "Treatment outcome of new culture positive pulmonary tuberculosis in Norway," *BMC Public Health*, vol. 5, article 14, 2005.

[10] M. Gegia, T. Cohen, I. Kalandadze, L. Vashakidze, and J. Furin, "Outcomes among tuberculosis patients with isoniazid resistance in Georgia, 2007–2009," *International Journal of Tuberculosis and Lung Disease*, vol. 16, no. 6, pp. 812–816, 2012.

[11] D. Menzies, A. Benedetti, A. Paydar et al., "Standardized treatment of active tuberculosis in patients with previous treatment and/or with mono-resistance to isoniazid: a systematic review and meta-analysis," *PLoS Medicine*, vol. 6, no. 9, Article ID e1000150, 2009.

[12] A. J. Hoopes, J. S. Kammerer, T. A. Harrington, K. Ijaz, and L. R. Armstrong, "Isoniazid-monoresistant tuberculosis in the United States, 1993 to 2003," *Archives of Internal Medicine*, vol. 168, no. 18, pp. 1984–1992, 2008.

[13] World Health Organization, "Anti-tuberculosis drug resistance in the world fourth global report," The WHO/IUATLD Global Project on Anti-tuberculosis Drug Resistance Surveillance, 2002–2007: WHO/HTM/TB/2008.394, World Health Organization, 2008.

[14] A. Pablos-Méndez, M. C. Raviglione, A. Laszlo et al., "Global surveillance for antituberculosis-drug resistance, 1994–1997. World Health Organization—International Union against tuberculosis and lung disease working group on anti-tuberculosis drug resistance surveillance," *The New England Journal of Medicine*, vol. 338, no. 23, pp. 1641–1649, 1998.

[15] W. Fox, G. A. Ellard, and D. A. Mitchison, "Studies on the treatment of tuberculosis undertaken by the British Medical Research Council Tuberculosis Units, 1946–1986, with relevant subsequent publications," *International Journal of Tuberculosis and Lung Disease*, vol. 3, pp. S231–S279, 1999.

[16] C. M. Nolan and S. V. Goldberg, "Treatment of isoniazid-resistant tuberculosis with isoniazid, rifampin, ethambutol, and pyrazinamide for 6 months," *International Journal of Tuberculosis and Lung Disease*, vol. 6, no. 11, pp. 952–958, 2002.

[17] World Health Organisation, *Guidelines for the Programmatic Management of Drug-Resistant Tuberculosis: Emergency Update*, WHO/HTM/TB/2008.402, WHO, Geneva, Switzerland, 2008.

[18] H. M. Blumberg, W. J. Burman, R. E. Chaisson et al., "American thoracic society/centers for disease control and

prevention/infectious diseases society of America: treatment of tuberculosis," *The American Journal of Respiratory and Critical Care Medicine*, vol. 167, no. 4, pp. 603–662, 2003.

[19] Centre for Disease Control, *Darwin Guidelines for the Control of Tuberculosis in the Northern Territory*, Northern Territory Government Department of Health and Community Services, 2002, http://health.nt.gov.au/library/scripts/objectifyMedia.aspx?file=pdf/25/05.pdf&siteID=1&str_title=Tuberculosis.

[20] L. Pinto and D. Menzies, "Treatment of drug-resistant tuberculosis," *Infection and Drug Resistance*, vol. 4, no. 1, pp. 129–135, 2011.

[21] R. Reves, C. M. Heilig, J. M. Tapy et al., "Intermittent tuberculosis treatment for patients with isoniazid intolerance or drug resistance," *International Journal of Tuberculosis and Lung Disease*, vol. 18, no. 5, pp. 571–580, 2014.

[22] A. Cattamanchi, R. B. Dantes, J. Z. Metcalfe et al., "Clinical characteristics and treatment outcomes of patients with isoniazid-monoresistant tuberculosis," *Clinical Infectious Diseases*, vol. 48, no. 2, pp. 179–185, 2009.

[23] S. S. Munsiff, D. Nilsen, and P. I. Fujiwara, *Tuberculosis Clinical Policies and Protocols*, Department of Health and Mental Hygiene, Bureau of Tuberculosis Control, New York, NY, USA, 4th edition, 2008.

[24] K. C. Chang, C. C. Leung, J. Grosset, and W. W. Yew, "Treatment of tuberculosis and optimal dosing schedules," *Thorax*, vol. 66, no. 11, pp. 997–1007, 2011.

[25] K. C. Chang, C. C. Leung, W. W. Yew, S. L. Chan, and C. M. Tam, "Dosing schedules of 6-month regimens and relapse for pulmonary tuberculosis," *The American Journal of Respiratory and Critical Care Medicine*, vol. 174, no. 10, pp. 1153–1158, 2006.

[26] D. C. Hadorn, D. Baker, J. S. Hodges, and N. Hicks, "Rating the quality of evidence for clinical practice guidelines," *Journal of Clinical Epidemiology*, vol. 49, no. 7, pp. 749–754, 1996.

[27] M. R. S. Rashid Ali, T. William, U. Parameswaran et al., "Mycobacterial viability: a prospective study in pulmonary tuberculosis in Malaysian Borneo using refrigerated, unpreserved sputum batched for up to 8 weeks," *International Journal of Tuberculosis and Lung Disease*, vol. 19, no. 5, 2015.

[28] T. William, U. Parameswaran, W. K. Lee, T. W. Yeo, N. M. Anstey, and A. P. Ralph, "Pulmonary tuberculosis in outpatients in Sabah, Malaysia: advanced disease but low incidence of HIV co-infection," *BMC Infectious Diseases*, vol. 15, no. 1, article 32, 2015.

[29] M. R. S. Rashid Ali, A. P. Ralph, and T. William, "Individualized second line antituberculous therapy for an extensively resistant pulmonary tuberculosis (XDR PTB) case in east Malaysia," *Malaysian Medical Journal*, Accepted.

[30] World Health Organization, *Multidrug and Extensively Drug-Resistant TB (M/XDR-TB) 2010 Global Report on Surveillance and Response*, WHO Library Cataloguing-in-Publication Data, WHO/HTM/TB/2010.3, 2010.

[31] G. Simpson, C. Coulter, J. Weston et al., "Resistance patterns of multidrug-resistant tuberculosis in Western Province, Papua New Guinea," *International Journal of Tuberculosis and Lung Disease*, vol. 15, no. 4, pp. 551–552, 2011.

[32] J. J. Kasthoori, C. K. Liam, and M. L. Wastie, "Lady Windermere syndrome: an inappropriate eponym for an increasingly important condition," *Singapore Medical Journal*, vol. 49, no. 2, pp. e47–e49, 2008.

[33] Y. S. Park, C. H. Lee, S. M. Lee et al., "Rapid increase of non-tuberculous mycobacterial lung diseases at a tertiary referral hospital in South Korea," *International Journal of Tuberculosis and Lung Disease*, vol. 14, no. 8, pp. 1069–1071, 2010.

[34] C.-Y. Chen, H.-Y. Chen, C.-H. Chou, C.-T. Huang, C.-C. Lai, and P.-R. Hsueh, "Pulmonary infection caused by nontuberculous mycobacteria in a medical center in Taiwan, 2005–2008," *Diagnostic Microbiology and Infectious Disease*, vol. 72, no. 1, pp. 47–51, 2012.

7

The Role of *Anethum graveolens* L. (Dill) in the Management of Diabetes

Mohammad Taghi Goodarzi,[1,2] Iraj Khodadadi,[1] Heidar Tavilani,[1] and Ebrahim Abbasi Oshaghi[1]

[1]*Department of Clinical Biochemistry, Medical School, Hamadan University of Medical Sciences, Hamadan, Iran*
[2]*Research Center for Molecular Medicine, Hamadan University of Medical Sciences, Hamadan, Iran*

Correspondence should be addressed to Ebrahim Abbasi Oshaghi; 7abbasi@gmail.com

Academic Editor: Carlos E. P. Corbett

Aim. There is evidence that *Anethum graveolens* (AG) has been used for centuries in Asian traditional medicine, and its constituents have useful effects on the control and management of diabetes and cardiovascular disorders. AG has many useful effects, including hypolipidemic and hypoglycemic effects, and it has been reported to reduce the incidence of diabetic complications. It acts mainly by affecting antioxidant capacity and change in some genes in glucose and lipid pathways. The aim of the present paper was to summarize pharmacological effects of AG in the management of diabetes. *Methods.* To prepare this review, a pharmacological and phytochemical literature survey was performed using Scopus, PubMed, and Web of Science. Also, some historical and ethnopharmacological literature sources were used. *Results.* This review plans to provide readers with an assessment of the pharmacological effects of AG, especially in diabetes. *Conclusion.* The paper highlights the therapeutic effects of AG which would aid in supporting their safe use in the management of diabetes and cardiovascular diseases.

1. Introduction

Diabetes mellitus is a chronic metabolic disorder that is distinguished by hyperglycemia, underutilization of blood glucose, and defects in the metabolism of macronutrients such as carbohydrates, fat, and protein, secondary to the disturbance in insulin action [1, 2]. Type 1 diabetes is caused as a result of insulin deficiency due to failure of pancreatic beta-cells. Therefore, diabetic patients need exogenous insulin injection, whereas patients with type 2, known as insulin independent, do not respond to insulin and consequently can be managed by lifestyle changes. Type 2 diabetes constitutes 90% of the diabetic cases in the world [3]. Next to cancer and heart disease, diabetes mellitus is the third most life-threatening disorder which has a high rate of morbidity and mortality worldwide. Prevalence of this disorder is quickly rising in every part of the world [4]. As a result, it is projected to affect 552 million people in 2030, rising sharply from 336 million in 2011 [3]. Signs of type 1 and 2 diabetes may include hyperglycemia, abnormal thirst, repeated urination, weight loss and severe hunger, nausea and vomiting, mood changes, and severe weakness and tiredness [1]. The purpose of this review was to identify *Anethum graveolens* L. (AG) as a valuable herbal plant, originating from Asian traditional medicine, in the management of diabetes. Conducted studies could allow representing the potential applications for future research. To complete the assumed task, traditional sources regarding the usage and the carried out investigation on *Anethum graveolens* L. are collected and explained. Essential assessments of the documented bioactive components particularly in terms of their correlation with recognized traditional use and current pharmacological knowledge are discussed. Phytochemical studies, antidiabetic properties, suggested mechanism, and the main compounds of AG that may be responsible for useful effects of AG are described too.

2. Materials and Methods

To prepare this review a pharmacological and phytochemical literature survey was performed using Scopus, PubMed, and Web of Science.

3. Results and Discussion

3.1. Blood Glucose and Lipid Profile in Diabetic Patients. Studies have shown that blood lipid peroxidation markedly rises in diabetes due to vascular injury, which is provoked by hyperglycemia and free radicals. This peroxidation can further aggravate the progress of diabetic complications and is thought to happen as a result of defects in insulin secretion by pancreatic β-cells. Diabetes also leads to an impaired lipid profile, including low levels of high-density lipoprotein (HDL) cholesterol and hypertriglyceridemia and raised oxidative stress [30, 31]. Diabetes also raises the risk of heart disease two- to fourfold. Therefore, uncontrolled hyperlipidemia leads to premature cardiovascular diseases (CVDs). CVD is the most common complication in diabetes, which is a common reason for premature mortality in diabetic patients. As a result, to reduce the risk of CVD, many studies potentially recommended control of dyslipidemia and hyperglycemia [1, 32–34].

In addition to dyslipidemia, hyperglycemia is known as a major risk factor for diabetic complications. Protein glycation is involved in the progress of complications such as retinopathy, neuropathy, nephropathy, dermopathy, and atherosclerotic lesions [1, 33, 35–37]. In the chronic state, excess glucose binds to free amino groups in tissue or blood proteins and body fluid and disturbs their functions [38–40]. This nonenzymatic reaction leads to formation of advanced glycosylation end products (AGEs). Glycation reaction leads to alteration in the structure and function of biomolecules particularly proteins. AGE formation is known as a key element in diabetes complications [41–46].

3.2. Free Radicals in Diabetes. In diabetic patients, reactive substances such as hydroxyl radicals ($^{\bullet}OH$), hydrogen peroxide (H_2O_2), lipid peroxyl radicals ($LOO^{\bullet}$), superoxide anion ($O_2^{\bullet-}$), and peroxyl radicals ($ROO^{\bullet}$) are mainly generated during the developing stage of diabetes. The reaction of these reactive species with polyunsaturated fatty acids (PUFAs) causes lipid peroxidation which is consequently implicated in early diabetes complications, especially premature cardiovascular disease [47, 48].

Enzymatic antioxidant mechanisms play an important role in the elimination of free radicals. For instance, superoxide dismutase (SOD) is known as one of the main endogenous enzymes that removes O_2^- and produces H_2O_2, which is then processed to water by the activity of catalase (CAT) and glutathione peroxidase (GPx). Hence, SOD can work as the chief protector against $O_2^{\bullet-}$ and it inhibits production of free radicals. CAT is an important enzyme involved in detoxification of hydrogen peroxide to water and oxygen. On the other hand, glutathione S-transferase (GST) and glutathione peroxidase (GPx) are other chief antioxidant enzymes [47, 49, 50]. GPx decreases free radical damage by preventing the production of extremely cytotoxic species, for instance, lipid peroxides and other organic hydroperoxides. GST is therefore believed to preserve the balance of cellular redox conditions [47, 49]. Lipid peroxidation naturally occurs on a small level in the body and plays a key role in diabetes and cardiovascular diseases pathogenesis. The reactive oxygen species such as hydroxyl radical and hydrogen peroxide attacks polyunsaturated fatty acids and causes lipid peroxidation. Iron ion and hydrogen peroxide in a known process, called Fenton reaction, lead to formation of hydroxyl radical which is a potent oxidative agent [15]. Oral administration of many herbal plants leads to a marked rise in the activities of SOD, CAT, GSH, GST, and GPx in diabetes [51, 52].

3.3. Diabetes Treatment. There are different ways for treatment and control of diabetes, including administration of insulin or hypoglycemic drugs, dietary control, and exercise [53, 54]. Furthermore, chemical drugs generally have low efficacy over time, are too expensive, and show severe side effects such that some patients cannot tolerate prolonged treatment or taking the high dosages of these drugs. In contrast, herbal medicines are regarded as potential sources for medication due to their useful effects, negligible side effects in clinical trials, and low cost [53–59].

3.4. Safety and Side Effects of Chemical Diabetic Medicines. People use different medicines such as sulfonylureas (glimepiride, glipizide, and glyburide), biguanides (metformin), thiazolidinediones (pioglitazone), alpha-glucosidase inhibitors (acarbose), meglitinides (nateglinide), and dipeptidyl peptidase 4 inhibitors (Januvia, Onglyza) for control and treatment of hyperglycemia. However, side effects can be seen in all diabetes drugs' usage. More than 10 to 20 percent of diabetic patients are known to eventually stop taking their medications because of the side effects. Some of the diabetes medicines can also cause hypoglycemia which is a harmful and potentially lethal side effect. Additional side effects of several antidiabetic drugs are weight gain, increased risk for fractures especially in women, and gastrointestinal disorders such as abdominal pain, gassiness, vomiting, nausea, diarrhea, and bloating. Edema and increased level of low-density lipoprotein cholesterol (LDL-C) were also reported by many patients. Uncommon side effects include congestive heart failure, allergic reactions, and anemia, which can be induced by chemical diabetic medicines [30, 31].

3.5. Role of Herbal Medicine in the Treatment of Diabetes Mellitus. Nowadays, many physicians prescribe insulin, thiazolidinediones, sulphonylureas, α-glucosidase inhibitors, and so forth, for treatment and control of diabetic complications [75]. Nevertheless, since adverse effects of these medicines are arguable, there is a need for novel agents in diabetes treatment. In this respect, some herbal medicines due to their lower side effects, low costs, useful properties such as antihyperglycemic, antihyperlipidemic, and antioxidant effects, and especially their natural origin have been proposed for potential management of diabetes [76, 77]. However, because of unknown mechanisms, only a small number of plants have

Table 1: Antidiabetic effects of AG in different studies.

Reference	Preparation	Study model and duration	Pharmacological properties
[5]	Alkaloid extracted from AG	Hypercholesterolemic rabbits, 4 weeks	(i) Hypolipidemic effect
[6]	Ethanolic extract of AG seed	Alloxan induced diabetic mice, 15 days	(i) Hypoglycemic effects
[7]	Hydroalcoholic extract of AG	Hypercholesterolemic rabbits, 3 days	(i) Significant reduced glucose levels, LDL-C, TC, AST, ALT, and fibrinogen (ii) The change in ApoB, factor VII, nitrite, and nitrate was not significant
[8]	Hydroalcoholic extract of AG	Hypercholesterolemic rabbits, 3 days	(i) Significantly declined TC, LDL-C, AST, ALT, and fibrinogen
[9]	Hexane extract of AG seed	High-fat-diet-induced hyperlipidemia and diabetic rat, 4 weeks	(i) Normalized blood lipid and glucose (ii) Increased blood adiponectin levels (iii) Significantly motivated FA oxidation by induced expression of FA oxidation-related genes (especially with activation of PPAR alpha) and also inhibited TG accumulation
[10]	Methanolic extract of AG	*In vitro*	(i) Antioxidant activity
[11]	Hydroalcoholic extract of AG	Patient with metabolic syndrome, 12 weeks	(i) Significantly reduced TG
[12]	Combined carnitine and hydroalcoholic extract of AG	Rat, 21 days	(i) AG does not improve serum lipids profiles
[13]	AG along with aerobic training	Type 2 diabetic patients, 4 weeks	(i) Hypoglycemic effects (ii) Hypolipidemic effect
[14]	AG leaves powder	Hyperlipidemic patients, 4 weeks	(i) Hypolipidemic effect
[15]	Ethanolic extract of AG	Hepatotoxicity induced by carbon tetrachloride in albino rats, 21 days	(i) Antioxidant and hepatoprotective activity
[16]	Ethanolic extract of AG	*In vitro*	(i) Antioxidant and antiradical and antityrosinase activity (ii) Inhibited lipid peroxidation
[17]	Aqueous extract of AG	Normal and scopolamine-induced amnestic rats, single dose	(i) Significant antistress and antioxidant memory enhancing and activity
[18]	AG tablet	STZ-induced diabetic mice, 21 days	(i) Significantly declined body weight, TG, and LDL-C and increased HDL (ii) The change of blood glucose was not significant
[19]	Ethanolic extract and oil of AG	*In vitro*	(i) Antioxidant activity (ethanolic extract had higher activity than essential oil)
[20]	AG powder	Hyperlipidemic rats, 30 days	(i) Significant antioxidant and radical scavenging activity (ii) Hypolipidemic effect
[21]	AG powder and essential oil	Hypercholesterolemic rat, 2 weeks	(i) Hypolipidemic effect
[22]	Hydroalcoholic extract of AG	Type 1 diabetic rats, 10 days	(i) Normalized blood lipids (ii) Hypoglycemic effects (similar to glybenclamide)
[23]	Hydroalcoholic extract of AG	Corticosteroid induced diabetic rats, 15 days	(i) Significantly declined both plasma glucose and insulin levels (ii) Antioxidant activity
[24]	Ethanolic extract of AG	Hyperlipidemic rats, 30 days	(i) Probably inhibited activity of HMG-CoA reductase (ii) Hypolipidemic effect
[25]	Hydroalcoholic extract of AG seed extract	Rat, 6–168 hrs	(i) Antioxidant and antiradical activity (ii) Significantly reduced liver enzymes

TABLE 1: Continued.

Reference	Preparation	Study model and duration	Pharmacological properties
[26]	*Anethum* tablet twice daily (650 mg)	Hyperlipidemic patients, 6 weeks	(i) Normalized blood lipids
[27]	*Anethum* tablet twice daily (650 mg)	Hyperlipidemic patients, one month	(i) Hypolipidemic effect
[28]	Hydroalcoholic extract of AG	Alloxan induced diabetic mice, 48 h	(i) Hypolipidemic effect (ii) Hypoglycemic effects
[29]	AG tablet	Hyperlipidemic patients, 1 month	(i) Hypolipidemic effect

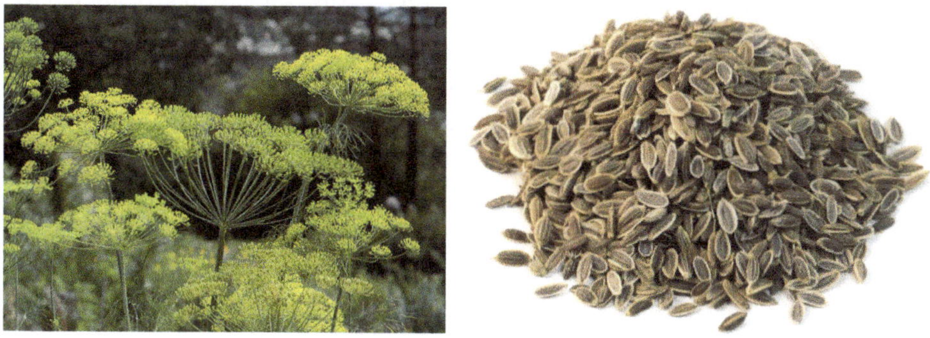

FIGURE 1: Plant and seed of AG.

been used for the management of diabetic complications [78]. Herbal plants contain many chemical components such as flavonoids (30%), terpenoids (17%), saponins (9%), polyphenols (6%), alkaloids (5%), tannins (4%), polysaccharides (3%), and miscellaneous compounds (17%), which are known to have remedial properties [78]. Interestingly, the World Health Organization (WHO) reported that about 80% of the world's people presently use herbal plants for treatment of different diseases [79]. Although many plants have been suggested for treatment of diabetes due to their antidiabetic properties, in this review, we will attempt to open a new window toward application of AG and its constituents in the management of type 2 diabetes.

3.6. Botanical Profile and Taxonomy of AG. The generic name of "*Anethum*" comes from the Greek word "anethon" and the colloquial name of dill is derived from the Old Norse word "dilla" that possibly means "to soothe." AG is the only species of the genus *Anethum*, still classified by several botanists related to *Peucedanum* genus as *Peucedanum graveolens* (L.) [80]. AG is an annual vertical plant with 50–150 cm stem belonging to the Apiaceae family. The fruits of AG are brown, flat, tiny, and oval in shape (Figure 1). This plant is cultivated in Mediterranean countries, in Asia, and in Europe. AG contains 36% carbohydrates, 15.68% proteins, 14.80% fiber, 9.8% ash, and 8.39% moisture as well as essential oils, fatty oil, minerals, and vitamins [80].

3.7. Traditional Uses of AG. AG is used in the traditional herbal medicine for the management and prevention of digestive disease, breath problem, motivation of lactation, and also reduction of cholesterol and glucose. Currently, many studies have established these properties; also, AG is recently known as anticancer, antimicrobial, antigastric irritation, anti-inflammatory, and antioxidant agent. In this respect, dill is produced as a hypolipidemic drug (*Anethum* tablet) in Iran which consists of *Anethum graveolens* (68%), *Cichorium intybus* (5%), *Fumaria parviflora* (5%), and lime (Citrus aurantifolia) (4%) [81].

3.8. Hypolipidemic and Hypoglycemic Properties of AG. Administration of different extractions of AG seed and leaf, as well as its essential oil, in diabetic models significantly reduced triglycerides, total cholesterol, low-density lipoprotein cholesterol (LDL-C), very-low-density lipoprotein cholesterol (VLDL-C), and glucose levels, whereas it increased HDL-C level [80]. On the other hand, many studies reported that AG has hypoglycemic and antioxidant activity [80]. The antioxidant activity of AG is due to its phenolic proanthocyanidins and flavonoids constituents [24]. It has also been shown that the extract from AG flowers had more antioxidant activity than either its seed or leaf extract [80]. Duration of treatment in different experiments was variable; for example, Koppula and Choi [17] used only single dose for one hour, while the treatment period in Mansouri et al.'s [11] study was 12 weeks. However, almost all of the experiments show that one month is an appropriate time for survey of antidiabetic properties of dill.

To survey the effects of AG on dyslipidemia, different animals were used. The rabbit is known as an animal model that has been commonly used for the study of hypercholesterolemia. Only few studies have been done on rabbits, whereas rats are an optional model for diabetes studies [7]. Therefore, as mentioned in Table 1, most of the studies used diabetic rats.

Some primary mechanisms have been proposed for hypolipidemic effects of AG. Inhibition of intestinal cholesterol absorption, binding to bile acids in the intestine, an increase in fecal excretion, and increasing production of bile acids might be the main mechanisms by which AG exerts its antidiabetic functions [80]. Yazdanparast et al. [24, 82] proposed that some components of AG such as carvone, limonene, or α-phellandrene are responsible for the hypolipidemic properties of AG, likely through reducing acyl CoA carboxylase or 3-hydroxy-3-methylglutaryl-CoA (HMG-CoA) reductase, the key enzymes in fatty acid and cholesterol metabolism. Other studies have suggested that AG components might rise liver LDL receptors, decrease fatty acid synthesis, and impact lipoprotein homeostasis mainly through improvement in lipoprotein metabolism [24]. Furthermore, some studies suggest that AG may improve the lipid profile by its antioxidant properties [10]. We have also observed that administration of 100 and 200 mg/kg of AG tablet and hydroalcoholic extract of AG in hypercholesterolemic hamsters resulted in significantly reduced HMG-CoA reductase activity and mRNA levels [83]. For the first time, we also showed that AG normalized the lipid profile by decreasing HMG-CoA reductase in the hypercholesterolemic hamsters and type 2 diabetic rats [83]. We have also shown that AG increased LDL receptor level in the liver resulting in stimulation of cholesterol clearance from the bloodstream (unpublished data). The results of Abbasi Oshaghi et al.'s [84] study showed that AG significantly increased cholesterol-7-alpha hydroxylase activity, the rate-limiting enzyme in bile acids biosynthesis [10]. Some studies have also reported that rutin and quercetin (components of dill) may decrease serum cholesterol and LDL-C levels and decrease liver cholesterol level. Other studies have also reported that quercetin reduces HMG-CoA reductase activity [24]. Histopathological experiments of Abbasi Oshaghi et al. [84] showed that treatment of diabetic rats with different extracts of AG normalized lipid deposits in the liver, pancreas, and heart. HPLC analysis showed that AG has high amounts of quercetin which may be responsible for the suppression of HMG-CoA reductase activity [10]. Numerous studies that have previously shown the antidiabetic effects of AG are listed in Table 1. Chemical compounds of AG extracts especially flavonoids, terpenoids, alkaloids, tannins, and phytosterols are probably responsible for its hypoglycemic effects [61]. We found that different extracts of AG reduce AGEs formation [85, 86]. Our study also showed that AG at the dose of 300 mg/kg had potential antioxidant and hypolipidemic effects [86]. Madani et al. [28] reported significant decline in fasting blood glucose level with 300 mg/kg hydroalcoholic extract of *Anethum graveolens*. Doses of AG up to 2 g/kg in a short period of time did not cause any death in animal models. Also, the AG doses up to 1000 mg/kg did not cause any toxic effect in short time experiments [87]. However, 50 mg/kg/day is the minimum and 1 g/kg/day is the maximum tolerated dose in a 45-day period [87]. Although different doses of AG were used in animal models, Ahmadi Mahmoudabadi [22] reported that the effective dose for metabolic properties is 300 mg/kg in animal models. Different studies showed that both high and low doses of AG have hypoglycemic and hypolipidemic effects. The doses less than 50 mg/kg could be known without adverse effect in rats and mice [87]. However, Piri et al. [18] demonstrated that 3-week administration of *Anethum* extract at the doses of 50, 100, and 200 mg/kg normalized blood lipid, and the change in blood glucose was not significant. The safe and effective dose in human studies is reported as 650 mg/kg [26]. In an *in vitro* study, Abbasi Oshaghi et al. [86] found that different extracts of AG at the concentrations of 0.032, 0.065, 0.125, 0.25, 0.5, and 1 mg/ml reduced AGEs formation; fructosamine level and carbonyl groups, also, raised thiol groups in type 2 diabetic animals. The components of AG are responsible for its antiglycation properties. Oxidation of carbonyl and thiol groups on blood proteins significantly reduces by *Anethum* in a dose dependent manner [28].

According to the study conducted by Adisakwattana et al. [88], polyphenolic compounds in plant extract may play a major role in the inhibition of AGEs formation. AGEs are recognized to contribute to the production of oxidative stress and inflammation, which are related to the diabetes complications. It has been reported that administration of AGE-rich diets in an animal model is associated with rising of blood and tissue AGEs and the conditions like atherosclerosis [89]. Mobasseri et al. [90] showed that administration of AG powder in type 2 diabetic patients reduced fasting blood glucose and normalized insulin resistance and lipid profiles. As mentioned above, AG is rich in antioxidant compounds; therefore, antioxidant and flavonoid components of AG probably are able to repair damaged β-cells and insulin secretion. It has been shown that AG significantly increases total antioxidants in the pancreas and also regenerates histopathological changes [84]. Therefore, AG with antioxidant activity likely increases insulin synthesis. Some researchers such as Madani et al. [28] and Mishra [6] reported that AG reduced blood glucose via the increase of insulin secretion. Takahashi et al. [91] have shown that AG extract normalized lipid profile in diabetic obese mice by activating peroxisome proliferator-activated receptor-α (PPAR-α) and increasing fatty acid oxidation-related genes expression.

Our colorimetric and HPLC analysis also showed that dill had a high amount of quercetin, phenol, flavonoid, tannin, saponin, and alkaloid [84]. All of these agents have hypoglycemic and hypolipidemic properties. Therefore, we can conclude that components of dill are responsible for its metabolic effects. Mishra [6] reported that aqueous extract of AG has a high amount of carvone, which is accountable for its antidiabetic activity. Carvone is able to cause decline in plasma glycoprotein components and motivate insulin secretion. The ethanolic extract of AG which is prepared in India showed very low antidiabetic properties [6]. On the other hand, Mudassir et al. [92] reported that the prepared ethanolic extract of AG in Pakistan significantly reduced blood glucose (34% reduction). They declared that hypoglycemic effects of AG might be due to the inhibition of intestinal glucose absorption [92].

In our laboratory, we have previously shown that AG has potential antioxidant activity [85]. Our results are in agreement with the results of a previous study by Bahramikia and Yazdanparast [20], indicating DPPH radical scavenging activity of AG. In our study, 1 mg/ml of AG water extract showed 96.04% scavenging of H_2O_2, whereas only 27.26% radical scavenging activity was reported for AG ethanolic extract [86]. AG also showed Fe^{2+} ion chelation which is known as a defense mechanism against oxidative damage by declining free radical production via Fenton reaction. In this reaction, iron(II) is oxidized by H_2O_2 to create potential free radicals such as hydroxyl radical. Nitric oxide scavenging activity has also been proposed for AG [20]. The results of a study by Bahramikia and Yazdanparast [20] showed that crude extract of AG exhibited a moderate NO scavenging activity. In line with this observation, we showed a nitric oxide scavenging activity of AG similar to the known radical scavengers, ascorbic acid and butylated hydroxytoluene (BHT) [86]. Interestingly, we showed that NO scavenging activity of AG is comparable with the activity of ascorbic acid and/or BHT. We showed that a 1 mg/ml solution of dill water extract has 90.41% NO scavenging activity which was much greater than that observed (78.49%) for ethanolic extract of AG by Orhan et al. [93]. We have also detected a greater antioxidant activity for AG water extract compared with methanolic extracts [85]. Interestingly, the antiradical and antioxidant properties of AG in all tests were similar to ascorbic acid and BHT [80]. The results of many studies established the notion that the particular parts of dill are often discriminated by significant diversity in their constituents' chemical compounds. It has been reported that ethanolic extract of AG has very low antidiabetic properties when compared with the aqueous extract [6]. However, Mishra reported that ethanolic extract of AG has hypoglycemic effects [6]. Concordant with the hypoglycemic function of AG ethanolic extract, other studies have reported that this extract significantly reduces blood lipids [24, 82]. Interestingly, we showed that different extracts of AG significantly reduced glucose level, but the reduction by water or hydroalcoholic extract was more as compared with the methanolic extract [86]. Furthermore, with review of the literature, we can find that different preparations such as hexane, ethanolic, water, and hydroalcoholic extracts of seed and leaf have been used in different studies (Table 1). However, the hydroalcoholic extract showed stronger antidiabetic effects compared with other extracts.

3.9. Chemical Composition. There is some diversity in the dill composition in different countries; for example, American dill oil has a high amount of alpha-phellandrene, while carvone and limonene are the main constituents of Asian and European dill [94]. In addition to essential oils especially carvone, limonene, and alpha-phellandrene, dill also contains fatty oil, proteins, carbohydrates, moisture, fiber, ash, vitamins (A and niacin), and mineral elements (calcium, potassium, magnesium, phosphorus, and sodium). This plant is known as a rich source of flavonoids, phenolic compounds, saponins, cardiac glycosides, and terpenes [80].

Jana and Shekhawat [80] reported that there are several volatile components of AG seeds and herb. For instance, carvone is the main odorant of AG seed and limonene, α-phellandrene, myristicin, and dill ether are the most vital odorants of AG herb. Larijani et al. [63] also reported that seeds and leaves of AG have different components and consequently have different therapeutic effects. Different parameters such as cultivating area, genotype, and environmental factors have huge effects on the composition of AG extracts [80]. Furthermore, Reichert et al. [95] reported that the different parts of AG have different compounds and these compounds may change depending on the stage of plant growth. For example, Sefidkon [96] reported that α-phellandrene and limonene are the major constituents of dill oil, while Singh [64] showed that carvone, dill apiole, limonene, trans- and cis-dihydrocarvone, and linalool are the main constituents. Consequently, the different components which are reported by the different studies also depend on the different plant growth stage, cultivating area, and the particular part of the plant that is used. Different compounds of AG have been described in the different published reports which are listed in Table 2.

3.10. Adverse Effects. However, it has been shown that AG administration is safe, and it may rarely lead to allergic reactions, vomiting, diarrhea, oral pruritus, urticaria tongue, and throat swelling [97]; furthermore, it is not suggested in pregnancy [97]. Mirhosseini et al. [98] reported that AG did not have any side effects, as compared with gemfibrozil, in treated patients. Other clinical trial studies did not report the side effect of AG [11, 13, 26, 27].

4. Conclusion

Herbal medicines have multiple key components such as flavonoids, terpenoids, saponins, polyphenols, tannins, alkaloids, and polysaccharides that have their individual remedial properties. The use of herbal medicines is not a novel matter. Herbal medicines especially AG have a lot of useful properties including antihyperlipidemic, antihypercholesterolemic, antidiabetic, anticancer, antioxidant, antistress, antisecretory, cardioprotective, antispasmodic, and diuretic effects. Moreover, epidemiologic experiments reported a converse relationship between AG consumption and risk of diabetes and CVD progression. Recent literature strongly supports the suggestion that consumption of AG has a significant antidiabetic effect in both humans and animals. According to the reported antidiabetic effects of dill, it can be suggested for the management of diabetic patients. However, the diverse preparations, dose of AG, period of AG consumption, and interaction with other drugs must be normalized. More studies are required to recognize the specific constituents of AG that are accountable for most of its valuable properties. Although all components of AG have antioxidant, hypoglycemic, and hypolipidemic effects, these components are at low levels in dill and possibly have synergic effects. Moreover, the findings suggest that activation of LDL-R, PPAR-alpha, and other FA oxidation-related genes and also inhibition of HMG-CoA reductase contribute to the hypolipidemic effects of AG.

Competing Interests

The authors have no competing interests to disclose.

TABLE 2: Components of AG in different studies.

References	Preparation	Components
[60]	Essential oil	Carvone, α-pinene, α-phellandrene, myrcene, dillapiole, anethole, p-cymene, limonene, dill ether, trans-dihydrocarvone, cis-dihydrocarvone, camphor
[61]	Dill seed oil	Carvone, limonene, gamma-terpinene, m-cymene, apiol, myristicin, trans-dihydrocarvone
[62]	Dill seed oil	Glycosides, reducing sugar, tannins, saponins, flavonoids, steroids, flavonosides, terpenoids
[63]	Dill seed oil	α-Phellandrene, sabinene bicycle, trans-caryophyllene, beta-santalene, eugenol, pentadecane, dill apiole, hexadecanol, methyl undecanoate, limonene, eudesmol, n-octane, mefranal, D-carvone, cyclohexasiloxane
[64]	Essential oil	α-Thujene, cyclohexane, β-myrcene, β-phellandrene, grandisol, thujyl alcohol, carvone, bis-1,2-benzenedicarboxylic acid, limonene
[65]	Essential oil	α-Pinene, β-pinene, α-thujene, β-phellandrene, α-cadinol, sabinene, (Z)-anethole, α-phellandrene, limonene, myristicin, γ-terpinene, β-myrcene, dimethyl phencone, phencone, linalool, dill ether, p-cymene, (Z)-dihydrocarvone, (E)-dihydrocarvone, (E)-carveol, carvone, apiole, phthalide isomer, D-germacrene, epi-bicyclosesquiphellandrene
[66]	Essential oil	α-Pinene, α-phellandrene, α-thujene, β-phellandrene, β-myrcene, carvone, dill ether, n-eicosane, limonene, n-eicosane, terpinolene, trans-dihydrocarvone, sabinol, apiole
[67]	Essential oil	Limonene, dill ether, α-thujene, sabinene, β-myrcene, α-pinene, p-cymene, α-phellandrene, cis-dihydrocarvone, carvone, cadinol, trans-dihydrocarvone, α-copaene, γ-muurolene, neophytadiene, n-nonadecane, n-docosane, n-heneicosane, n-tricosane, n-tetracosane, n-eicosane, n-pentacosane, n-heptacosane, n-hexacosane
[68]	Essential oil	Limonene, linalool, D-carvone, carvacrol, sabinene, dihydrocarvone, β-myrcene, ρ-cymene, γ-terpinene, E-limonene oxide, estragole, α-pinene, terpineol, cumin aldehyde, β-caryophyllene, D-germacrene, α-phellandrene, thymol, dill apiole, myristicin
[69]	Dill flower extract	Gentisic acid, kaempferol, gallic acid, catechin, chlorogenic acid, luteolin, epicatechin, p-coumaric acid, sinapic acid, benzoic acid, p-anisic acid, myricetin, quercetin, caffeic acid, total phenolic acid, apigenin, proanthocyanidins, total flavonoid
[70]	Dill seed oil	cis-Dihydrocarvone, farnesene, m-carveol, dihydrocarvone, D-carvone, myristicin, cis-dihydrocarveol, 3,5-dimethylcyclohexen-1-one, limonene, diplaniol, 1,2-diethoxyethane, α-phellandrene, β-myrcene, limonene, ethylacetate, sabinene, α-humulene, carvone, cis-carvone
[21]	Dill weed oil	Dill ether, limonene, α-phellandrene, α-pinene
[71]	Dill oil and acetone extract	α-Pinene, α-ylangene, α-thujene, foeniculin, sabinene, myrcene, p-cymene, sylvestrene, isocaryophyllene, terpinolene, linalool, trans-carveol, camphor, dill ether, cis-dihydrocarvone, trans-dihydrocarvone, undecane, isodihydrocarveol, geranyl acetate, carvone, limonene, α-humulene, D-germacrene, β-caryophyllene, β-selinene, trans-guaiene, α-cadinene, β-bisabolene, trans-isocroweacin, dill apiole, apiole, elemicin, trans-anethole, eugenol, p-anisaldehyde, lauric aldehyde, trans-bergamotene, nonadecanone, myristicin, trans-muurolol, heptadecane, neophytadiene, palmitic acid, linoleic acid, γ-terpinene
[72]	Essential oil	α-Thujene, α-phellandrene, camphene, sabinene, α-pinene, myrcene, p-cymene, limonene, β-phellandrene, (Z)-β-ocimene, (E)-β-ocimene, terpinolene, α-p-dimethyl styrene, carvone, bornyl acetate, D-germacrene, β-bisabolene, myristicin, T-cadinol, phthalide isomer, farnesol, apiole, n-octadecane, n-heptadecane, n-nonadecane
[73]	Essential oil	Glycosides, saponins, tannins, terpenoids, steroids, flavonoids, phlobatannin, cardiac glycoside, anthraquinone
[74]	Fruit essential oil	Carvacrol, D-carvone, cis-carveol, trans-carveol, cis-dihydrocarvone, trans-dihydrocarvone, limonene, terpinene-4-ol, d-dihydrocarveol, l-dihydrocarveol, a- and g-terpinene, thymol, a-phellandrene, b-terpineol, p-cymene

References

[1] M. Ståhlman, B. Fagerberg, M. Adiels et al., "Dyslipidemia, but not hyperglycemia and insulin resistance, is associated with marked alterations in the HDL lipidome in type 2 diabetic subjects in the DIWA cohort: impact on small HDL particles," *Biochimica et Biophysica Acta (BBA)—Molecular and Cell Biology of Lipids*, vol. 1831, no. 11, pp. 1609–1617, 2013.

[2] M. Rabkin, Z. Melaku, K. Bruce et al., "Strengthening health systems for chronic care: leveraging HIV programs to support diabetes services in Ethiopia and Swaziland," *Journal of Tropical Medicine*, vol. 2012, Article ID 137460, 6 pages, 2012.

[3] D. R. Whiting, L. Guariguata, C. Weil, and J. Shaw, "IDF diabetes atlas: global estimates of the prevalence of diabetes for 2011 and 2030," *Diabetes Research and Clinical Practice*, vol. 94, no. 3, pp. 311–321, 2011.

[4] S. Wild, G. Roglic, A. Green, R. Sicree, and H. King, "Global prevalence of diabetes: estimates for the year 2000 and projections for 2030," *Diabetes Care*, vol. 27, no. 5, pp. 1047–1053, 2004.

[5] A. J. Al-Fartosy, S. A. Zearah, and N. A. Alwan, "Total antioxidant capacity and antihyperlipidemic activity of alkaloid extract from aerial part of *Anethum graveolens* L. plant," *European Scientific Journal*, vol. 9, no. 33, pp. 413–423, 2013.

[6] N. Mishra, "Haematological and hypoglycemic potential Anethum graveolens seeds extract in normal and diabetic Swiss albino mice," *Veterinary World*, vol. 6, no. 8, pp. 502–507, 2013.

[7] M. Setorki, M. Rafieian-Kopaei, A. Merikhi et al., "Suppressive impact of anethum graveolens consumption on biochemical risk factors of atherosclerosis in hypercholesterolemic rabbits," *International Journal of Preventive Medicine*, vol. 4, no. 8, pp. 889–895, 2013.

[8] M. Setorkil, N. Shahinfard, R. Ansari, Z. Foronzandeh, S. Asgharzadeh, and M. Rafieian-Kopaei, "Comparison between the effects of hydroalcoholic extract of dill and statins on lipid profile," *Journal of Kerman University of Medical Sciences*, vol. 20, no. 2, pp. 158–168, 2013.

[9] N. Takahashi, L. Yao, M. Kim et al., "Dill seed extract improves abnormalities in lipid metabolism through peroxisome proliferator-activated receptor-α (PPAR-α) activation in diabetic obese mice," *Molecular Nutrition & Food Research*, vol. 57, no. 7, pp. 1295–1299, 2013.

[10] H. Edziri, S. Ammar, L. Souad et al., "In vitro evaluation of antimicrobial and antioxidant activities of some Tunisian vegetables," *South African Journal of Botany*, vol. 78, pp. 252–256, 2012.

[11] M. Mansouri, N. Nayebi, A. Keshtkar, S. Hasani-Ranjbar, E. Taheri, and B. Larijani, "The effect of 12 weeks Anethum graveolens (dill) on metabolic markers in patients with metabolic syndrome; A randomized double blind controlled trial," *DARU Journal of Pharmaceutical Sciences*, vol. 20, no. 1, article 47, 2012.

[12] A. K. Rezapour and H. H. Maleki, "The effect of combined carnitine and dill extract complementation on serum lipids of male fat rats," *International Journal of Agronomy and Plant Production*, vol. 3, no. 12, pp. 638–641, 2012.

[13] A. Rashid Lamir and S. A. A. Hashemi Javaheri, "The effect of 4-weeks aerobic training according with the usage of Anethum Graveolens on blood sugar and lipoproteins profile of diabetic women," *Annals of Biological Research*, vol. 3, no. 9, pp. 4313–4319, 2012.

[14] A. S. Sahib, I. H. Mohammad, and A. AlGareeb, "Effects of Anethum graveolens leave powder on lipid profile in hyperlipidemic patients," *Spatula DD*, vol. 2, no. 2, pp. 153–158, 2012.

[15] R. Tamilarasi, D. Sivanesan, and P. Kanimozhi, "Hepatoprotective and antioxidant efficacy of *Anethum graveolens* Linn in carbon tetrachloride induced hepatotoxicity in Albino rats," *Journal of Chemical and Pharmaceutical Research*, vol. 4, no. 4, pp. 1885–1888, 2012.

[16] M. Dadashpour, I. Rasooli, F. Sefidkon, M. B. Rezaei, and S. Danish Alipour Astaneh, "Lipid peroxidation inhibition, superoxide anion and nitric oxide radical scavenging properties of Thymus daenensis and Anethum graveolens essential oils," *Journal of Medicinal Plants*, vol. 1, no. 37, pp. 109–120, 2011.

[17] S. Koppula and D. K. Choi, "*Anethum Graveolens* linn (*Umbelliferae*) extract attenuates stress-induced urinary biochemical changes and improves cognition in scopolamineinduced amnesic rats," *Tropical Journal of Pharmaceutical Research*, vol. 10, no. 1, pp. 47–54, 2011.

[18] M. Piri, M. Shahin, and S. Oryan, "The effects of Anethum on plasma lipid and lipoprotein in normal and diabetic rats fed high fat diets," *Journal of Shahrekord University of Medical Sciences*, vol. 11, no. 4, pp. 15–25, 2010.

[19] A. Kamkar, "The study of antioxidant activity of essential oil and extract of Iranian Anethum graveloens," *The Horizon of Medical Sciences*, vol. 15, no. 2, pp. 11–16, 2009.

[20] S. Bahramikia and R. Yazdanparast, "Efficacy of different fractions of *Anethum graveolens* leaves on serum lipoproteins and serum and liver oxidative status in experimentally induced hypercholesterolaemic rat models," *The American Journal of Chinese Medicine*, vol. 37, no. 4, pp. 685–699, 2009.

[21] V. Hajhashemi and N. Abbasi, "Hypolipidemic activity of *Anethum graveolens* in rats," *Phytotherapy Research*, vol. 22, no. 3, pp. 372–375, 2008.

[22] N. Ahmadi Mahmoudabadi, "The effects of hydroalcoholic extracts of dill (Anethum graveolens L.) and artichoke (Cynara scolymus L.) against type 1 diabetes mellitus," *Iranian Journal of Medicinal And Aromatic Plants*, vol. 24, no. 3, pp. 333–341, 2008.

[23] S. Panda, "The effect of *Anethum graveolens* L. (dill) on corticosteroid induced diabetes mellitus: involvement of thyroid hormones," *Phytotherapy Research*, vol. 22, no. 12, pp. 1695–1697, 2008.

[24] R. Yazdanparast and S. Bahramikia, "Evaluation of the effect of *Anethum graveolens* L. crude extracts on serum lipids and lipoproteins profiles in hypercholesterolaemic rats," *DARU Journal of Pharmaceutical Sciences*, vol. 16, no. 2, pp. 88–94, 2008.

[25] M. Taher and A. G. R. Karmiyan, "Effects of volatile oil extracts of Anethum graveolens L. and Apium graveolens L. seeds on activity of liver enzymes in rat," *The Journal of Qazvin University of Medical Sciences*, vol. 11, no. 2, pp. 8–12, 2007.

[26] J. Kojuri, A. R. Vosoughi, and M. Akrami, "Effects of anethum graveolens and garlic on lipid profile in hyperlipidemic patients," *Lipids in Health and Disease*, vol. 6, article 5, pp. 1476–1512, 2007.

[27] T. Kazemi, M. Kashanian, and H. Akbari, "Effect of Dill pearl on serum lipids," *Arak Medical University Journal*, vol. 8, no. 3, pp. 35–41, 2006.

[28] H. Madani, N. Ahmady Mahmoodabady, and A. Vahdati, "Effects of hydroalchoholic extract of Anethum graveolens (Dill) on plasma glucose an lipid levels in diabetes induced rats," *Iranian Journal of Diabetes and Metabolism*, vol. 5, no. 2, pp. 109–116, 2005.

[29] K. Yazdanpanah, "Effects of dill juice on serum low density lipoprotein, triglyceride and high density lipoprotein in patients with hyperlipidemia," *Scientific Journal of Kurdistan University of Medical Sciences*, vol. 5, no. 3, p. 1, 2001.

[30] P. Barter, A. M. Gotto, J. C. LaRosa et al., "HDL cholesterol, very low levels of LDL cholesterol, and cardiovascular events," *The New England Journal of Medicine*, vol. 357, no. 13, pp. 1301–1310, 2007.

[31] J. van Olmen, F. Schellevis, W. Van Damme, G. Kegels, and F. Rasschaert, "Management of chronic diseases in sub-Saharan Africa: cross-fertilisation between HIV/AIDS and diabetes care," *Journal of Tropical Medicine*, vol. 2012, Article ID 349312, 10 pages, 2012.

[32] A. Mohammadi, M. R. Bazrafshani, and E. Abbasi Oshaghi, "Effect of garlic extract on some serum biochemical parameters and expression of npc1l1, abca1, abcg5 and abcg8 genes in the intestine of hypercholesterolemic mice," *Indian Journal of Biochemistry & Biophysics*, vol. 50, no. 6, pp. 500–504, 2013.

[33] J. Shahryari, M. Poormorteza, A. Noori Sorkhani et al., "The effect of concomitant ethanol and opium consumption on lipid profiles and atherosclerosis in golden syrian Hamster's aorta," *Addiction & Health*, vol. 5, no. 3-4, p. 83, 2013.

[34] A. Mohammadi, E. A. Oshaghi, A. N. Sorkhani, F. Oubari, R. H. Kia, and A. Rezaei, "Effect of opium on lipid profile and expression of liver X receptor alpha (LXRα) in normolipidemic mouse," *Food and Nutrition Sciences*, vol. 3, no. 2, pp. 249–254, 2012.

[35] C. Wekesa, G. Asiki, I. Kasamba et al., "Atherogenic risk assessment among persons living in rural uganda," *Journal of Tropical Medicine*, vol. 2016, Article ID 7073894, 8 pages, 2016.

[36] A. Mohammadi, F. Mirzaei, M. Jamshidi et al., "Influence of flaxseed on lipid profiles and expression of LXRα, in intestine of diabetic rat," *International Journal of Biology*, vol. 5, no. 4, pp. 23–29, 2013.

[37] A. Mohammadi, F. Mirzaei, M. N. Moradi et al., "Effect of flaxseed on serum lipid profile and expression of NPC1L1, ABCG5 and ABCG8 genes in the intestine of diabetic rat," *Avicenna Journal of Medical Biochemistry*, vol. 1, no. 1, pp. 1–6, 2013.

[38] M. T. Goodarzi, S. Ghahramany, and M. Hossien, "Glycation of human IgG induces structural alterations leading to changes in its interaction with anti-IgG," *Iranian Journal of Immunology*, vol. 2, no. 1, pp. 36–42, 2005.

[39] M. T. Goodarzi, S. Ghahramany, and M. H. Mirmomeni, "In vitro glycation of human IgG and its effect on interaction with anti-IgG," *Iranian Journal of Allergy, Asthma and Immunology*, vol. 3, no. 4, pp. 181–188, 2004.

[40] M. T. Goodarzi, M. Rezaei, H. Piry, and S. Amiry, "Effect of in vitro glycation of human placental collagen (Type IV) on platelet aggregation," *Pakistan Journal of Biological Sciences*, vol. 8, no. 9, pp. 1203–1206, 2005.

[41] M. T. Goodarzi, M. Rezaei, E. Moadel, S. Homayounfar, and M. R. Safari, "Changes in sialylation of low-density lipoprotein in coronary artery disease," *European Journal of Lipid Science and Technology*, vol. 110, no. 4, pp. 302–306, 2008.

[42] M. T. Goodarzi, A. A. Navidi, M. Rezaei, and H. Babahmadi-Rezaei, "Oxidative damage to DNA and lipids: correlation with protein glycation in patients with type 1 diabetes," *Journal of Clinical Laboratory Analysis*, vol. 24, no. 2, pp. 72–76, 2010.

[43] M. T. Goodarzi, H. Babaahmadi-Rezaei, M. Kadkhodaei-Eliaderani, and S. Haddadinezhad, "Relationship of serum adiponectin with blood lipids, HbA1c, and hs-CRP in type II diabetic postmenopausal women," *Journal of Clinical Laboratory Analysis*, vol. 21, no. 3, pp. 197–200, 2007.

[44] N. Ahmed, "Advanced glycation endproducts—role in pathology of diabetic complications," *Diabetes Research and Clinical Practice*, vol. 67, no. 1, pp. 3–21, 2005.

[45] K. Adeli, C. Taghibiglou, S. C. Van Iderstine, and G. F. Lewis, "Mechanisms of hepatic very low-density lipoprotein overproduction in insulin resistance," *Trends in Cardiovascular Medicine*, vol. 11, no. 5, pp. 170–176, 2001.

[46] I. Lubitz, J. Ricny, D. Atrakchi-Baranes et al., "High dietary advanced glycation end products are associated with poorer spatial learning and accelerated Aβ deposition in an Alzheimer mouse model," *Aging Cell*, vol. 15, no. 2, pp. 309–316, 2016.

[47] A. C. Maritim, R. A. Sanders, and J. B. Watkins III, "Diabetes, oxidative stress, and antioxidants: a review," *Journal of Biochemical and Molecular Toxicology*, vol. 17, no. 1, pp. 24–38, 2003.

[48] A. Mohammadi, F. Mirzaei, M. Jamshidi et al., "The in vivo biochemical and oxidative changes by ethanol and opium consumption in syrian hamsters," *International Journal of Biology*, vol. 5, no. 4, p. 14, 2013.

[49] R. Rahimi, S. Nikfar, B. Larijani, and M. Abdollahi, "A review on the role of antioxidants in the management of diabetes and its complications," *Biomedicine & Pharmacotherapy*, vol. 59, no. 7, pp. 365–373, 2005.

[50] F. Mirzaeipour, N. Azdaki, G. A. Mohammadi, and E. Addasi, "The effects of opium addiction through different administration routes on inflammatory and coagulation factors," *Journal of Kerman University of Medical Sciences*, vol. 20, no. 3, pp. 292–300, 2013.

[51] M. Modak, P. Dixit, J. Londhe, S. Ghaskadbi, and T. P. A. Devasagayam, "Indian herbs and herbal drugs used for the treatment of diabetes," *Journal of Clinical Biochemistry and Nutrition*, vol. 40, no. 3, pp. 163–173, 2007.

[52] A. Mohammadi, P. Norouzian, M. Jamshidi et al., "Effect of garlic (Allium sativum) on lipid profiles, antioxidant activity and expression of scavenger receptor class B type I (SR-BI) in liver and intestine of hypercholesterolemic mice," *Journal of Advances in Chemistry*, vol. 5, no. 3, pp. 784–791, 2013.

[53] V. Somsak, S. Chachiyo, U. Jaihan, and S. Nakinchat, "Protective effect of aqueous crude extract of neem (*Azadirachta indica*) leaves on *Plasmodium berghei*-induced renal damage in mice," *Journal of Tropical Medicine*, vol. 2015, Article ID 961205, 5 pages, 2015.

[54] G. Alvarez-Uria, M. Midde, R. Pakam, P. S. Yalla, P. K. Naik, and R. Reddy, "Short-course induction treatment with intrathecal amphotericin B lipid emulsion for HIV infected patients with cryptococcal meningitis," *Journal of Tropical Medicine*, vol. 2015, Article ID 864271, 6 pages, 2015.

[55] P. Modi, "Diabetes beyond insulin: review of new drugs for treatment of diabetes mellitus," *Current Drug Discovery Technologies*, vol. 4, no. 1, pp. 39–47, 2007.

[56] J. P. Overington, B. Al-Lazikani, and A. L. Hopkins, "How many drug targets are there?" *Nature Reviews Drug Discovery*, vol. 5, no. 12, pp. 993–996, 2006.

[57] S. Parvazi, S. Sadeghi, M. Azadi et al., "The effect of aqueous extract of cinnamon on the metabolome of *Plasmodium falciparum* using ^{1}HNMR spectroscopy," *Journal of Tropical Medicine*, vol. 2016, Article ID 3174841, 5 pages, 2016.

[58] A. Mohammadi, S. A. Vafaei, M. N. Moradi, M. Ahmadi, M. Pourjafar, and E. Abbasi Oshaghi, "Combination of ezetimibe and garlic reduces serum lipids and intestinal Niemann-Pick C1-like 1 expression more effectively in hypercholesterolemic mice," *Avicenna Journal of Medical Biochemistry*, vol. 3, no. 1, pp. 1–5, 2015.

[59] M. Abbas, N. Mohammadi, N. Nader et al., "Influence of flaxseed on some biochemical factors, antioxidant activity and expression of ABCG5 and ABCG8 genes in the liver of diabetic rat," *British Journal of Medicine and Medical Research*, vol. 4, no. 18, pp. 3571–3580, 2014.

[60] F. S. Sharopov, W. Michael, I. S. Gulmurodov, and J. Salomiddin, "Composition and bioactivity of the essential oil of Anethum graveolens L. from Tajikistan," *International Journal of Medicinal and Aromatic Plants*, vol. 3, no. 2, pp. 125–130, 2013.

[61] R. A. Babri, I. Khokhar, Z. Mahmood, and S. Mahmud, "Chemical composition and insecticidal activity of the essential oil of *Anethum graveolens* L.," *Science International (Lahore)*, vol. 24, no. 4, pp. 453–455, 2012.

[62] P. Dahiya and S. Purkayastha, "Phytochemical analysis and antibacterial efficacy of dill seed oil against multi-drug resistant clinical isolates," *Asian Journal of Pharmaceutical and Clinical Research*, vol. 5, no. 2, pp. 62–64, 2012.

[63] K. Larijani, M. J. Shakouri, N. Pishbin, S. Mansourbahmani, and A. A. Heidari, "The essential oils of Dill (*Anethum graveblens* L.) collected from Gilan, Iran," *Annals of Biological Research*, vol. 3, no. 2, pp. 1010–1013, 2012.

[64] S. Singh, "Chemical constituents of essential oil from Anethum sowa Kurz. seed," *Journal of Chemical and Pharmaceutical Research*, vol. 4, no. 9, pp. 4156–4160, 2012.

[65] R. Vokk, T. Lõugas, K. Mets, and M. Kravets, "Dill (*Anethum graveolens* L.) and parsley (*Petroselinum crispum* (Mill.) Fuss) from Estonia: seasonal differences in essential oil composition," *Agronomy Research*, vol. 9, no. 2, pp. 515–520, 2011.

[66] B. Andalibi, S. Zehtab Salmasi, K. Ghassemi Gholezani, and J. Saba, "Changes in essential oil yield and composition at different parts of dill (*Anethum graveolens* L.) under limited irrigation conditions," *Journal of Agricultural Science*, vol. 21, no. 2, pp. 11–22, 2011.

[67] V. Rădulescu, M. L. Popescu, and D.-C. Ilieş, "Chemical composition of the volatile oil from different plant parts of Anethum graveolens L. (Umbelliferae) cultivated in Romania," *Farmacia*, vol. 58, no. 5, pp. 594–600, 2010.

[68] F. Oyoughi, M. Barzegar, M. Sahari, and H. N. Badi, "Effect of some of plant extracts on the growth of two *Aspergillus* species," *Iranian Journal of Medicinal Plants*, vol. 2, pp. 1–13, 2009.

[69] Y.-S. Shyu, J.-T. Lin, Y.-T. Chang, C.-J. Chiang, and D.-J. Yang, "Evaluation of antioxidant ability of ethanolic extract from dill (*Anethum graveolens* L.) flower," *Food Chemistry*, vol. 115, no. 2, pp. 515–521, 2009.

[70] A. Yili, H. A. Aisa, V. V. Maksimov, O. N. Veshkurova, and S. I. Salikhov, "Chemical composition and antimicrobial activity of essential oil from seeds of anethum graveolens growing in uzbekistan," *Chemistry of Natural Compounds*, vol. 45, no. 2, pp. 280–281, 2009.

[71] G. Singh, S. Maurya, M. P. De Lampasona, and C. Catalan, "Chemical constituents, antimicrobial investigations, and antioxidative potentials of Anethum graveolens L. essential oil and acetone extract—part 52," *Journal of Food Science*, vol. 70, no. 4, pp. M208–M215, 2005.

[72] A. Orav, T. Kailas, and A. Jegorova, "Bioactivities of l-carvone, d-carvone, and dihydrocarvone toward three stored product beetles," *Estonian Academy of Sciences*, vol. 52, no. 4, 2003.

[73] P. A. G. Santos, A. C. Figueiredo, P. M. L. Lourenço et al., "Hairy root cultures of Anethum graveolens (dill): establishment, growth, time-course study of their essential oil and its comparison with parent plant oils," *Biotechnology Letters*, vol. 24, no. 12, pp. 1031–1036, 2002.

[74] M. Miyazawa and H. Kameoka, "Constitution of the volatile oil from dill seed," *Japan Oil Chemists Society*, vol. 23, p. 746, 1974.

[75] H. Javad, H.-Z. Seyed-Mostafa, O. Farhad et al., "Hepatoprotective effects of hydroalcoholic extract of *Allium hirtifolium* (Persian shallot) in diabetic rats," *Journal of Basic and Clinical Physiology and Pharmacology*, vol. 23, no. 2, pp. 83–87, 2012.

[76] G. Y. Yeh, D. M. Eisenberg, T. J. Kaptchuk, and R. S. Phillips, "Systematic review of herbs and dietary supplements for glycemic control in diabetes," *Diabetes Care*, vol. 26, no. 4, pp. 1277–1294, 2003.

[77] M. O. Nafiu, T. A. Abdulsalam, and M. A. Akanji, "Phytochemical analysis and antimalarial activity aqueous extract of *Lecaniodiscus cupanioides* root," *Journal of Tropical Medicine*, vol. 2013, Article ID 605393, 4 pages, 2013.

[78] C. J. Bailey and C. Day, "Traditional plant medicines as treatments for diabetes," *Diabetes Care*, vol. 12, no. 8, pp. 553–564, 1989.

[79] F. O. A. Ajose, "Some Nigerian plants of dermatologic importance," *International Journal of Dermatology*, vol. 46, supplement 1, pp. 48–55, 2007.

[80] S. Jana and G. Shekhawat, "Anethum graveolens: an indian traditional medicinal herb and spice," *Pharmacognosy Reviews*, vol. 4, no. 8, pp. 179–184, 2010.

[81] E. A. Oshaghi, I. Khodadadi, H. Tavilani, and M. Goodarzi, "Effect of dill tablet (*Anethum graveolens* L) on antioxidant status and biochemical factors on carbon tetrachloride-induced liver damage on rat," *International Journal of Applied and Basic Medical Research*, vol. 6, no. 2, pp. 111–114, 2016.

[82] R. Yazdanparast and M. Alavi, "Antihyperlipidaemic and antihypercholesterolaemic effects of Anethum graveolens leaves after the removal of furocoumarins," *Cytobios*, vol. 105, no. 410, pp. 185–191, 2000.

[83] E. Abbasi Oshaghi, I. Khodadadi, M. Saidijam et al., "Lipid lowering effects of hydroalcoholic extract of *Anethum graveolens* L. and dill tablet in high cholesterol fed hamsters," *Cholesterol*, vol. 2015, Article ID 958560, 7 pages, 2015.

[84] E. Abbasi Oshaghi, S. Arash Noori, and R. Ali, "Effects of walnut on lipid profile as well as the expression of sterol-regulatory element binding protein-1c (SREBP-1c) and peroxisome proliferator activated receptors α (PPARα) in diabetic rat," *Food and Nutrition Sciences*, vol. 3, no. 2, pp. 255–259, 2012.

[85] E. Abbasi Oshaghi, I. Khdadadi, H. Tavilani, and M. T. Goodarzi, "Aqueous extract of Anethum Graveolens L. has potential antioxidant and antiglycation effects," *Iranian Journal of Medical Sciences*, vol. 41, no. 4, pp. 328–333, 2016.

[86] E. Abbasi Oshaghi, H. Tavilani, I. Khodadadi, and M. T. Goodarzi, "Dill tablet: a potential antioxidant and anti-diabetic medicine," *Asian Pacific Journal of Tropical Biomedicine*, vol. 5, no. 9, pp. 720–727, 2015.

[87] B. S. Arbabi, E. Taheri, H. Baher, and P. Ziarati, "Safety evaluation of oral anethum graveolens L total hydroalcoholic extract in mice," *Journal of Pharmaceutical & Health Sciences*, vol. 1, no. 2, pp. 61–67, 2011.

[88] S. Adisakwattana, T. Thilavech, and C. Chusak, "*Mesona chinensis* Benth extract prevents AGE formation and protein oxidation against fructose-induced protein glycation in vitro," *BMC Complementary and Alternative Medicine*, vol. 14, no. 1, article 130, pp. 1–9, 2014.

[89] R.-Y. Lin, R. P. Choudhury, W. Cai et al., "Dietary glycotoxins promote diabetic atherosclerosis in apolipoprotein E-deficient mice," *Atherosclerosis*, vol. 168, no. 2, pp. 213–220, 2003.

[90] M. Mobasseri, L. Payahoo, A. Ostadrahimi, Y. K. Bishak, M. A. Jafarabadi, and S. Mahluji, "Anethum graveolens supplementation improves insulin sensitivity and lipid abnormality in type 2 diabetic patients," *Pharmaceutical Sciences*, vol. 20, no. 2, pp. 40–45, 2014.

[91] Y. Takahashi, N. Inaba, S. Kuwahara, and W. Kuki, "Antioxidative effect of citrus essential oil components on human low-density lipoprotein in vitro," *Bioscience, Biotechnology and Biochemistry*, vol. 67, no. 1, pp. 195–197, 2003.

[92] H. A. Mudassir, M. B. Azmi, and S. A. Qureshi, "Phytochemical investigation of ethanolic seed extract of anethum graveolens and its effect on glucose tolerance in rabbits," *FUUAST Journal of Biology*, vol. 1, no. 2, p. 41, 2011.

[93] I. E. Orhan, F. S. Senol, N. Ozturk, S. A. Celik, A. Pulur, and Y. Kan, "Phytochemical contents and enzyme inhibitory and antioxidant properties of *Anethum graveolens* L. (dill) samples cultivated under organic and conventional agricultural conditions," *Food and Chemical Toxicology*, vol. 59, pp. 96–103, 2013.

[94] J. Bailer, T. Aichinger, G. Hackl, K. de Hueber, and M. Dachler, "Essential oil content and composition in commercially available dill cultivars in comparison to caraway," *Industrial Crops and Products*, vol. 14, no. 3, pp. 229–239, 2001.

[95] S. Reichert, D. Fischer, S. Asche, and A. Mosandl, "Stable isotope labelling in biosynthetic studies of dill ether, using enantioselective multidimensional gas chromatography, online coupled with isotope ratio mass spectrometry," *Flavour and Fragrance Journal*, vol. 15, no. 5, pp. 303–308, 2000.

[96] F. Sefidkon, "Essential oil composition of anethum graveolens," *Pajouhesh-va-Sazandegi*, vol. 3, no. 2, pp. 73–77, 2012.

[97] A. E. Al-Snafi, "The pharmacological importance of *Anethum graveolens*—a review," *International Journal of Pharmacy and Pharmaceutical Sciences*, vol. 6, no. 4, pp. 11–13, 2014.

[98] M. Mirhosseini, A. Baradaran, and M. Rafieian-Kopaei, "Anethum graveolens and hyperlipidemia: a randomized clinical trial," *Journal of Research in Medical Sciences*, vol. 19, no. 8, pp. 758–761, 2014.

8

Cytokine Profiles and Cell Proliferation Responses to Truncated ORF2 Protein in Iranian Patients Recovered from Hepatitis E Infection

Reza Taherkhani,[1,2] Fatemeh Farshadpour,[1,2] Manoochehr Makvandi,[3] Hamid Rajabi Memari,[4] Ali Reza Samarbafzadeh,[3] Nasrin Sharifi,[5] Behrouz Naeimi,[1,2] Saeed Tajbakhsh,[1,2] and Samad Akbarzadeh[2]

[1] *Department of Microbiology and Parasitology, School of Medicine, Bushehr University of Medical Sciences, Bushehr 7514633341, Iran*
[2] *Persian Gulf Tropical Medicine Research Centre, Bushehr University of Medical Sciences, Bushehr 7514633341, Iran*
[3] *Health Research Institute, Infectious and Tropical Disease Research Centre, Ahvaz Jundishapur University of Medical Sciences, Ahvaz 6135715794, Iran*
[4] *Department of Agronomy and Plant Breeding, Faculty of Agriculture, Ahvaz Shahid Chamran University, Ahvaz 6135715794, Iran*
[5] *Department of Nutrition, School of Medicine, Kashan University of Medical Sciences, Kashan 8715988141, Iran*

Correspondence should be addressed to Fatemeh Farshadpour; f.farshadpour@yahoo.com

Academic Editor: Susana A. Laucella

Background. The aim of this study was to evaluate *hepatitis E virus* (HEV) specific cellular immune responses to truncated ORF2 protein in Iranian patients recovered from HEV infection. Information about HEV-specific immune responses could be useful in finding an effective way for development of HEV vaccine. *Methods.* A truncated form of HEV ORF2 protein containing amino acids 112-608 was used to stimulate peripheral blood mononuclear cells (PBMCs) separated from HEV-recovered and control groups. Finally, the levels of four cytokines, IFN-γ ELISPOT, and cell proliferative responses following stimulation with the truncated ORF2 protein were assessed in the both groups. *Results.* The truncated ORF2 protein was able to induce IFN-γ ELISPOT and cell proliferation responses and to produce significant amounts of IFN-γ and IL-12 cytokines, but low amounts of IL-10 and IL-4 cytokines *in vitro*. These responses were significantly higher in the recovered group compared to the control group. These results indicate the antigenic nature of the truncated ORF2 protein and production of T helper type 1 cytokines. *Conclusion.* The truncated ORF2 protein can effectively induce significant cellular immune responsesand can be introduced as a potential vaccine candidate. However, further studies are required to evaluate this protein *in vivo*.

1. Introduction

Hepatitis E virus (HEV) is a nonenveloped virus with a nonsegmented positive-sense RNA genome containing three open reading frames (ORFs) [1, 2]. HEV belongs to the family Hepeviridae and the genus *Hepevirus* [3]. The genus *Hepevirus* has two species including mammalian HEV and avian HEV. The mammalian HEV, which infects humans and several mammalians, is classified into four major genotypes, namely, genotypes 1, 2, 3, and 4 [4]. The HEV genotypes share highly conserved immunodominant domains that are serologically cross-reactive [5].

HEV causes large outbreaks of acute hepatitis in developing countries where sanitary conditions are inadequate and the infection is enterically transmitted by the fecal-oral route especially contaminated water [6, 7]. The zoonotic spread of the disease is also possible especially in developed countries where the sporadic cases of the infection have been reported [2, 4]. Although the infection is usually asymptomatic or acute self-limiting in general population, but it can progress to lethal fulminant hepatitis in pregnant women and chronic hepatitis in immunosuppressed and organ transplant patients [5, 8]. The general mortality rate of HEV infection is between

1% and 15%, and this level may reach up to 30% due to fulminate hepatic failure during pregnancy, which may lead to high rate of spontaneous abortion and premature birth [5, 9]. Consequently, HEV has become a serious public-health concern especially in endemic areas, and control and prevention of this infection are necessary [2]. So far, no effective treatment or commercial vaccines for HEV infection are available, and the only way to reduce incidence of the infection is prevention [2, 10].

Currently, the focus for development of HEV vaccine is on ORF2 protein. ORF2 encodes capsid protein that comprises 660 amino acids. HEV capsid protein has several immune-dominant conserved epitopes that can induce long-lived immunity; therefore, it has been studied for vaccine development [11]. However, the full-length capsid protein is not suitable for vaccine production. Since it is hydrophobic and insoluble and its immunoreactive epitopes are masked, much attention has been drawn to the truncated or short forms of ORF2 protein as protective vaccines [12, 13].

The truncated ORF2 protein, containing amino acids 112 to 660 of the ORF2 protein, self assembles into virus-like particles and can induce strong immunity [14]. Moreover, 52 amino acids from the C terminus and 111 amino acids from the N terminus of the ORF2 protein do not have any antigenic domain, and most antigenic domains have located within 268 amino acids of C terminal of the ORF2 protein [5]. Also, the truncated ORF2 protein containing amino acids 459 to 607 is needed to produce anti-HEV antibodies; therefore, it seems that antigenic epitopes are conformational [5]. Anti-HEV antibodies from all genotypes cross-react with the ORF2 protein of genotype 1 [5]; therefore, production of a broadly protective vaccine seems to be possible by expression the truncated ORF2 protein of genotype 1 [13].

In the present study, the cellular immune responses to the truncated ORF2 protein were evaluated in the peripheral blood mononuclear cells (PBMCs) of individuals recovered from hepatitis E infection.

2. Materials and Methods

2.1. Ethics Statement. This study (with research project number D/574) was approved by the Jundishapur University Ethical Committee, and informed consent was taken from all the participants.

2.2. Study Group. Forty anti-HEV IgG positive subjects (24, 60% males and 16, 40% females; mean age ± SD, 35.12 ± 9.66 years) and forty-eight anti-HEV IgG negative subjects (28, 58.3% males and 20, 41.7% females; mean age ± SD, 33.06 ± 10.70 years) were randomly selected as HEV-recovered and control groups to study the immunogenicity of the truncated ORF2 protein. The presence of anti-HEV IgG antibody was detected by the commercial ELISA kit (HEV IgG ELISA kit, DIA.PRO, Milan, Italy). All the participants were negative for anti-HEV IgM antibody, anti-HAV IgM antibody, anti-HCV antibodies, and hepatitis B surface antigen (HEV IgM ELISA kit, HAV IgM ELISA kit, HCV Ab ELISA kit, HBs Ag ELISA kit, DIA.PRO, Milan, Italy) and had normal ALT level.

2.3. Preparation of Peripheral Blood Mononuclear Cells. Ficoll-Hypaque (Lymphoflot, Biotest Diagnostics, Germany) and density gradient centrifugation method were used to separate peripheral blood mononuclear cells (PBMCs) from 10 mL heparinized venous blood sample of the each individual. Then the cells were washed twice by RPMI 1640 medium and resuspended in RPMI 1640 plus 10% FCS (Invitrogen, Carlsbad, CA, USA). Trypan blue staining was used to evaluate the cells viability.

2.4. Preparation of Truncated ORF2 Protein. A truncated form of HEV ORF2 protein containing amino acids 112–608 was produced as described previously [15]. Briefly, a truncated ORF2 gene encoding amino acids 112–660 of Sar-55 strain from HEV genotype 1 was optimized for expression in *E. coli* and synthesized and cloned into pBluescript II SK(+) vector by Biomatik Company (Biomatik Corporation, Cambridge, Canada). The truncated gene was subcloned into expression vector pET-30a(+) and the recombinant plasmid pET30a-ORF2$_{(aa\ 112-660)}$ was constructed. Then, a 193-nucleotide fragment was removed from the nucleotide sequence of the truncated ORF2 gene by digestion with NheI restriction enzyme and another truncated form of ORF2 gene encoding amino acids 112–608 was constructed. The recombinant plasmid pET-30a-ORF2$_{(aa\ 112-608)}$ was transformed into *E. coli* BL21 (DE3) using electroporation. Expression of the truncated ORF2 protein containing amino acids 112–608 was induced by adding 1 mM IPTG to the bacterial culture followed by 4 hr incubation at 37°C. The expressed truncated ORF2 protein was purified by Ni2+-chelate-affinity chromatography (Qiagen, Hilden, Germany). Refolding of the purified protein was done by dialysis in PBS + 10% glycerol at 4°C for 4 hr. Amicon Ultra-4 Centrifugal Filter Unit (EMD Millipore, Billerica, MA, USA) was used to improve the concentration and purity of the target protein. To remove endotoxin contamination that may be obtained during protein purification, endotoxin was extracted from the protein by Toxin Eraser Endotoxin Removal kit (GenScript, Piscataway, NJ, USA).

2.5. Cell Proliferation Assay. The cell proliferation was carried out by the colorimetric assay using MTT (3-(4,5-dimethylthiazol-2-yl)-2,5-diphenyl tetrazolium bromide) as described previously [16]. For each sample, approximately 1×10^5 PBMCs/well in RPMI 1640 plus 10% FCS were added to 3 wells of 96-well plates in final volume of 180 μL/well. The first well was stimulated with 10 μg/mL of truncated ORF2 protein in final volume 20 μL. 20 μL/well of phytohemagglutinin (PHA) (5 μg/mL) (Sigma–Aldrich, St. Louis, MO, USA) was used as positive control in the second well and the third well remained unstimulated as negative control. Blanking was done by putting RPMI 1640 (20 μL) alone in the well. The optimal concentrations of truncated ORF2 protein and PHA and the optimum stimulation duration were determined based on preliminary experiments. The plate was incubated in the presence of 5% CO_2 at 37°C for 4 days, and then 10 μL of MTT solution (5 mg/mL) was added to each well. After incubation at 37°C for 4 hr and centrifugation in 1000 ×g

Table 1: Results of cytokine, lymphocyte proliferation, and ELISPOT assays in response to truncated ORF2 protein in HEV recovered individuals and control group.

Parameter	Control group (n = 48)	Recovered group (n = 40)	p value
IFN-γ	17.12 ± 6.93	143.40 ± 52.33	<0.001
IL-12	18.33 ± 9.04	112.75 ± 43.26	<0.001
IL-10	18.72 ± 8.55	27.80 ± 19.55	0.100 (NS)
IL-4	4.30 ± 1.53	4.90 ± 1.49	0.067 (NS)
ELISPOT	4.39 ± 5.51	65.92 ± 58.99	<0.001
Cell proliferation	1.50 ± 0.17	2.01 ± 0.28	<0.001

Cytokine values are represented as picograms per milliliter (pg/mL), the results of ELISPOT assay are expressed as spot forming cells per 10^5 cells (SFC/10^5 cells), and the results of cell proliferation assay are shown as proliferation index (PI).
All data are shown as mean ± SD.
NS = nonsignificant.

for 10 min, the supernatant was discarded and 100 μL of DMSO was added to each well and mixed by pipetting. The absorbance of the wells was measured using an ELISA reader at 570 nm within an hour. The results were expressed as proliferation index (PI). PI was defined as OD570 stimulated sample/OD570 unstimulated sample.

2.6. IFNγ ELISPOT Assay. The IFNγ ELISpot assay was performed by Human IFN-γ ELISPOT Ready-SET-Go kit (eBioscience, San Diego, CA, USA) to determine HEV-specific IFN-γ-producing cells. According to manufacturer's structure, a PVDF bottomed ELISPOT plate (Millipore, Bedford, MA, USA) was coated with Capture Antibody solution (100 μL/well) overnight at 4°C. For each sample, approximately 1×10^5 PBMCs/well in RPMI 1640 plus 10% FCS were added to 3 wells of the 96-well ELISPOT plate in final volume of 150 μL/well. The first well was stimulated with 10 μg/mL truncated ORF2 protein. Five μg/mL of PHA was used as positive control in the second well, and the third well remained unstimulated as negative control. The optimal count of PBMC in each well, the optimal concentrations of truncated ORF2 protein and PHA, and the optimum duration of stimulation were determined based on preliminary experiments. The plate was incubated at 37°C for 24 hr. Then, the cells and medium were removed and the wells were washed 3 times with ELISPOT Wash Buffer. The plate was incubated with Biotinylated Detection Antibody (100 μL/each well) at 4°C overnight and washed 4 times with ELISPOT Wash Buffer. In the next step, the plate was incubated with 100 μL/well of Avidin-Horseradish Peroxidase reagent at room temperature for 45 min and washed with ELISPOT Wash Buffer and 1x PBS. Finally, the dark purple spots were developed by adding 100 μL/well AEC (3-amino-9-ethylcarbazole), followed by incubation at room temperature. The plate was washed 3 times with 200 μL/well distilled water and dried at room temperature, and then a dissection stereoscope was used to count the number of spots. The results were shown as spot forming cells (SFCs) per 10^5 cells, while each spot was considered as one HEV-specific IFN-γ secreting cell.

2.7. Cytokine Assay. PBMCs of each sample were stimulated with the truncated ORF2 protein (10 μg/mL) at 37°C. In addition, five μg/mL PHA was used as positive control. The optimal concentrations of truncated ORF2 protein and PHA and the optimum stimulation duration were determined based on preliminary experiments. Culture supernatants were harvested after 1-2 days and used to measure amounts of four cytokines (IL-4, IL-12 p70, IFN-γ, and IL-10). Cytokine assay was performed by commercially available ELISA kits (eBioscience, San Diego, CA, USA) according to the manufacturer's instructions. The results were shown as picograms per milliliter (pg/mL). The limits of sensitivity of the assays were 1.3 pg/mL for IL-4, 1.0 pg/mL for IL-10, 2.1 pg/mL for IL-12 p70, and 0.99 pg/mL for IFN-γ.

2.8. Statistical Analysis. SPSS 17 Package program (SPSS Inc., Chicago, USA) was used for statistical analysis, and p values below 0.05 indicated statistical significance. The data were analyzed and compared by the Mann-Whitney U test or independent t-test. All data were expressed as mean ± SD.

3. Results

3.1. Cell Proliferative Response to Truncated ORF2 Protein. Proliferation of PBMCs in response to the truncated ORF2 protein was measured in the control and HEV-recovered groups. The cell proliferative responses to truncated ORF2 protein in the control and HEV-recovered groups were 1.50 ± 0.17 and 2.01 ± 0.28, respectively. The corresponding figures following stimulation with PHA were 2.91 ± 0.37 and 2.81 ± 0.33 in the control and recovered groups, respectively (p = NS). Overall, the recovered group showed significantly higher cell proliferation compared to the control group ($p < 0.001$) (Table 1, Figure 1).

3.2. IFN-γ ELISPOT Responses to the Truncated OR2 Protein. The frequencies of IFN-γ-secreting cells in PBMCs of HEV-recovered and control groups were assessed in response to truncated ORF2 protein by ELISPOT assay. IFN-γ ELISPOT responses following stimulation with the truncated ORF2 protein in the control and HEV-recovered groups were 4.39 ± 5.51 and 65.92 ± 58.99, respectively. ELISPOT responses to PHA in the control and recovered groups were 223.41 ± 94.58 and 228.25 ± 123.41, respectively (p = NS). Overall, IFN-γ ELISPOT responses were significantly higher in the recovered

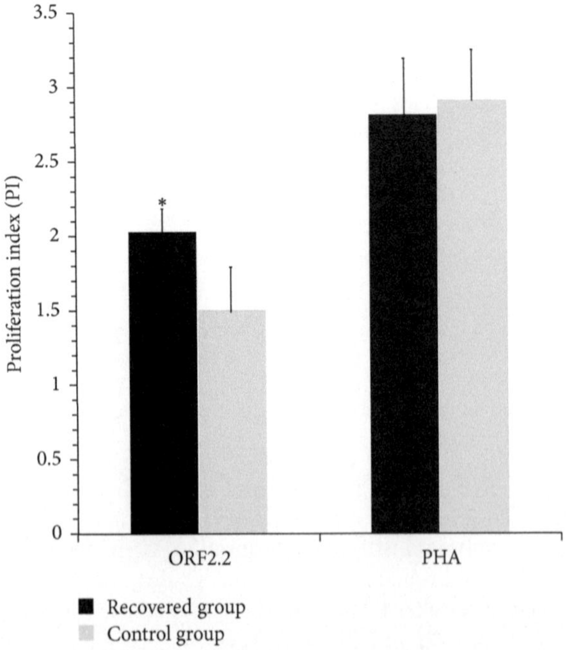

FIGURE 1: Cell proliferative responses in HEV-recovered individuals and control group. Proliferative responses to the truncated ORF2 protein are significantly higher in HEV-recovered group compared to the control group, while both groups showed good nonspecific stimulation with PHA. The results are shown as proliferation index (mean ± SD PI).

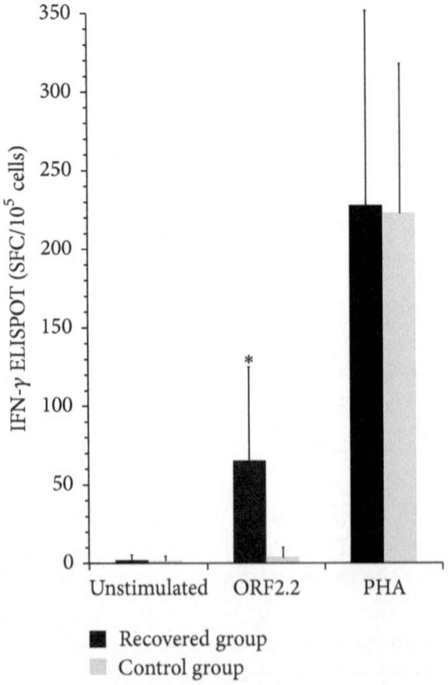

FIGURE 2: IFN-γ ELISPOT responses in HEV-recovered and control groups. IFN-γ ELISPOT responses to the truncated ORF2 protein are significantly higher in the recovered group compared to the controls, while both groups showed good nonspecific stimulation with PHA. The results are shown as spot forming cells per 10^5 cells (SFC/10^5 cells).

group compared to the control group ($p < 0.001$) (Table 1, Figure 2).

3.3. Cytokine Production in Responses to Truncated ORF2 Protein. Significant amounts of IFN-γ and IL-12 cytokines but low amounts of IL-10 and IL-4 cytokines were produced following stimulation with the truncated ORF2 protein. Comparison between the two groups revealed no significant differences in the levels of IL-10 ($p = 0.100$) and IL-4 ($p = 0.067$), while IFN-γ and IL-12 p70 were significantly higher in the recovered group compared to the control group ($p < 0.001$). Stimulation with PHA resulted in almost similar expression of all cytokines in the control and recovered groups, including 11.96 ± 4.55 and 11.29 ± 3.9 for IL-4 (p = NS), 199.45 ± 108.43 and 204.97 ± 103.61 for IL-10 (p = NS), 109.91 ± 32.86 and 103.22 ± 25.9 for IL-12 (p = NS), and 410.37 ± 46.96 and 418.37 ± 75.65 for IFN-γ (p = NS), respectively (Table 1, Figure 3).

4. Discussion

HEV causes self-limited acute hepatic infection worldwide and especially in developing countries where the disease is endemic and 30% to 80% of the adult population has anti-HEV antibody [17]. The infection is more severe in pregnant women and patients with underlying liver problems and may progress to lethal fulminant hepatitis [5, 8]. Information about HEV specific cellular immune responses could be useful in finding an effective way for development of HEV vaccine, in particular as any protective vaccine for HEV infection is not still licensed [2, 9]. However, some studies have evaluated HEV-specific cellular immune responses among different groups [6, 18–20], but current information on cellular immune responses against HEV is not sufficient to prevent HEV infection. Therefore, this study aimed to evaluate HEV-specific cellular immune responses to the truncated ORF2 protein in the recovered individuals from HEV infection.

In the present study, a significant increase in the cell proliferation and IFN-γ ELISPOT responses following stimulation with the truncated ORF2 protein were found in the HEV-recovered subjects, while both groups showed good nonspecific stimulation with PHA. Therefore, the increase in responses induced by truncated ORF2 protein was specific in the recovered group. These results indicate the antigenic nature of the truncated ORF2 protein. Suneetha et al. reported a similar increase in the HEV-specific T-cell responses by PBMCs obtained from recovered individuals from HEV infection. The stimulating antigen in their study was overlapping peptide pools and not the whole HEV ORF2 protein [20]. Regarding the full length ORF2 protein, Husain et al. presented similar results in acute hepatitis E patients compared to the controls [21]. It has been shown that ORF2 protein has several HTL (helper T-lymphocyte) dominant immunogenic regions and therefore it is a good antigen to elicit high and long-lasting specific anti-HEV immune responses [22]. The HEV-specific T-helper cell responses, especially against capsid protein, play a critical role in

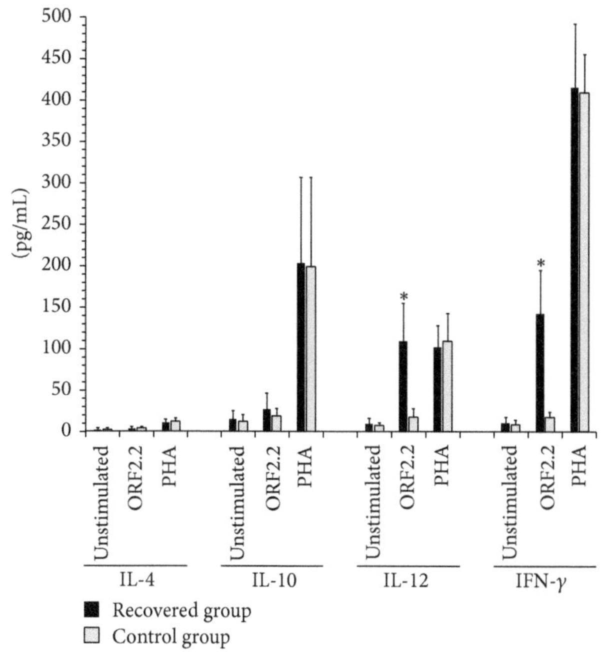

Figure 3: The levels of IL-4, IL-10, IL-12 p70, and IFN-γ cytokines in HEV-recovered and control groups following stimulation with the truncated ORF2 protein. Significant amounts of IFN-γ and IL-12 cytokines but low amounts of IL-10 and IL-4 cytokines were produced. IL-12 p70 and IFN-γ cytokines production following stimulation with the truncated ORF2 protein was significantly higher in the recovered group compared to the control group, while there were no significant differences in the levels of IL-10 and IL-4 between the two groups. Both groups showed almost similar expression of all cytokines following stimulation with PHA. Results are shown as mean ± SD pg/mL.

clearing and controlling viral infections, either directly through cytokines production or indirectly by activating cytotoxic T cells [1].

Production of T-helper type 1 (Th1) cytokines such as IFN-γ, TNF-α/β, IL-2, IL-3, and IL-12 have been implicated in viral clearance or resistance to infection, while production of Th2 cytokines such as IL-4, IL-5, IL-13, IL-6, and IL-10 cytokines is associated with progression of the infection or viral persistence [23–28]. In the present study, the truncated ORF2 protein could significantly stimulate PBMCs to produce IFN-γ and IL-12 but little or no IL-4. These results demonstrate that the Th1 responses are induced against the truncated ORF2 protein. The results of this study being consistent with those of others suggest that viral proteins that can shift immune responses to Th1, rather than Th2, may have a better chance of success as a vaccine candidate against HEV infection [29]. All participants in control and recovered groups showed almost similar expression of all cytokines following stimulation with PHA. Therefore, the increase in production of IFN-γ and IL-12 cytokines following stimulation with truncated ORF2 protein was specific in the recovered group.

The results of the previous studies have shown that the production of Th1 cytokines such as IL-12 and IFN-γ during HEV infection results in self-limiting hepatitis E, suggesting the role of these cytokines in the recovery and clearance of hepatitis E, while the Th2 cytokines increase in fatal fulminant hepatitis E, especially during pregnancy [18, 27, 30, 31]. In Saravanabalaji et al. study, levels of IFN-γ and IL-12 cytokines following stimulation of PBMCs by recombinant ORF2 protein were higher in recovered patients than those with fatal fulminant hepatitis E, while IL-10 was higher in fatal patients [30]. In Pal et al. study, high levels of IL-4 and IL-10 were observed in pregnant women with acute hepatitis E following stimulation of PBMCs with different peptides of HEV ORFs, while the level of IFN-γ was low in this group [27]. In Srivastava et al. study, the IFN-γ production following stimulation with ORF2 protein was higher in patients with acute HEV infection compared to control [6].

In this study, antigenic properties of the expressed ORF2 protein in *E. coli* BL21 cell were evaluated. Among the various microorganisms and systems available for protein production, *E. coli* BL21 containing pET-derived plasmids has become the most commonly used expression system because of its high expression capabilities, protein production with high purity, low cost, simple and fast cultivation, its well-known genetics, and therefore ease of genetic manipulation [32]. However, there are a variety of factors that affect the expression level as well as the solubility and especially biological function of overexpressed proteins. One of the ways to improve the expression of foreign protein in *E. coli* is codon optimization, which results in selection of host favorite codons and elimination of high GC contents [33, 34]. By evaluating the antigenic properties and immunogenicity of the truncated ORF2 protein, it was indicated that this protein has biological function and can stimulate specific anti-HEV immune responses.

In conclusion, the truncated ORF2 protein is able to induce significant cellular immune responses and production of Th1 cytokines *in vitro* and therefore can be introduced as a potential vaccine candidate for HEV infection. However further studies are required to evaluate this protein *in vivo*.

Conflict of Interests

The authors declare there is no conflict of interests in the content of this study.

Authors' Contribution

Fatemeh Farshadpour takes responsibility for the accuracy of the data. Reza Taherkhani and Fatemeh Farshadpour contributed equally to the design and performance of the study. Fatemeh Farshadpour and Manoochehr Makvandi drafted the paper. Nasrin Sharifi performed the statistical analysis. Ali Reza Samarbafzadeh, Saeed Tajbakhsh, Behrouz Naeimi, and Samad Akbarzadeh participated in the laboratory evaluation. Hamid Rajabi Memari performed the literature review. All authors have read and approved the paper.

Acknowledgments

The authors would like to acknowledge Grant no. 91111 supported financially by Deputy Research and Affairs of Ahvaz

Jundishapur University of Medical Science, Ahvaz, Iran. The study was supported financially by the grant (no. 91111) provided by the Infectious and Tropical Diseases Research Center of Ahvaz Jundishapur University of Medical Sciences, Ahvaz, Iran.

References

[1] R. Aggarwal, R. Shukla, S. Jameel et al., "T-cell epitope mapping of ORF2 and ORF3 proteins of human hepatitis e virus," *Journal of Viral Hepatitis*, vol. 14, no. 4, pp. 283–292, 2007.

[2] N. J. de Oya, E. Escribano-Romero, A.-B. Blázquez et al., "Characterization of hepatitis E virus recombinant ORF2 proteins expressed by vaccinia viruses," *Journal of Virology*, vol. 86, no. 15, pp. 7880–7886, 2012.

[3] T. Yamashita, Y. Mori, N. Miyazaki et al., "Biological and immunological characteristics of hepatitis E virus-like particles based on the crystal structure," *Proceedings of the National Academy of Sciences of the United States of America*, vol. 106, no. 31, pp. 12986–12991, 2009.

[4] R. H. Purcell and S. U. Emerson, "Hepatitis E: an emerging awareness of an old disease," *Journal of Hepatology*, vol. 48, no. 3, pp. 494–503, 2008.

[5] L. Xing, J. C. Wang, T.-C. Li et al., "Spatial configuration of hepatitis E virus antigenic domain," *Journal of Virology*, vol. 85, no. 2, pp. 1117–1124, 2011.

[6] R. Srivastava, R. Aggarwal, S. Jameel et al., "Cellular immune responses in acute hepatitis E virus infection to the viral open reading frame 2 protein," *Viral Immunology*, vol. 20, no. 1, pp. 56–65, 2007.

[7] F. Farshadpour, R. Taherkhani, and M. Makvandi, "Prevalence of hepatitis E virus among adults in south-west of Iran," *Hepatitis Research and Treatment*, vol. 2015, Article ID 759589, 5 pages, 2015.

[8] F.-C. Zhu, J. Zhang, X.-F. Zhang et al., "Efficacy and safety of a recombinant hepatitis E vaccine in healthy adults: a large-scale, randomised, double-blind placebo-controlled, phase 3 trial," *The Lancet*, vol. 376, no. 9744, pp. 895–902, 2010.

[9] R. Taherkhani, F. Farshadpour, and M. Makvandi, "Design and production of a multiepitope construct derived from hepatitis E virus capsid protein," *Journal of Medical Virology*, vol. 87, no. 7, pp. 1225–1234, 2015.

[10] L. Wang and H. Zhuang, "Hepatitis E: an overview and recent advances in vaccine research," *World Journal of Gastroenterology*, vol. 10, no. 15, pp. 2157–2162, 2004.

[11] S. U. Emerson and R. H. Purcell, "Recombinant vaccines for hepatitis E," *Trends in Molecular Medicine*, vol. 7, no. 10, pp. 462–466, 2001.

[12] M. Zhang, S. U. Emerson, H. Nguyen et al., "Immunogenicity and protective efficacy of a vaccine prepared from 53 kDa truncated hepatitis E virus capsid protein expressed in insect cells," *Vaccine*, vol. 20, no. 5-6, pp. 853–857, 2001.

[13] R. Taherkhani and F. Farshadpour, "A new strategy for development of hepatitis E vaccine: epitope-based vaccines," *Pathogen & Infectious Disease*, vol. 1, no. 1, article e933, 2015.

[14] T.-C. Li, N. Takeda, T. Miyamura et al., "Essential elements of the capsid protein for self-assembly into empty virus-like particles of hepatitis E virus," *Journal of Virology*, vol. 79, no. 20, pp. 12999–13006, 2005.

[15] R. Taherkhani, M. Makvandi, and F. Farshadpour, "Development of enzyme-linked immunosorbent assays using 2 truncated ORF2 proteins for detection of IgG antibodies against Hepatitis E virus," *Annals of Laboratory Medicine*, vol. 34, no. 2, pp. 118–126, 2014.

[16] M. Majumdar, R. Ratho, Y. Chawla, and M. P. Singh, "Evaluation of antigenicity and cell mediated immunity of hepatitis E virus patients: using non radioactive MTT assay," *Indian Journal of Medical Microbiology*, vol. 31, no. 1, pp. 64–68, 2013.

[17] J. H. Hoofnagle, K. E. Nelson, and R. H. Purcell, "Hepatitis E," *The New England Journal of Medicine*, vol. 367, no. 13, pp. 1237–1244, 2012.

[18] A. S. Tripathy, R. Das, S. B. Rathod, and V. A. Arankalle, "Cytokine profiles, CTL response and T cell frequencies in the peripheral blood of acute patients and individuals recovered from hepatitis E infection," *PLoS ONE*, vol. 7, no. 2, Article ID e31822, 2012.

[19] S. B. Rathod and A. S. Tripathy, "Hepatitis E rORF2p stimulated and unstimulated peripheral expression profiling in patients with self-limiting hepatitis E infection," *Journal of Immunology Research*, vol. 2014, Article ID 565284, 10 pages, 2014.

[20] P. V. Suneetha, S. Pischke, V. Schlaphoff et al., "Hepatitis E virus (HEV)-specific T-cell responses are associated with control of HEV infection," *Hepatology*, vol. 55, no. 3, pp. 695–708, 2012.

[21] M. M. Husain, R. Aggarwal, D. Kumar, S. Jameel, and S. Naik, "Effector T cells immune reactivity among patients with acute hepatitis e," *Journal of Viral Hepatitis*, vol. 18, no. 10, pp. e603–e608, 2011.

[22] T. Wu, J. Zhang, Z.-J. Su et al., "Specific cellular immune response in hepatitis E patients," *Intervirology*, vol. 51, no. 5, pp. 322–327, 2009.

[23] X. G. Fan, W. E. Liu, C. Z. Li et al., "Circulating Th1 and Th2 cytokines in patients with hepatitis C virus infection," *Mediators of Inflammation*, vol. 7, no. 4, pp. 295–297, 1998.

[24] M. Clerici and G. M. Shearer, "A $T_H1 \rightarrow T_H2$ switch is a critical step in the etiology of HIV infection," *Immunology Today*, vol. 14, no. 3, pp. 107–111, 1993.

[25] X. G. Fan, J. Yakoob, X. J. Fan, and P. W. N. Keeling, "Enhanced T-helper 2 lymphocyte responses: immune mechanism of *Helicobacter pylori* infection," *Irish Journal of Medical Science*, vol. 165, no. 1, pp. 37–39, 1996.

[26] R. L. Modlin and T. B. Nutman, "Type 2 cytokines and negative immune regulation in human infections," *Current Opinion in Immunology*, vol. 5, no. 4, pp. 511–517, 1993.

[27] R. Pal, R. Aggarwal, S. R. Naik, V. Das, S. Das, and S. Naik, "Immunological alterations in pregnant women with acute hepatitis E," *Journal of Gastroenterology and Hepatology*, vol. 20, no. 7, pp. 1094–1101, 2005.

[28] C. Ptaschinski, S. Mukherjee, M. L. Moore et al., "RSV-induced H3K4 demethylase KDM5B leads to regulation of dendritic cell-derived innate cytokines and exacerbates pathogenesis in vivo," *PLoS Pathogens*, vol. 11, no. 6, Article ID e1004978, 2015.

[29] A. J. MacDonald, M. Duffy, M. T. Brady et al., "CD4 T helper type 1 and regulatory T cells induced against the same epitopes on the core protein in hepatitis C virus-infected persons," *The Journal of Infectious Diseases*, vol. 185, no. 6, pp. 720–727, 2002.

[30] S. Saravanabalaji, A. S. Tripathy, R. R. Dhoot, M. S. Chadha, A. L. Kakrani, and V. A. Arankalle, "Viral load, antibody titers and recombinant open reading frame 2 protein-induced Th1/Th2 cytokines and cellular immune responses in self-limiting and fulminant hepatitis E," *Intervirology*, vol. 52, no. 2, pp. 78–85, 2009.

[31] R. Srivastava, R. Aggarwal, S. Sachdeva, M. I. Alam, S. Jameel, and S. Naik, "Adaptive immune responses during acute uncomplicated and fulminant hepatitis E," *Journal of Gastroenterology and Hepatology*, vol. 26, no. 2, pp. 306–311, 2011.

[32] M. Fakruddin, R. Mohammad Mazumdar, K. S. Bin Mannan et al., "Critical factors affecting the success of cloning, expression, and mass production of enzymes by recombinant *E. coli*," *ISRN Biotechnology*, vol. 2013, Article ID 590587, 7 pages, 2013.

[33] F. Farshadpour, R. Taherkhani, M. Makvandi et al., "Codon-optimized expression and purification of truncated ORF2 protein of hepatitis E virus in *Escherichia coli*," *Jundishapur Journal of Microbiology*, vol. 7, no. 7, Article ID e11261, 2014.

[34] C. Elena, P. Ravasi, M. E. Castelli, S. Peirú, and H. G. Menzella, "Expression of codon optimized genes in microbial systems: current industrial applications and perspectives," *Frontiers in Microbiology*, vol. 5, article 21, 2014.

9

Parasitological Indices of Malaria Transmission in Children under Fifteen Years in Two Ecoepidemiological Zones in Southwestern Burkina Faso

Aristide S. Hien,[1] Ibrahim Sangaré,[2] Sanata Coulibaly,[1] Moussa Namountougou,[2] Léa Paré-Toé,[1] Anicet Georges Ouédraogo,[2] Abdoulaye Diabaté,[1] Brian D. Foy,[3] and Roch K. Dabiré[1]

[1]*IRSS/Centre Muraz, Bobo-Dioulasso, Burkina Faso*
[2]*Université Polytechnique de Bobo-Dioulasso, Bobo-Dioulasso, Burkina Faso*
[3]*Colorado State University, Fort Collins, CO, USA*

Correspondence should be addressed to Aristide S. Hien; aristide.hien@yahoo.fr and Roch K. Dabiré; dabire_roch@hotmail.com

Academic Editor: Jean-Paul J. Gonzalez

Twenty years after the latest publications performed on the parasitological indices of malaria transmission in northwest of the second city of Burkina Faso, it was important to update the epidemiological profile of malaria in children under the age of 15 years. The objective of this study was to determine and compare the parasitological parameters of malaria transmission by season, area, and age in the two zones (rice and savanna) in the northwest of Bobo-Dioulasso, Burkina Faso. Overall, the results showed that there was no significant difference in the parasitological indices of malaria transmission within children under fifteen years between the rice site and the savannah site and whatever the season ($P > 0.05$). The profound environmental modifications that occurred in the rice zone would have led to changes in vector behavior and consequently to changes in the epidemiological profile of malaria, contrary to the results obtained since the last publications. An entomological study correlated with this study is therefore necessary for effective decision-making for the malaria control in both areas. Future research must now focus on the impact that these profound environmental modifications of rice area are having on malaria control in Burkina Faso.

1. Background

Febrile illness is the most common and important component of malaria syndrome in sub-Saharan Africa [1]. Children under 5 years of age and pregnant women constitute the major groups for developing life-threatening malaria [2]. In Burkina Faso, malaria is both endemic and hyperendemic [2] and remains a major public health problem. Malaria control policies in Burkina Faso include free distribution of insecticide-treated bed nets (ITNs), Intermittent Preventive Treatment (IPT) for pregnant women, and treatment of malaria cases with artemisinin-based combination therapy (ACT). Seasonal Malaria Chemoprevention (SMC) was adopted as policy in 2012 according to the WHO recommendations and a national plan for introducing SMC has been implemented because clinical trials in Mali and Burkina Faso have shown a strong protective effect of SMC against clinical malaria and severe malaria even in areas with high net coverage [3]. But despite recent efforts in scaling up these interventions, coverage of ITNs and access to treatment with ACTs remain relatively low [4].

Furthermore, Burkina Faso, like many other African countries, is also facing major food security challenges. The solution to this challenge has been a policy to promote the development of irrigated crops including rice and is based on water management and the development of irrigation schemes. Although hydroagricultural works can provide enormous benefits, it is also acknowledged that population health can be negatively influenced by them through profound changes in the ecosystem. Indeed, irrigation promotes the proliferation of mosquito breeding sites and affects both the duration and speed of replication of *Anopheles* mosquitoes. The landscaped perimeter of "Vallée du Kou" was realised within the framework of cooperation between the Volta (today Burkina Faso) and China in 1969 and construction began in 1970 on 1000 hectares. This perimeter led to health consequences by promoting the proliferation of *Anopheles* mosquitoes; in particular, the density of *Anopheles gambiae*, the major vector of malaria transmission in the area, multiplied 20-fold and this was followed by a doubling of the rate of malaria transmission [5]. The annual number of infectious bites has increased significantly in the valley compared to the neighboring savannah [5, 6].

However, while past results have been focused on the evaluation of entomological parameters of malaria transmission, few studies have focused on the evaluation of parasitological parameters of malaria transmission in both the rice-growing area and the surrounding savannah.

Twenty years have passed since the last publications were published on the parasitological indices of malaria transmission in the area [7, 8]. This study was performed to update our knowledge of parasitological indices in the area. There are continuing questions about whether irrigated perimeters are more or less suitable to malaria compared to the savanna area and if parasitological indices are higher or lower in the rice-growing area than in the savanna area. This study was initiated to answer these questions and provide new information to update the data on the parasitological parameters of malaria transmission in these two different ecoepidemiological areas with a focus on the most vulnerable group of the community, children under fifteen years. Our objective was to determine and compare the parasitological parameters of malaria transmission by season, area, and age range in both zones (rice and savanna) in northern-west Bobo-Dioulasso, Burkina Faso.

2. Methods

2.1. Study Area. The District of Dandé is located in the northern-west of Bobo-Dioulasso (Figure 1). The climat is of Sudano-Guinean type, alternating with a wet season and a dry season unevenly distributed throughout the year. The dry season occurs from November to June and the rainy season from June to October with peak maximum rainfall in August-September. The average annual rainfall is about 1000 mm. April is the hottest month (39°C) and December is the coldest month (23°C). The minimum and maximum temperatures range from 20°C to 27 (average 23°C) and 33°C to 39°C (average 37°C), respectively. The rainy season is the most suitable for mosquito breeding and transmission of malaria in the area, which extends from June to November, but residual malaria transmission can last beyond this period in some places. *An. gambiae* s.l. is the major vector of malaria in the study area, with *Anopheles gambiae* predominating in some places while *Anopheles coluzzii* is predominant in the rice-growing area; *An. funestus* and *An. arabiensis* are present in small proportions and frequencies increase towards the end of the rainy season [5, 9].

Two localities from this district were retained as our study sites as representative of two ecoepidemiological areas. Study sites in rice and savanna areas are, respectively, the Kou Valley 1 (VK1) (11°22′56, 4″N; 4°25′13, 1″W) and Samandeni (11°28′22, 7″N; 4°28′30, 8″W). These two localities are separated by 15 km and are located on the Bobo-Faramana-Mopti road. The populations of the two study sites are composed of about fifteen ethnic groups and the main spoken language is Dioula. Populations are engaged in subsistence agriculture in the savanna area; however in the rice area the main activity is the cultivation of rice. According to the data from Dandé District in 2014, the two localities counted about 4018 and 10555 inhabitants in VK1 and Samandeni, respectively. Children and adolescents (0–14 years) represented 45.1% of the population. The prevalence of malaria in children 0 to 14 years old one year before the start of the survey based on rapid diagnostic tests (RDTs) and reported by the respective health facilities was 29.8% in VK1 and 15% and in Samandeni.

2.2. Sample Size and Study Populations. We have carried out a random sampling by relying on subjects who were present at the time of our passage in each site until we reached the estimated number of subjects planned for the study. based on a random sampling of 80 to 110 children from 0 to under fifteen per passage, we conducted six passages, three passages in the dry season (November, January, and April) and three passages in the rainy season (June, August, and October) in each study site. The objective was to reach at least 300 children per season and per site required for the study, considering prevalence of 29.8% in the savanna zone and 15% in the rice zone in rainy season with an accuracy of 10%, standard deviation (1.96) corresponding to the risk of error 5% and 10% of nonrespondents.

The study included all children in the village aged between 0 and under 15 years whose parents gave their consent. Those excluded were study children whose parental consent was not obtained and children not residing in the two sites selected. Also, subjects who received antimalarial treatment during the last 14 days are excluded.

The study was conducted for one year, from November 2014 to October 2015.

2.3. Thin and Thick Smears. Blood samples were collected monthly by the standard finger-prick method according to the season. The thin and thick blood smears were air dried. Thereafter, the thin and thick smears were fixed in ethanol, then stained with 10% Giemsa (Sigma) in phosphate buffer (pH 7.0) for 30 minutes, and examined using oil immersion magnification (100x). Each slide was examined by two microscopists, who estimated the parasite density by counting the number of asexual *P. falciparum* parasites in fields containing 200 white blood cells and multiplied that number by 25 to estimate the number of asexual *P. falciparum* parasites per μL (based on an average white blood cells count of 8000 per μL [10]). Slides were considered positive or negative after two readers examined fields containing 200 white blood cells. Slides on which there was disagreement were examined by a third microscopist to confirm the result. Random checks were carried out on the slide counts (to include at least 10% of all slides) by independent microscopists to ensure quality control. An individual was considered positive if malaria parasites were detected in the blood smear.

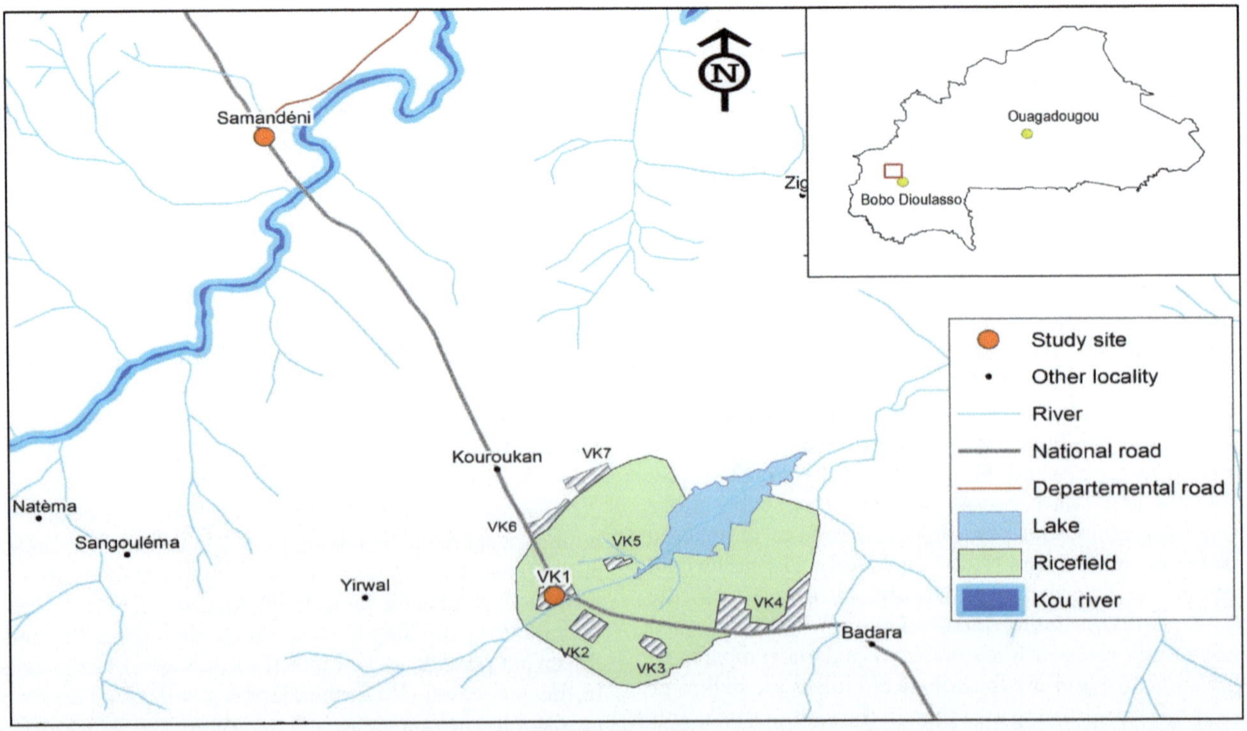

Figure 1: Location of study sites. Colored red points represent the two study sites located on the Bobo-Faramana-Mopti road colored in black. VK1 is the study site in rice area and Samandeni is study site in savannah area. The plot colored green shows the rice field with different rice-growing sites (VK1–VK7).

The parasite carriage rate or the plasmodic index (PI) was estimated by the proportion of positive numbers from examined thick smears and the gametocytemic index (GI) by the proportion of subjects presenting sexual forms or gametes in the thick smear. Parasite densities of sexual and asexual forms were expressed as the mean number of parasites per microliter (μL) of blood. Parasite densities obtained by the study site were classified and annotated as follows: 1: less than 1000 parasites/μL; 2: 1,000–5,000 parasites/μL; 3: 5,001–10,000 parasites/μL; and 4: more than 10,000 parasites/μL.

2.4. Clinical Examination. Axillary temperatures were measured by skilled health personnel in order to detect any temperature greater than 38°C (the pyrogenic threshold considered in our study). Any child who had fever above 38°C was considered clinically ill if he/she had fever (a core body temperature $\geq$ 38°C) and malaria parasites identified from the blood smear. Any child that was clinically ill at the survey date was taken to the nearest public health facility for treatment free of charge. The temperature was taken using an electronic thermometer (Ormon^{R}).

2.5. Ethical Approval. Ethical approval of the study was obtained of ethic committee from Centre Muraz (Bobo-Dioulasso). After its approval, each participant was then informed about the protocol; care was given to all study participants. Oral informed assent was then obtained from each participant. All the study participants considered clinically ill were examined and treated in line with the national malaria guidelines of Ministry of Health, Burkina Faso.

2.6. Data Analysis. Excel and GraphPad Prism 5 software were used, respectively, for entry and analysis data. The malariological indices were determined and compared by site, season, and age range to determine the variations between the two ecoepidemiological areas. The nonparametric Wilcoxon signed-rank test was used to compare longitudinal samples throughout season and the Mann-Whitney test for mean comparison between areas with an alpha of 0.05.

3. Results

3.1. Participant Recruitment. The census of children under fifteen years of selected households in the two study sites counted 1,121 children of both sexes eligible for this study. There were 555 children from VK1 and 566 children from Samandeni. Their distribution according to sex by site ranged from 242 females to 313 males from VK1 and 246 females to 320 males from Samandeni (Table 1). However, the distribution according to age group showed that 36 children (6.48%) in VK1 compared to 31 (5.47%) in Samandeni were aged less than one year; 116 (20.9%) compared to 183 (32.33%) between 1 and 5 years of age; 249 (44.86%) compared to 226 (39.92%) were between 5 and 10 years of age, and 154 (27.74%) compared to 126 (22.26%) were between 10 and 15 years of

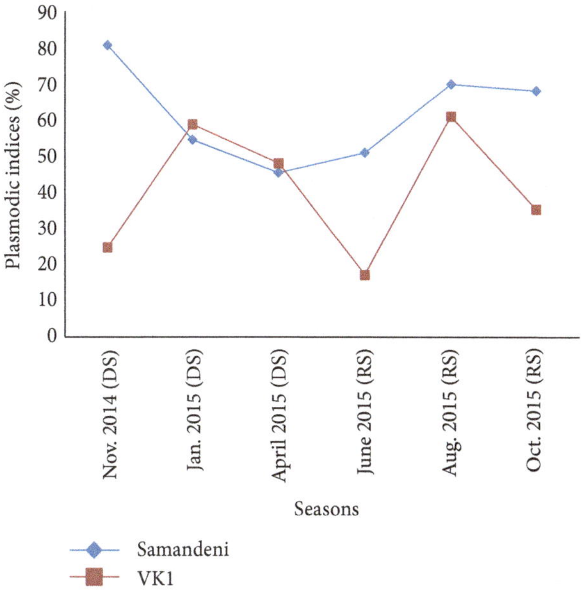

FIGURE 2: Seasonal variation of plasmodic indices of study sites. DS: dry season; RS: rainy season; the blue curve: seasonal variation of Samandeni children's plasmodic index; the red curve: seasonal variation of the VK1 children's plasmodic index.

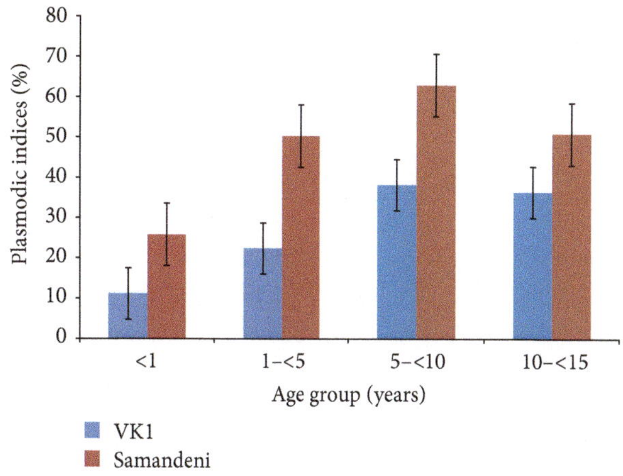

FIGURE 3: Plasmodic indices with standard errors bars (SEM) according to age (means ± SEM). When standard error bars (SEM) do not overlap, this means that the difference between two means is statistically significant ($P < 0.05$).

age. There was no statistically significant difference in the representation of the two sexes and age groups in the study site ($P > 0.05$).

3.2. Plasmodic Index by Site. A total of 1121 thick and thin smears were performed during the study period and examined. 558 of them were carriers of malaria parasites and the mean plasmodic index was 49.77% (CI: 34.99–58.01). The plasmodic index was 40.85% (95% CI: 21.89–59.81) and 61.66% (95% CI: 47.55–75.76), respectively, in the rice zone and in the savanna zone. It was higher in the savanna zone and lower in the rice zone, but this difference was not statistically significant ($P > 0.05$).

3.3. Seasonal Variations of the Plasmodic Index and Plasmodium Species. Overall, seasonal variations in plasmodic index were not significant in the different ecoepidemiological zones ($P > 0.05$). But it was higher in Samandeni (savanna zone) than in VK1 (rice area) at the beginning of the dry seasons (November 2014: mean PI 80.72% versus 24.69%) and rainy season (June: mean PI 51% versus 17.18%) ($P < 0.05$). However the evolution of the plasmodic index according to the dry season months showed a higher parasitaemia in January and April in the rice zone compared to the savanna zone ($P > 0.05$) (Figure 2).

Plasmodium falciparum was the most prevalent in the dry season, as well as in the rainy period, but with a higher proportion in the rainy season whatever the site. Three species of malaria parasites have been observed during the rainy season in the savanna area while two species (*P. falciparum* and *P. malariae*) were detected only during the dry season in the rice zone. Mixed infections (*P. falciparum* and *P. malariae*) were observed in positive slides only during the rainy season in the rice zone and in both seasons in the savanna zone. Three cases of mixed infections were found in the rice area compared to 15 cases in the savannah area. No cases of triparasitism were found in either site.

3.4. Variations of the Plasmodic Index according to Age Ranges. The plasmodic index increased with age, as it was very low in toddlers and reached a maximum in children between 5 and 10 years old, but it then decreased in children >10 years old, regardless of the study site. The children between 5 and 10 years old were the most infected and had plasmodic index of 62.33% in Samandeni and 38.15% in VK1 (Figure 3). The least infected children were those <1 year old in VK1 (11%) in contrast to those of Samandeni where a quarter of this age group were infected. The proportion of children aged 2 to 9 had a plasmodic index of 53.48% and 55.6% (Table 1), respectively, in the rice and savannah zone.

For the two biogeographic zones, the plasmodic index showed no significant differences between the different age groups by site ($P > 0.05$) and between the two study sites ($P = 0.11$).

3.5. Gametocytemic Index. Of the 551 thick smears examined for the rice-growing area, twenty-one of these showed gametocytes of *Plasmodium falciparum*, thus a gametocytic index of 3.78% (21/551). In the savanna zone, gametocytic index was 1.94% (11/566). This difference in the gametocyte rate found between the two sites was statistically significant ($P < 0.05$). Gametocytes were found in the positive slides, whatever the period and the study site but with a higher proportion in the rainy season in the rice zone (2.70%) compared to the savanna zone (0.5%). The subjects likely to infect vectors became more important in the population during the rainy season in the rice-growing area.

For all 1,121 specimens examined, the mean gametocytemic index was 2.85%.

Table 1: Study participant's characteristics.

Characteristic	Rice site	Savanna site	P value
Sex			
Male	242 (43.6)	246 (43.5)	>0.05
Female	313 (56.4)	320 (56.5)	>0.05
Age			
Mean ± SD	8.625 ± 2.905	6.804 ± 4.242	0.06
Range	1-14.8	0.8–14.9	
Age group			
<1 year	36	31	>0.05
1–<5 years	116	183	
5–<10 years	249	226	
10–<15 years	154	126	
2–9 years	285	329	
Temperature (°C)			
Mean ± SD	36.41 ± 0.7646	36.68 ± 0.6816	0.0786
Range	34.5–37.60	35–39.20	
Plasmodic index			
Mean ± SD	40.85 ± 18.07	61.66 ± 13.44	0.0931
Range	17.18–61	45.45–80.72	
2–9 years	53.48%	55.6%	
GMPD			
Mean ± SD	2706 ± 252	2742 ± 189	0.93
Range	2335–3000	2414–2912	

SD: standard deviation. GMPD: geometric mean parasite density and numbers in brackets represent percentages. There were no significant differences between participant's characteristics of two study sites.

3.6. Distribution of Parasite Densities in the Different Ecoepidemiological Zones. The lowest parasite density was 16 parasites/μL of blood and the highest was 471,889 parasites/μL, all observed in Samandeni during the dry season (November 2014 and January 2015). For a better interpretation of parasite density in order to compare the two study populations, we expressed parasite densities by the geometric mean parasite density (GMPD) in children from 0 to 15 years, taking into consideration the positive and negative slides examined. The difference in geometric mean parasite densities between the rice area (2706; 95% CI: 2441–2970) and the savanna (2742; 95% CI: 2543–2940) was not significant ($P = 0.68$; mean square = 3888, Df = 1). However, geometric means have evolved significantly in each study site ($P = 0.03$). In contrast, they were comparable whatever the season in the two study sites ($P < 0.05$).

Parasite densities less than 1000 parasites/μL of blood were most frequently encountered in children aged 5 to 10 years, 36.75% in Samandeni (208/566) and 22% in VK1 (122/555) at both sites ($P = 0.01$). There were 4% against 5% of subjects, respectively, in rice and savannah areas who had parasite densities above 10,000 parasites/μL.

3.7. Relationship between Body Temperature and Infection Prevalence of Malaria. Of a total of 555 children examined in VK1, 217 were carriers of malaria parasites and 140 were febrile (25.22%). Of the 140 participants with fever, 43.57% were carriers of malaria parasites compared to 56.43% who were not carrying *Plasmodium*. This difference is not statistically significant ($P > 0.05$).

The presence of fever in VK1 was not related to the presence of asexual malaria parasites in the blood (OR < 1). Contrary to VK1, the presence of asexual malaria parasites was strongly related to the presence of fever in Samandeni (OR = 28.61 with 95% CI: 3.60–158.80), with 53.07% of participants having both fever and *Plasmodium* compared to 46.92% with fever but no *Plasmodium* (Table 2). In both sites, as age increased, so did the number of participants carrying malaria parasites who also had fever: 0% in children less than one year old, 7.69% for children 1–5 years old, 34.61% for children between 5 and 10 years old, and 57.69% in children 10–15 years old ($P < 0.001$).

The risk of having a febrile attack increased with parasite density group in VK1. This risk became significant ($P < 0.01$) with a parasite density > 10,000 parasites/μL (odds ratio of 1.5 for PD > 10,000; 95% CI: 0.96–5.6). However, there was no variation in the different parasite density groups in Samandeni, but the risk of having a febrile attack was higher in the lowest parasite density group ($1000 \leq DP < 5000$).

4. Discussion

The assessment of parasite prevalence provides indications on the extent of transmission and the state of circulation of parasites in a community.

TABLE 2: Relation between presence of fever and malaria-carrying parasite.

Parasitemia	Status of fever		Total	Odds ratio
	No fever	Fever		
VK1				
Positive thick smears	151	61	217	0.93 $0 \leq OR \leq 2.1$
Negative thick smears	257	79	338	
Total	408	140	555	
Samandeni				
Positive thick smears	241	69	310	28.61 $3.60 \leq OR \leq 158.8$
Negative thick smears	195	61	256	
Total	436	130	566	

The plasmodic index indicates the percentage of subjects carrying *Plasmodium* in the peripheral blood. This index, in subjects less than one year old, may be a good indication of the intensity of transmission. In adolescents and adults, it provides information on the degree of immunity of this population. The mean rates of the plasmodic indices in the two localities were all greater than 10%. This confirms the presence of endemic and stable malaria in two localities. Moreover, at the 3rd African Conference on Malaria, held in Yaoundé, Cameroon, in July 1962, it was decided to retain this terminology (hypo-, meso-, and holoendemic) using the criterion of the plasmodic index in children aged 2 to 9 years. The plasmodic indices (PI) obtained confirm in this study area the presence of hyperendemic malaria according to the plasmodic indices observed in children aged 2 to 9 years in the two study sites.

Stable malaria is referred to when the transmission season is very long and there is little change in incidence during the year and from year to year. In such conditions, climate change is too insignificant to influence anopheline transmission activity, temperature ensures a rapid sporogonic cycle, the vector is highly anthropophilic, and vector survivorship is long. Stable malaria is most often due to *P. falciparum* malaria in Africa, and there is a very high degree of immune protection in the population. In our study, the predominant plasmodial species in both localities was *P. falciparum*. This confirms the literature data that report that this species is most common in West Africa [11–13]. The dominance of this species, according to Gaye et al. [14], is likely due to better efficiency of transmission of its sporozoites. Also, the results of the study remain consistent with this hypothesis, whereby all children carried *Plasmodium* either alone (95%) or in association with *P. malariae* (1–4%) or *P. ovale* (about 1%). These prevalence rates were higher than those of Meetselaar and Van Thiel [11], in the city of Bobo-Dioulasso which is located 25 km from the study area. No infections occurred with all three species together, and no infections with *P. vivax* were observed, which was congruent with historical epidemiological studies [15]. In addition, there was no seasonal variation in the plasmodic indices. They were also comparable in the two study sites. This could be explained by the profound environmental changes in this rice-growing region. In the past in this rice zone, rice was grown according to a well-defined calendar with two growing periods, one in the dry season and the other in the rainy season. The abundance of malaria vectors was also closely linked to this cultural rhythm of rice harvesting. But today it is no longer the case. There is no calendar and therefore vectors can be found at any time of the year as in the savanna zone. This could explain why there is no difference in the evolution of the plasmodic indices and the parasitic loads in the rice zone as in the savanna zone. Instead, they show that plasmodic indices are stable throughout the year in Samandeni but falls into VK1. But this difference in the plasmodic indices was not significant. This suggests that children in the rice area are exposed to malaria in the same way as children in the savanna zone and explains why we did not find any significant difference in the variation of the plasmodic indices between the age groups and the site. This result is the same with the parasite carriage portage. Indeed, the parasitic densities were comparable whatever the time of the year between the two sites. The age group most susceptible to malaria was children aged 5–10 years, in contrast to other studies that have demonstrated the most susceptible children are those less than five years old [15–17]. Indeed, the national malaria control policy of the Burkina Faso promotes the use of insecticide-treated nets among the most vulnerable groups in the community, who are defined to be pregnant women and children under five years of age. This approach has an additional benefit in reducing malaria in this age group in these study sites. The fact that children aged 5 to 10 years are not receiving these needed benefits as those less than one year could lead to high exposure to mosquito bites in both localities. This could contribute to increased parasite densities in this age range. Moreover, our study found a higher gametocytemic index in VK1 (3.78%) than in the savannah zone (1.94%). The profound environmental changes observed in the rice area could explain these results. Ecological changes that occurred in the rice-growing areas are one possible reason for the strong gametocytemic index that was observed. This would help to maintain permanent transmission until the dry season, as shown by the results of the study.

5. Conclusion

This study investigated the epidemiological profile of malaria in ecologically different environments in children under 15 years in Burkina Faso. In Burkina Faso, as in most of the developing countries, food security is crucial and requires water storage and management. The intensification of irrigated crops is a response to this challenge. Our study suggests that hydroagricultural developments in the northwest of the city of Bobo-Dioulasso influences malaria prevalence and morbidity rates in the region. Indeed, the morbidity rate was comparable between rice area and savanna area. We think that the development of irrigated crops, in particular rice cultivation in Sudan zones as in Burkina Faso, has encouraged the proliferation of mosquitoes, some of which are malaria vectors which would lead to increased number of malaria cases. The once stated theory of the "paradox of Vallée du Kou" seems to have changed over time, and now the rice cultivation zone has similar ecoepidemiological characteristics of the nearby savannah zone.

Competing Interests

The authors declare that they have no competing interests.

Authors' Contributions

Roch K. Dabiré conceived and designed the study. Aristide S. Hien performed the field study, analyzed the data, and drafted the manuscript and contributed also to the study design. Sanata Coulibaly assured the laboratory analyses. Ibrahim Sangaré, Moussa Namountougou, Léa Paré-Toé, Anicet Georges Ouédraogo, Abdoulaye Diabaté, and Brian D. Foy reviewed the first draft of the article. Roch K. Dabiré is guarantor of the study. All authors contributed to the drafts and read and approved the final manuscript.

Acknowledgments

The authors express their sincere gratitude to nurses and community health workers for their availability and support throughout the study period. They thank warmly the inhabitants of the two study sites for having accepted the implementation of the study in their villages. This study was financially supported by the PRIPA Project 10463-009 of IDRC and partially by the DawaPlus Project implemented in Centre Muraz.

References

[1] B. M. Greenwood, K. Bojang, C. J. M. Whitty, and G. A. T. Targett, "Malaria," *The Lancet*, vol. 365, no. 9469, pp. 1487–1498, 2005.

[2] World Malaria Report 2015, http://www.who.int/iris//bitstream/10665/200018/1/9789241565158_eng.pdf.

[3] A. L. Wilson, "A systematic review and meta-analysis of the efficacy and safety of intermittent preventive treatment of malaria in children (IPTc)," *PLoS ONE*, vol. 6, no. 2, Article ID e16976, 2011.

[4] M. De Allegri, V. R. Louis, J. Tiendrébeogo et al., "Moving towards universal coverage with malaria control interventions: achievements and challenges in rural Burkina Faso," *International Journal of Health Planning and Management*, vol. 28, no. 1, pp. 102–121, 2013.

[5] T. Baldet, A. Diabaté, and T. R. Guiguemdé, "Etude de la transmission du paludisme en 1999 dans la zone rizicole de la Vallée du Kou (Bama) Burkina Faso," *Cahiers Santé*, vol. 13, no. 1, pp. 1–6, 2003.

[6] A. Diabaté, *Paludisme au Burkina Faso: Etude de la transmission et répartition géographique de la résistance d'Anopheles gambiae sl. aux pyréthrinoïdes [Ph.D. thesis]*, Université de Montpellier, 2003.

[7] V. Robert, P. Gazin, C. Boudin, J. F. Molez, V. Ouedraogo, and P. Carnevale, "The transmission of malaria in a wooded savannah area and a rice-growing area around Bobo-Dioulasso (Burkina Faso)," *Annales de la Societe Belge de Medecine Tropicale*, vol. 65, no. 2, pp. 201–214, 1985.

[8] P. Gazin, V. Robert, and P. Carnevale, "Longitudinal study of malaria indices in 2 villages of the Bobo Dioulasso region (Burkina Faso)," *Annales de la Societe Belge de Medecine Tropicale*, vol. 65, supplement 2, pp. 181–186, 1985.

[9] K. R. Dabiré, A. Diabaté, L. Djogbenou et al., "Dynamics of multiple insecticide resistance in the malaria vector *Anopheles gambiae* in a rice growing area in South-Western Burkina Faso," *Malaria Journal*, vol. 7, article 188, 2008.

[10] D. Payne, "Use and limitations of light microscopy for diagnosing malaria at the primary health care level," *Bulletin of the World Health Organization*, vol. 66, no. 5, pp. 621–626, 1988.

[11] D. Meetselaar and P. H. Van Thiel, "Classification of malaria," *Tropical and Geographical Medicine*, vol. 11, no. 2, pp. 157–161, 1959.

[12] P. Gazin, V. Robert, and P. Carnevale, "Longitudinal study of malaria indices in 2 villages of the Bobo Dioulasso region (Burkina Faso)," *Annales de la Societe Belge de Medecine Tropicale*, vol. 65, pp. 181–186, 1985.

[13] R. Benasseni, P. Gazin, P. Carnevale, and D. Boudon, "Le paludisme urbain a Bobo Dioulasso (Burkina Faso) Etude de la morbidité palustre," *Cahiers ORSTOM Série Entomologie Médicale et Parasitologie*, vol. 25, no. 3, pp. 165–170, 1987.

[14] O. Gaye, I. B. Bah, E. Bengue, S. Diallo, and O. Faye, "Morbidité palustre en milieu urbain. Etude de 353 accèsfébriles," *Medecine Tropicale*, vol. 49, no. 4, pp. 401–404, 1989.

[15] T. R. Burkot, P. M. Graves, J. A. Cattan, R. A. Wirtz, and F. D. Gibson, "The efficiency of sporozoite transmission in the human malarias, *Plasmodium falciparum* and *Plasmodium vivax*," *Bulletin of the World Health Organization*, vol. 65, no. 3, pp. 375–380, 1987.

[16] M. C. Baldé, M. Camara, A. O. Barry et al., "Etude de la prévalence du paludisme dans 24 villages de la Guinée," *Bulletin de la Société de Pathologie Exotique*, vol. 95, no. 2, supplement 4, pp. 192–194, 2001.

[17] G. I. Olasehinde, A. A. Ajay, S. O. Taiwo, B. T. Adekeye, and O. A. Adeyeba, "Prevalence and management of Falciparium malaria among infants and children in Ota, Ogun state, Southwestern Nigeria," *African Journal of Clinical and Experimental Microbiology*, vol. 11, no. 3, pp. 159–163, 2010.

10

Knowledge, Attitude, and Practice of Health Workers in a Tertiary Hospital in Ile-Ife, Nigeria, towards Ebola Viral Disease

Samuel Anu Olowookere, Emmanuel Akintunde Abioye-Kuteyi, Olusegun Kayode Adepoju, Oluwaseun Taiwo Esan, Temitope Michael Adeolu, Tolulope Kola Adeoye, Adesola Adebayo Adepoju, and Adedayo Titilayo Aderogba

Department of Community Health, College of Health Sciences, Obafemi Awolowo University, Ile-Ife, Nigeria

Correspondence should be addressed to Samuel Anu Olowookere; sanuolowookere@yahoo.com

Academic Editor: Peter Leggat

Background. Health workers are more prone to Ebola viral disease (EVD) than the general population. This study assessed the preparedness of health workers in the control and management of EVD. *Methods.* A descriptive cross-sectional study. Consenting 400 health workers completed a semistructured questionnaire that assessed participants' general knowledge, emergency preparedness, and control and management of EVD. Data were analysed using descriptive and inferential statistics. *Results.* The mean age (SD) was 34.5 ± 8.62 years ranging from 20 to 59 years. Most participants were medical doctors (24.6%) and nurses (52.2%). The majority had practised <10 years (73.8%) and were aware of the EVD outbreak in the West African subregion (85.5%). Colleagues (40%) and radio (37.2%) were their major sources of information. Only 42% had good knowledge while 27% knew that there was no vaccine presently to prevent EVD. About one-quarter (24.2%) had low risk perception. The majority (89%) felt the hospital infection control policy was inadequate to protect against EVD. The only predictor of good knowledge was participants' occupation. *Conclusion.* There is knowledge gap and poor infection control preparedness among respondents. Thus, knowledge and practices of health workers towards EVD need improvement.

1. Introduction

Ebola viral disease (EVD) is an acute febrile illness caused by the Ebola virus, a member of the family of Filoviridae. EVD is associated with a high mortality rate in humans and non-human primates since its initial recognition in the Democratic Republic of the Congo in 1976 [1, 2]. The Filoviruses are thread-like RNA viruses that cause haemorrhagic fever. The Ebola virus causes severe disease in humans with an extremely high case fatality rate ranging from 25 to 90%, depending on the viral subtype and the availability of medical care. Haemorrhagic symptoms occur in about 30–50% of described human cases [1]. Four Ebola viral subtypes (Zaire, Sudan, Ivory Coast, and Uganda) and the Marburg virus cause illness in humans, and the subtypes Zaire and Ivory Coast and the Marburg virus are known to cause illness in non-human primates. One Ebola subtype (Reston) causes illness in non-human primates but has induced only asymptomatic disease in humans [3]. The natural reservoir of the Ebola viruses remains unknown. The incubation period of Ebola virus is 2–21 days and it is transmitted majorly through direct contact with body fluid including blood, urine, excreta, vomit, saliva, sweat, mother's breast milk, organs, body parts, secretions, and seminal fluid. A rare mode of transmission is contact with the unknown natural reservoir or infected animals. Routes of infection are oral, the conjunctivae, mucous-membrane exposure (e.g., nose and mouth), sexual intercourse, and a break in the skin, a penetrating object infected with body fluids of a patient (e.g., needles or razor blades). Infections occur when health staff or relatives are taking care of a patient without proper protection. Contact with infected corpses (human or animal) put people at high risk to become infected with EVD. Nosocomial transmissions of EVD do occur when appropriate precautions are not taken [1].

The latest outbreak which affects Guinea, Liberia, Sierra Leone, and Nigeria in West Africa is the worst in EVD history with 2127 reported cases out of which 1145 died by August 15, 2014 [4]. Health workers were included among the infected and the dead from EVD while caring for people infected with this highly fatal disease. EVD prevention and control in the region raises a number of challenges for healthcare workers practising in countries where health systems and infrastructures are weak; healthcare financing is poor and health insurance coverage is limited [5]. Very few studies on EVD had been conducted among health workers in Nigeria [6]. It is therefore imperative to assess the preparedness of health workers in the control and management of EVD.

2. Methods

The study was conducted at the Obafemi Awolowo University Teaching Hospital Complex (OAUTHC), Ile-Ife, Nigeria, in the month of July, 2014. It is a 576-bedded hospital with referrals from neighbouring states such as Oyo, Ondo, Ekiti, Kogi, Kwara, and beyond.

The study population included the clinical members of staff, namely, medical doctors, nurses, pharmacists, medical laboratory technologists, community health workers (CHEW), medical records officer, and physiotherapists.

The sample size of 352 was calculated using an appropriate statistical formula for estimating the minimum sample size in descriptive health studies [$n = Z^2 pq/d^2$] [7], where 64.4% of health care workers knew that EVD had no cure [8]. A sample size of 400 was used after nonresponders being taken into consideration.

The number allocated to each group of clinical staff was determined proportionately using the formula $n/N \times 400$, where n is the number of occupational groups and N is the total number of clinical staff [9].

Consenting health workers completed a pretested semi-structured self-administered questionnaire that assessed participants' general knowledge, emergency preparedness, and control and management of EVD. The questionnaires were distributed consecutively to members of each occupational group during the break period. The respondents were allowed to fill the questionnaire in their spare time at their convenience. Questionnaire information was anonymised.

Ethical approval to conduct the study was obtained from Ife Central Local Government Ethical Review Committee. Written informed consent was taken from the respondents while they were reassured of the confidentiality of the information obtained. The data collected were entered and kept in a password protected computer.

The data obtained were analysed using SPSS version 16. Simple descriptive and inferential statistics were done. Knowledge score was computed for a 41-item question on knowledge of EVD. Each item was assigned "+1" for correct knowledge and "0" for incorrect knowledge. The knowledge score was graded as good or appropriate (if respondent scored ≥ 27 points) and not good or not appropriate (if score was <27 points) using the mean score as the break-off point. Test of significance was conducted using appropriate statistical methods. Multivariate analysis was performed using logistic regression to evaluate sociodemographic variables and other variables that are independently associated with good knowledge of EVD. Adjusted odd ratio (AOR) and 95% CI were presented and used as measures of the strength of association. Significant level was put at $p < 0.05$.

Table 1: Sociodemographic characteristics of participants.

Variable	Frequency	%
Age group (years)		
20–29	135	33.8
30–39	164	41
≥40	101	25.2
Sex		
Male	159	39.8
Female	241	60.2
Marital status		
Single	137	34.2
Married	263	65.8
Occupation		
Medical doctor	98	24.6
Nurse	209	52.2
Pharmacist	25	6.3
Medical laboratory technologist	23	5.8
Community health officers	19	4.7
Medical records officer	17	4.2
Physiotherapist	9	2.2
Duration of employment (years)		
<10	295	73.8
≥10	105	26.2

3. Results

Four hundred completed questionnaires were analysed. The mean age (SD) of the respondents was 34.5 ± 8.62 years (range 20–59 years). Most participants were medical doctors (24.6%) and nurses (52.2%). The majority were females (60.2%), were married (65.8%), and had practised <10 years (73.8%) (Table 1).

The majority 342 (85.5%) were aware of the on-going EVD outbreak in the West African subregion. Colleagues (40%) and radio (37.2%) were their major sources of information (Table 2).

Only 42.3% had good knowledge of EVD (Figure 1). Most knew that EVD is a viral infection (93.2%) that is deadly (91.5%). Also, majority knew that EVD can be transmitted from person to person (87.8%) and animal to person (86.2%) while only 46.8% knew it can be transmitted from inanimate objects to persons (Table 3).

Although the majority of participants knew that EVD is transmissible through body fluids, below half knew that the causative agent penetrates broken skin (Table 4).

Most health workers knew high grade fever (78.2%) and unexplained bleeding (73.4%) as common presentation

TABLE 2: EVD awareness and source of information on the outbreak.

Variable	Frequency	%
Aware of EVD epidemic in West Africa		
Yes	342	85.5
No	58	14.5
*Source of information		
Colleagues	160	40.0
Radio	149	37.2
Internet	114	28.4
Television	93	23.3
Newspapers	92	23.1
Notice boards/pamphlets	44	10.9

*Multiple responses.

TABLE 3: EVD knowledge of clinical variables.

Variable	Frequency	%
Ebola fever is a viral disease		
Yes	373	93.2
No	27	6.8
Incubation period last from 2 to 21 days		
Yes	247	61.8
No	153	38.2
The reservoir is usually bats		
Yes	270	67.5
No	130	32.5
Infection with the organism is usually deadly		
Yes	366	91.5
No	34	8.5
Ebola can be transmitted from person to person		
Yes	351	87.8
No	49	12.2
Ebola can be transmitted from animal to person		
Yes	345	86.2
No	55	13.8
Ebola can be transmitted from inanimate objects to person		
Yes	187	46.8
No	213	53.2

in EVD patients while fewer health workers knew that gastrointestinal symptoms and shock (27%) could occur in these patients (Table 5).

Although majority of participants knew some treatment and prevention of EVD, about three-quarter did not know that EVD has no vaccine presently (Table 6). Most respondents were not aware of the process for EVD reporting (Table 7). Most respondents had poor risk perception and negative attitude to EVD diagnosis, management, and prevention. About 11% felt that the infection control policy of the hospital is adequate to protect health workers against EVD (Table 8).

Medical doctors (54.1%) and nurses (42.6%) had appropriate knowledge compared to other health workers and this association was statistically significant (Table 9).

The only predictor of good/appropriate knowledge was participants' occupation (Table 10).

TABLE 4: Knowledge of EVD mode of transmission.

Variable	Frequency	%
Ebola can be transmitted through saliva		
Yes	274	68.5
No	126	31.5
Ebola can be transmitted through blood		
Yes	331	82.8
No	69	17.2
Ebola can be transmitted through seminal/vagina fluid		
Yes	222	55.5
No	178	44.5
Causative agent penetrates broken skin		
Yes	186	46.5
No	214	53.5
Bodies of dead cases constitute a potential hazard		
Yes	300	75
No	100	25
Cases cease to be infectious after the acute phase of the disease		
Yes	107	26.8
No	293	73.2

TABLE 5: Knowledge of EVD clinical presentation.

EVD cases are characterized by fever >38°C		
Yes	313	78.2
No	87	21.8
Unexplained bleeding could be diagnostic		
Yes	294	73.4
No	106	26.6
Vomiting, diarrhoea, and shock are rarely observed in hospitalized patients		
Yes	292	73.0
No	108	27.0
Fever refractory to treatment and unexplained mucosal bleeding is a sign		
Yes	296	74.0
No	104	26.0

Table 6: EVD knowledge of treatment and prevention.

Variable	Frequency	%
*Drug use for treatment		
Antipyretics	343	85.8
IV fluids	339	84.8
Corticosteroids	212	53.0
Uses of vaccine protect from EVD infection		
Yes	292	73.0
No	108	27.0
Environmental sanitation protects from infection		
Yes	350	87.5
No	50	12.5
Safe sex protects from infection		
Yes	248	62.0
No	152	38.0
Barrier nursing protects from infection		
Yes	333	83.2
No	67	16.8
Cases can be confirmed without laboratory assistance		
Yes	125	31.2
No	275	68.8

*Multiple responses.

Table 7: Knowledge of EVD reporting.

Variable	Frequency	%
Critical number of cases must occur before reporting		
True	174	43.5
False	150	37.5
Not sure	76	19.0
Suspected cases qualify for reporting		
True	322	80.5
False	20	5.0
Not sure	58	14.5
Cases should be reported weekly for administrative efficiency		
True	227	56.8
False	67	16.8
Not sure	106	26.4
*Tertiary health facilities should notify directly		
Federal ministry of health	290	72.5
State ministry of health	211	52.8
Local ministry of health	208	52.0

*Multiple responses.

Table 8: Risk perception and attitude to EVD.

Variable	Frequency	%
Consider self to be at risk		
Agree	156	39.0
Disagree	173	42.8
Undecided	71	18.2
Health workers are prone to having EVD		
Agree	303	75.8
Disagree	51	12.7
Undecided	46	11.5
It is possible to prevent EVD spread		
Agree	318	79.5
Disagree	35	8.7
Undecided	47	11.8
There is no risk in living with EVD patient		
Agree	20	5.0
Disagree	332	83.0
Undecided	48	12.0
Infection control policy of the hospital is inadequate		
Agree	109	27.3
Disagree	42	10.5
Undecided	249	62.2

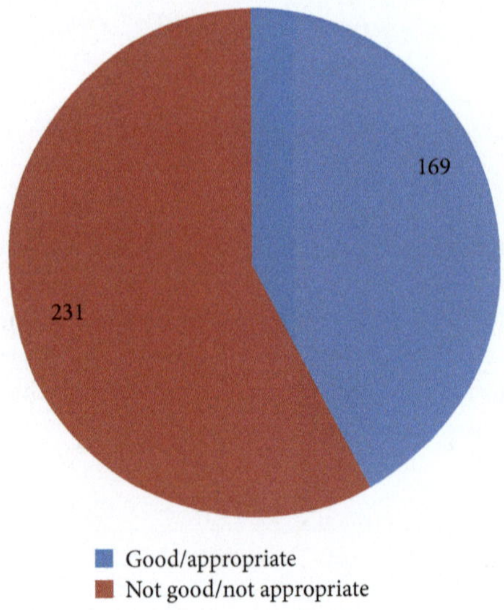

Figure 1: Graded score on EVD knowledge.

4. Discussion

This study assessed the knowledge, attitude, and practice of health workers in a tertiary hospital in the south-western part of Nigeria towards EVD. The health workers that participated included medical doctors, nurses, pharmacists, medical

TABLE 9: Association between respondents' characteristics and knowledge of EVD.

Variable	Knowledge		χ^2	p value
	Appropriate	Not appropriate		
Age (years)				
20–29	58 (43.0)	77 (57.0)		
30–39	78 (47.6)	86 (52.4)	5.720	0.057
≥40	33 (32.7)	68 (67.3)		
Sex				
Male	70 (44.0)	89 (56.0)	0.341	0.559
Female	99 (41.1)	142 (58.9)		
Marital status				
Currently married	111 (42.2)	152 (57.8)	0.001	0.980
Not currently married	58 (42.3)	79 (57.7)		
Occupation				
Medical doctor	53 (54.1)	45 (45.9)		
Nurse	89 (42.6)	120 (57.4)	12.291	0.002
Other health workers	27 (29.0)	66 (71.0)		
Duration of employment (years)				
<10	132 (44.7)	163 (55.3)	2.869	0.090
≥10	37 (35.2)	68 (64.8)		

TABLE 10: Binary logistic regression of respondents' characteristics and EVD knowledge.

Variable	AOR	95% CI	p value
Occupation			
Medical doctor	2.879	1.582–5.239	0.001
Nurse	1.813	1.072–3.065	0.026
Other health workers (ref.)	1		

laboratory technologists, medical record officers, physiotherapists, and community health workers. All these health workers come into contact with patients or their body fluids in the work place. Hence this baseline study determines their preparedness towards EVD. Most participants were young, were females, were married, and had practised less than 10 years. This implies that the participants still had more years to work and hence the necessity to remain healthy in order to perform their health care duties. Also, these health workers could be a source of spread of this life threatening infection to coworkers, their families, and community.

Although most respondents were aware of the EVD epidemic in the West African subregion, some were not aware. This is not acceptable as every health worker should be aware to ensure necessary precautions are taken to reduce the ongoing epidemic and control it whenever such spreads to the facility. This will ensure early diagnosis, management, control, and reporting of such cases to appropriate authority whenever they occur. Colleagues and radio were identified by the participants as their major sources of information. This shows the importance of peers and media in information management. Studies in Nigeria and elsewhere had reported the radio as a valid means of spreading current information to hospital workers as well as the general populace [8, 9].

Over half of the respondents had poor knowledge of EVD. This is probably because as at the time this study commenced, no case was reported in Nigeria. EVD was seen by most respondents as too far away to be a problem. However, this perception about a dangerous infectious disease such as EVD could result in uncontrollable epidemics; hence attitudinal change will be necessary if this must be averted. The World Health Organization had reported several cases of EVD outside the epidemic zone with Nigeria reporting its first case on July 20, 2014 [10]. This study reported that most respondents knew that EVD is caused by a deadly virus while they did not know it can penetrate broken skin. Also, most respondents did not know that EVD has no vaccine presently and were not aware of the process for EVD reporting. This shows the gap in knowledge that must be filled urgently.

Most participants felt that the infection control policy of the hospital was inadequate to protect health workers against EVD. This implies that the hospital authorities must do all that is required to develop a policy targeting EVD.

Occupation was found to be the only predictor of EVD knowledge with medical doctors and nurses having better knowledge more than other health workers. This reflects the training undergone by these groups of workers and the need to strengthen the capacity of other health workers with adequate knowledge of preventing, diagnosing, and managing EVD cases. All health workers need continuous education on EVD. Also, the training should focus on the concept of universal precautions, which must be observed by every health care worker while interacting with every patient [11].

This baseline study is limited by its cross-sectional design and the fact that some respondents could have given socially acceptable answers to some questions. However, this study will serve as a guide for planning and implementing interventions targeted at controlling possible epidemics in the study area.

5. Conclusion

In conclusion, most health workers had inappropriate knowledge about EVD; hence continuous medical education focusing on the concept of universal precautions should target all health workers. Also, an infection control policy targeting EVD is urgently required and emergency preparedness towards possible EVD epidemic is necessary.

Conflict of Interests

The authors declare that they had no competing interests.

Acknowledgments

The authors are grateful to the management of Obafemi Awolowo University Teaching Hospitals and health workers that participated in this study. The authors thank Mr. Anthony Adejuwon for editing this paper.

References

[1] E. Sterk, *MSF Ebola & Marburg Outbreak Control Guidance Manual*, 2008.

[2] C. Comoro and J. Sivalon, "Ebola: fear of the unknown," *Tanzania Health Research Bulletin*, vol. 3, no. 2, pp. 1–4, 2001.

[3] J. Changalucha, "EBOLA: haemorrhagic fever outbreak in Uganda: the Mwanza region experience," *Tanzania Journal of Health Research*, vol. 3, no. 2, pp. 4–6, 2001.

[4] World Health Organization, *Global Alert and Response (GAR): Ebola Virus Disease Update—West Africa*, 2014, http://www.who.int/csr/don/2014_08_15_ebola/en/.

[5] A. Yakubu, M. O. Folayan, N. Sani-Gwarzo, P. Nguku, K. Peterson, and B. Brown, "The Ebola outbreak in Western Africa: ethical obligations for care," *Journal of Medical Ethics*, 2014.

[6] Center for Public Policy Alternatives, *Study on the Ebola Virus Disease (EVD) Knowledge, Attitudes and Practices of Nigerians in Lagos State*, Center for Public Policy Alternatives, 2014.

[7] L. Kish, *Survey Sampling*, John Wiley & Sons, New York, NY, USA, 1965.

[8] V. S. Cozma, *Attitudes and Practices (KAP) Survey on the Ebola Virus Disease (EVD)—Kailahun and Kenema Districts, Sierra Leone*, International Federation of Red Cross and Red Crescent Societies, Geneva, Switzerland, 2014.

[9] O. Adekanle, D. A. Ndububa, S. A. Olowookere, O. Ijarotimi, and K. T. Ijadunola, "Knowledge of hepatitis B virus infection, immunization with hepatitis B vaccine, risk perception, and challenges to control hepatitis among hospital workers in a Nigerian Tertiary Hospital," *Hepatitis Research and Treatment*, vol. 2015, Article ID 439867, 6 pages, 2015.

[10] D. Grady, "With Ebola cases still few, populous Nigeria has chance to halt its outbreak," *The New York Times*, 2014, http://nyti.ms/1mSQTu2.

[11] S. A. Olowookere, A. A. Fatiregun, O. O. Gbolahan, and E. G. Adepoju, "Diagnostic proficiency and reporting of Lassa fever by physicians in Osun State of Nigeria," *BMC Infectious Diseases*, vol. 14, article 344, 8 pages, 2014.

11

Determinants of Adherence with Malaria Chemoprophylactic Drugs Used in a Traveler's Health Clinic

Ibrahim Shady

Community Medicine Department, Faculty of Medicine, Mansoura University, Mansoura 35516, Egypt

Correspondence should be addressed to Ibrahim Shady; ebrshady@hotmail.com

Academic Editor: Marcel Tanner

Background. The WHO recommends mefloquine, atovaquone/proguanil, and doxycycline for malaria chemoprophylaxis. Adherence to a drug is determined by many factors. *Objective.* To detect the determinants of travelers' adherence to malaria chemoprophylaxis. *Methods.* A prospective comparative study was conducted from January 2012 to July 2013 that included travelers (928 travelers) to malaria endemic countries who visited the THC. They were classified into 3 groups: the 1st is the mefloquine group (396 travelers), the 2nd is the doxycycline group (370 travelers), and finally those who did not receive any drugs (162 travelers). The participants from the 1st and 2nd groups enrolled in the study. *Results.* Univariate and multivariate analyses were performed. The predictors for adherence in the mefloquine group were travel to an African destination [OR = 51 (6.8–2385)], higher than a secondary school education [OR = 21 (4.1–144.2)], organized travel [OR = 4 (2.1–6.5)], traveling for leisure [OR = 2.1 (1.1–0.4)], and nationality [OR = 2 (1.11–4.00)]. In the doxycycline group, the predictors included higher than a secondary education [OR = 20.1 (4.5–125.1)], organized travel [OR = 11.4 (5.5–20.9)], travel for leisure [OR = 7 (2.3–22.9)], travel to an African destination [OR = 6.1 (0.41–417)], and nationality [OR = 4.5 (2.3–9.5)]. *Conclusion.* Adherence with malaria chemoprophylaxis could be affected by many factors such as nationality, education, and organized travel.

1. Background

Malaria is an important threat to tourists, employees, and international travelers traveling or working in endemic areas due to the potentially rapid onset of infection and the severity of the disease. International travelers should be protected from malaria by chemoprophylaxis and prophylactic measures against mosquito bites. Chemoprophylaxis is a key component of malaria prevention because none of the vector protection measures completely protect against mosquito bites during night time activities. However, the effectiveness of chemoprophylaxis is limited by lack of compliance with drug intake [1–3].

Malaria chemoprophylaxis has been shown to have a low cost-benefit ratio compared to other prophylactic interventions for travelers [4], and several studies have suggested that increased risks of malaria may occur in noncompliant travelers [5–8]. Among travelers to endemic areas, compliance regarding malaria chemoprophylaxis is generally poor, ranging from 32 to 74% depending on the definitions used [9, 10].

Risk factors that predict noncompliance are important, as they may be used to increase compliance by improving pretravel information. Such risk factors have been studied among European and North American travelers on return flights from Kenya and several West African countries and have included young age, longer travel duration, previous travel to tropical destinations, visits to friends or family as the travel purpose, occurrence of adverse reactions, and use of the drugs [11, 12].

Kuwait is considered a high income country, and its inhabitants commonly travel during the summer period due to hot weather, as the temperature may reach as high as 50°C. Malaria is not endemic in Kuwait but, with a large expatriate population, the number of imported infections increased every year compared with the increased number of recruiting expatriates. However, malaria infection risk is still very low due to the absence of the vector for malaria transmission [13, 14].

Only one traveler's health clinic is available in Kuwait to provide travel health services, which include immunizations, chemoprophylaxis for malaria, and health advice/information about the prevalent diseases/health hazards in the destination country [15].

Two drugs are used for malaria chemoprophylaxis. These drugs include mefloquine hydrochloride (250 mg tab) (generic: mefloquine or lariam), which is given on weekly basis (i.e., every week starting one week before travel and completed at least 4 weeks after leaving the malaria endemic area), and doxycycline (100 mg caps) (generic: vibramycin or doxydar), which is given on daily basis (i.e., one capsule every day starting one day before travel and completed 4 weeks after leaving the malaria endemic area) [16–20].

Many studies have been conducted to identify factors that influence compliance with medications, most of which have focused on treatments to cure, the ability to reduce or delay complications and symptoms caused by chronic diseases. Only a few studies have assessed compliance in the context of chemoprophylaxis. Recently, the concept of adherence has supplanted compliance, as adherence implies that the patient agrees with the prescribed recommendations rather than passively obeying them [11].

The main objectives of this study are to explore the determinants and risk factors affecting the adherence of travelers visiting the THC to malaria chemoprophylactic drugs.

2. Subjects and Methods

Our study is a prospective comparative (analytical) study that included all travelers to malaria endemic areas who visited the THC (928 travelers) to obtain malaria prophylaxis. The study period was from January 2012 to July 2013.

We interviewed 928 travelers who visited the THC to receive their malaria chemoprophylaxis. They consisted of Kuwaitis and residents from other nationalities, mainly Egyptians and Indians, to lesser extent Arabians other than Egyptians, Europeans, Americans, and Asians, and rarely those from South and West African countries. This was consistent with the population demography in Kuwait [21, 22].

All of the 928 travelers were classified on the basis of malaria chemoprophylactic drugs into 3 groups: the 1st group consisted of travelers who received mefloquine (396 travelers, 42.7%), the 2nd group consisted of travelers who received doxycycline (370 travelers, 39.9%), and the last group consisted of travelers who refused to receive malaria drugs or had contraindications to the drugs (162 travelers, 17.5%). The choice of drug was based on many factors, including the traveler's health status, past history of taking the drug without problems, contraindications, and the traveler's decision as reported by Senn et al., 2007, who reported many causes behind travelers' choice of malaria chemoprophylactic drug and the factors that influenced their final decision [19].

Malaria chemoprophylactic drugs were given to all travelers free of charge according to the rules set by the managing department.

All travelers enrolled on this study were interviewed by the same travel health team (physician and/or nurse) and asked to complete a predeparture health questionnaire [20] that included sociodemographic data that consisted of contact information (mobiles, landlines, and emails), travel journey data, and malaria prophylactic drugs.

Fortunately, Kuwait has well-developed communication infrastructure which is cheap and widespread. This communication system enables nearly all of its inhabitants to have more than one mean of communications (emails, mobiles, and landlines). The government holds the control over the landline system which is provided with accepted annual fees for the subscribers. In addition, there are three large mobile providing companies that provide mobile lines in reasonable fees covering all over the country. Also, Internet access is available and it is widely distributed.

We used mobile lines as the first line of communication, followed by landlines and then the Internet. Luckily, most of travelers responded to the mobile contact which is used by some researchers for monitoring the malaria and its treatment [23].

We contacted all of the 766 travelers (there were no defaulters or drop-out cases) who obtained malaria chemoprophylaxis twice after their return (after the 1st week and at the end of the 4th week after their return). They were asked about the regularity with which they took the drug during and after their return. Only those who answered "no" were subjected to another set of questions to determine the factors related to their nonadherence.

Adherence to the chemoprophylaxis regimen was recorded retrospectively according to self-reported use and defined as regular and uninterrupted use of both drugs until the posttravel communication with the travelers [18].

The operational definition of regular and uninterrupted use was not having missed more than one day dose per week on average for the daily dose drug and not having missed any dose of the weekly dose drug. However, the term adherence has recently supplanted compliance, as adherence implies that the patient agrees with the prescribed recommendations rather than passively obeying them [11].

We designed two versions of the questionnaire (Arabic and English). Individuals below 6 years of age were helped by their parents or older brothers/sisters, and individuals who could not understand or complete the questionnaire were assisted in its completion.

Informed consent was obtained from every individual in this study. We obtained approval to conduct our study from the ethical and approval committee of Traveler's Health Board and the head of the department.

The terms adherence and compliance were used interchangeably in this study as compliance constitutes an element of adherence.

2.1. Date Collection and Analyses. Data were collected and analyzed using SPSS for Windows version 17.0 (SPSS, Chicago, IL). Continuous data are expressed as the mean ± SD. Comparisons of the continuous data between the two groups were performed using independent Student's t-tests. All categorical data are expressed in number and percent and were compared between the two groups using Pearson's and Fisher's exact χ^2 tests. The 95% confidence intervals (CI) for the differences in means were calculated. Statistical significance was set at $p < 0.05$. Multivariate analysis was performed to determine the factors that affect adherence to the drug regimens, and the variables of the multivariate analysis were selected from the most significant variables in the univariate analysis.

3. Results and Comments

The sociodemographic and travel-related data of the 928 subjects enrolled initially in this study were obtained and are described in Table 1, which shows that males represent slightly less than 2/3 of individuals in the groups that received mefloquine (group 1) and doxycycline (group 2), but this proportion was inverted for the no chemoprophylaxis group (group 3). Nonnationals represented approximately 60% of the 3 groups. Most travelers in groups 1 and 2 were educated above the secondary level; however, for the 3rd group, postgraduate education was higher. Most of the travelers in the 3 groups were working (80.8% to 87.7%). Many people were travelling for leisure purposes (59.6% to 70.4%) followed by work purposes and then for family visits. Organized trips were more prevalent than independent trips. African countries were the destination of choice for groups 1, 2, and 3 (73.7%, 78.4%, and 59.3%, resp.), followed by Asian countries and Latin countries. The mean age of the travelers was between 32 and 38.5 years, and the mean travel duration was 3.5 to 4.1 weeks.

3.1. Use of Chemoprophylaxis and Adherence. Of the 928 subjects initially enrolled on the study, only 82.5% obtained the chemoprophylactic drugs against malaria, and these individuals were classified into 2 groups; the 1st group was the mefloquine group, and the 2nd group was the doxycycline group. The rates of nonadherence for groups 1 and 2 were 18.4% and 20.5%, respectively [Figure 1]. In the 1st group, most of the nonadherence occurred after finishing travel (27.4% dropped out after the 1st week and 28.8% dropped out after the 4th week) as opposed to the 2nd group (13.2% dropped out after the 1st week and 14.5% dropped out after the 4th week), and the differences were statistically significant ($p = 0.03$). However, a larger proportion of the second group dropped out during travel (32.9%) in contrast to the 1st group (6.8%), and the difference was highly statistically significant ($p = 0.0001$).

3.2. Factors Affecting Adherence to Malaria Chemoprophylaxis. Tables 3 and 4 show the univariate analysis of adherence for the mefloquine and doxycycline groups with the risk factors of interest. Some risk factors were significantly associated with nonadherence in both groups. Nationality significantly affected the degree of adherence, specifically by 2.25-fold in group 1 and 5.1-fold in group 2. Regarding education, after using noneducated individuals as a reference value for comparison, we found that the level of education maximally affected the degree of adherence for individuals with higher than a secondary level of education (24.6- and 22.3-fold for group 1 and group 2, resp.), and the differences were statistically significant ($p = 0.0001$). However, nonadherence was maximal among university educated individuals in groups 1 and 2 (27.4% and 30.3%, resp.), and the differences were statistically significant ($p = 0.005$). Regarding occupation, after using the nonworking group as a reference value for comparison, we found that nonadherence was increased among blue collar workers for groups 1 and 2 (35.6% and 25%, resp.) and the differences were statistically significant ($p = 0.0001$). Additionally, the domestic helper occupation category showed significant nonadherence tendencies in both groups. Traveling for leisure was a very important factor in determining adherence in groups 1 and 2 (71.8% and 67.7%, resp., $p = 0.0001$). Additionally, travel that was organized by an agent affected the tendency for adherence more than travel that was arranged independently, and the difference was statistically significant for both groups ($p = 0.0001$). Travel destination to African countries was a significant factor for adherence and compliance to the drug and its dosing for the complete regimen and produced 53-fold higher adherence for the mefloquine group (group 1) and 8.6-fold higher adherence for the doxycycline group (group 2). The travel duration was also a significant factor for adherence to the given drug ($p = 0.0001$).

Table 5 shows the multivariate analysis for selected risk factors that predicted good adherence for both groups. We

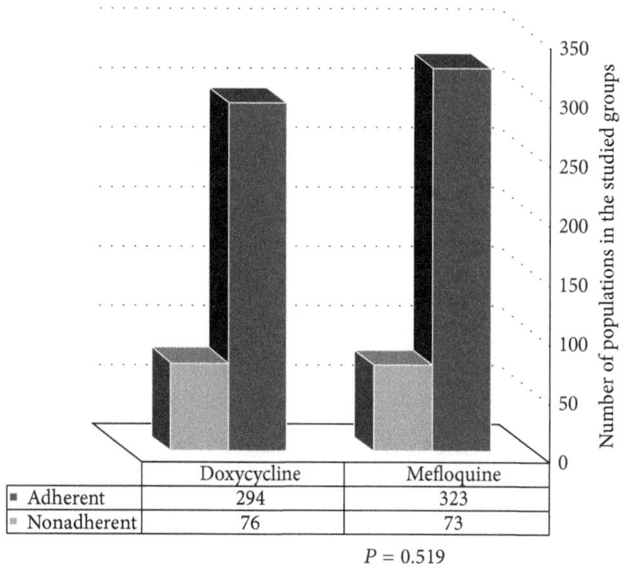

Figure 1: Comparison between the mefloquine and doxycycline groups according to adherence.

TABLE 1: Sociodemographic characteristics of the studied groups.

Characteristic	Mefloquine group		Doxycycline group		No chemoprophylaxis	
	N	(%)	*N*	(%)	*N*	(%)
Total = 928 (100)	**396**	**100**	**370**	**100**	**162**	**100**
Sex						
Male	247	62.4	231	62.4	71	43.8
Female	149	37.6	139	37.6	91	56.2
Nationality						
Non-Kuwaiti	241	60.9	222	60.0	101	62.3
Kuwaiti	155	39.1	148	40.0	61	37.7
Education						
Not educated	11	2.8	15	4.1	5	3.1
Primary, secondary	89	22.5	78	21.1	32	19.8
Above secondary	159	40.2	122	33.0	35	21.6
University	73	18.4	59	16.0	12	7.4
Postgraduate	64	16.2	96	26.0	81	50
Occupation						
Not working	73	18.4	71	19.2	20	12.3
White collar	189	47.7	2.3	54.9	88	54.3
Blue collar	57	14.4	33	8.9	21	13
Domestic helper	77	19.4	63	17	33	20.4
Travel purpose						
Leisure	236	59.6	242	65.4	114	70.4
Family visit	52	13.1	28	7.6	12	7.4
Work	108	27.3	100	27	36	22.2
Travel style						
Independent	120	30.3	96	25.9	36	22.2
Organized	276	69.7	274	74.1	126	77.8
Destination						
Africa	292	73.7	290	78.4	96	59.3
Asia	96	24.2	77	20.8	24	14.8
South America	8	2.1	3	0.8	42	25.9
	Mean	SD	Mean	SD	Mean	SD
Age (years)	38.5	11.9	37.5	12.4	32.6	13.2
Travel duration (W)	4.0	1.0	4.1	1.2	3.5	1.1

TABLE 2: Nonadherence types among the studied groups.

Types of nonadherence	Mefloquine group	Doxycycline group	*P* value	OR ± 95 CI
Not started	12 (16.4)	5 (6.6)	0.05	
Irregular use	15 (20.5)	25 (32.9)	0.08	052 ± (0.25–1.11)
Dropped during travel	5 (6.8)	25 (32.9)	0.0001	0.5 ± (0.05–0.4)
Dropped after 1st week of return	20 (27.4)	10 (13.2)	0.03	2.5 ± (1.1–2.9)
Dropped after 4th week of return	21 (28.8)	11 (14.5)	0.03	2.4 ± (1.1–5.5)
Total	**73 (100)**	**76 (100)**		**149 (100)**

TABLE 3: Univariate analysis of mefloquine group between adherent and nonadherent individuals.

Characteristic	Nonadherent		Adherent		*P* value	OR ± 95 CI
	N	(%)	*N*	(%)		
Total = 149 (100)	**73**	**100**	**323**	**100**		
Sex						
Male	45	61.7	202	62.5	0.4	0.96 (0.57–1.63)
Female	28	38.3	121	37.5		
Nationality						
Non-Kuwaiti	55	75.3	186	57.6	0.002	2.25 (1.28–4.08)
Kuwaiti	18	24.7	137	42.4		
Education						
Not educated*	8	11	3	0.9		
Primary, secondary	17	23.3	72	22.3	0.0005	10.9 (2.32–70.6)#
Above secondary	15	20.5	144	44.6	0.0001	24.6 (5.23–159.3)#
University	20	27.4	53	16.4	0.005	6.87 (1.46–44.3)#
Postgraduate	13	17.8	51	15.8	0.001	10.3 (2.43–45.04)#
Occupation						
Not working*	6	8	67	20.7		
White collar	25	34.2	164	50.8	0.13	0.6 (0.21–1.44)
Blue collar	26	35.6	31	9.5	0.0001	0.11 (0.04–0.28)
Domestic helper	16	21.9	61	18.9	0.01	0.34 (0.12–0.92)
Travel purpose						
Family visit*	18	24.7	34	10.5		
Leisure	34	46.6	232	71.8	0.0001	3.6 (1.8–7.1)
Work	21	28.8	87	26.9	0.01	2.18 (1.03–4.63)
Travel style						
Independent	43	58.9	77	23.8	0.0001	4.6 (2.7–7.8)
Organized	30	41.1	246	76.2		
Destination						
South America*	7	9.5	1	0.3		
Asia	33	45.2	63	19.5	0.004	13.05 (1.57–611.5)#
Africa	33	45.2	259	80.2	0.0001	53.6 (7.96–2485)#
	Mean	SD	Mean	SD	*t*-test	
Age (years)	38.5	11.9	42.6	10.3	0.003	
Travel duration (W)	4.0	1.0	5.2	1.1	0.0001	

*Reference value for comparison.
#Fisher's exact test (chi square).

found that predictors of good adherence for the mefloquine group included travel to an African destination, education above a secondary level, organized travel, traveling for leisure, and Kuwaiti nationality.

However, in the doxycycline group, the predictors included higher than a secondary level of education, followed by organized travel, and then travel for leisure, travel to an African destination, and Kuwaiti nationality.

TABLE 4: Univariate analysis of doxycycline group between adherent and nonadherent individuals.

Characteristic	Nonadherent		Adherent		P value	OR ± 95 CI
	N	(%)	N	(%)		
Total = 396 (100)	**76**	**100**	**294**	**100**		
Sex						
Male	53	69.7	178	60.5	0.07	1.5 (0.87–1.61)
female	23	30.1	116	39.5		
Nationality						
Non-Kuwaiti	65	85.5	157	53.4	0.0001	5.1 (2.66–10.58)
Kuwaiti	11	14.5	137	46.6		
Education						
Not educated*	12	15.8	3	1.0		
Primary, secondary	16	21.1	62	21.1	0.0001	14.9 (3.5–92.1)#
Above secondary	18	23.7	104	35.4	0.0001	22.3 (5.33–135.1)#
University	23	30.3	36	12.2	0.004	6.1 (1.4–37.4)#
Postgraduate	7	9.2	89	30.3	0.0001	46.9 (9.9–320.7)#
Occupation						
Not working*	10	13.2	61	20.7		
White collar	20	26.3	183	63.3	0.2	1.5 (0.63–3.35)
Blue collar	19	25	14	4.8	0.0001	0.12 (0.05–0.32)
Domestic helper	27	35.5	36	12.2	0.0001	0.22 (0.09–0.5)
Travel purpose						
Family visit*	21	27.6	7	2.4		
Leisure	43	56.6	199	67.7	0.0001	13.7 (5.6–36.6)
Work	12	15.8	88	29.9	0.0001	21.1 (7.6–64.3)
Travel style						
Independent	52	68.4	44	15.0	0.00001	12.2 (6.9–22.1)
Organized	24	31.6	250	85.0		
Destination						
South America*	2	2.6	1	0.3		
Asia	20	26.3	57	19.4	0.06	5.6 (0.27–343)#
Africa	54	71.1	236	80.3	0.09	8.6 (0.44–517.1)#
	Mean	SD	Mean	SD	t-test	
Age (years)	37.5	12.4	40.6	9.6	0.02	
Travel duration (W)	4.1	1.2	5.0	1.2	0.0001	

*Reference value for comparison.
#Fisher's exact test (chi square).

TABLE 5: Multivariate analysis of some risk factors in both groups.

Variables	Group			
	Mefloquine group		Doxycycline group	
	Adj. OR	P	Adj. OR	P
Kuwaiti nationality	2 (1.11–4.0)	<0.05	4.5 (2.3–9.5)	<0.001
Above secondary	21 (4.1–144.2)	<0.001	20.1 (4.5–125.1)	<0.001
White collars	0.11 (0.04–0.33)	>0.05	1 (0.5–2.1)	>0.05
Leisure travel	2.1 (1.1–3.4)	<0.05	7 (2.3–22.9)	<0.05
Organized travel	4 (2.1–6.5)	<0.05	11.4 (5.5–20.9)	<0.001
African destination	51 (6.8–2385)	<0.001	6.1 (0.41–417)	=0.05

4. Discussion

This study identified both collective and individual determinants of correct adherence to malaria chemoprophylaxis among individuals travelling to malaria endemic areas and visiting the THC during the period from January 2012 to July 2013.

4.1. Use of Chemoprophylaxis and Adherence. Of the 928 subjects initially enrolled on the study, only 82.5% received chemoprophylactic drugs against malaria due to many factors such as refusing to take the antimalarial drugs due to bad previous experience and/or contraindications to the drugs [19, 24, 25]. Individuals who received the drugs were classified into 2 groups; the 1st group was the mefloquine group, and the 2nd group was the doxycycline group (Table 2).

The rate of adherence for groups 1 and 2 was 81.6% and 79.5%, respectively, as shown in Figure 1. This rate is higher than that reported in the study by Frank G. J. and Anne L. K. (1991-1992), which examined adherence to malaria chemoprophylaxis among Dutch travelers [26] and reported an overall adherence of 59%. This difference may be due to differences in the types of subjects enrolled in the study, as we enrolled all individuals who visited the THC for travel health advice and measures; however, the Dutch study was a part of larger cohort study of health risks among travelers. In addition, our adherence results were higher than those reported by other studies [26–33]. In our study the rates of nonadherence to both drugs were nearly the same which might be due to travelers' beliefs that they had a lower risk of malaria infection on returning to Kuwait due to the fact that malaria is not endemic in Kuwait [14]. Other causes that lead to nonadherence included simply forgetting, fear of long term side effects, discontinuation due to occurrence of unpleasant side effects [such as neuropsychiatric (nightmares, vivid dreams, anxiety, insomnia, and depression), gastrointestinal (heart burns, colic, nausea, and vomiting), and musculoskeletal (easy fatigability, muscle pains, and lassitude)], and busy life style.

In the 1st group, most of the nonadherence occurred after finishing travel (27.4% dropped out after the 1st week and 28.8% dropped out after the 4th week) in contrast to the 2nd group (13.2% dropped out after the 1st week and 14.5% dropped out after the 4th week), and the differences were statistically significant ($p = 0.03$). However, for the second group, more individuals dropped out during travel (32.9%) than in the 1st group (6.8%), and the difference was highly statistically significant ($p = 0.0001$). Our results regarding the mode of nonadherence are much lower than those reported by the Dutch study [26], which indicated that half of all noncompliance was due to early discontinuation after return. More than half of the travelers had stopped their chemoprophylaxis because they found that it was unnecessary to continue the treatments. However, in our study, the lower rate of nonadherence as well as the lower rate of discontinuation, either early or late after return, may be attributed to the travel-related information provided to the travelers during their visits to the THC. Nonadherent individuals reported that they found it inconvenient to continue to take the medications for 4 weeks after return due to their busy schedules. Others believed that they were not exposed to malaria during their travels; however, some individuals experienced unpleasant side effects, as reported in some studies [24, 25].

4.2. Factors Affecting Adherence to Malaria Chemoprophylaxis. A univariate analysis was conducted to determine which factors affect the traveler's adherence to the chemoprophylactic drugs (mefloquine group, Table 3, and doxycycline group, Table 4).

Tables 3 and 4 show the factors of both groups of travelers. Nationality increases the degree of adherence in both groups (by 2.25-fold in the mefloquine group and 5.1-fold in the doxycycline group) which could be attributed to the fact that some non-Kuwaiti individuals usually travel during the holidays to their home countries and they believe that they are not at risk for acquiring malaria. The nationality of the travelers affected the adherence rate through factors such as the belief that malaria is not endemic in the country due to the absence of the vector transmitting it. So, Kuwaitis tended to be nonadherent especially when they return to their home country. Non-Kuwaitis who come from areas where malaria is endemic know the impact of malaria on their health as well as the long duration of treatment so their adherence rate is higher. Non-Kuwaitis from developed countries have a high amount of health information about travel-related health hazards leading them to be more adherent.

Education significantly affected the degree of adherence for both groups, and the maximum difference was observed in individuals with higher than a secondary level of education (24.6-fold and 22.3-fold); however, a university level of education significantly increased the degree of nonadherence in both groups. This could be because those educated above secondary level usually adhere to advice to take a drug due to their psychological condition regarding their health. Also, those educated above secondary level showed an increased level of awareness of antimalarial chemoprophylaxis, which served to motivate them to adhere to the prescribed drug regimens. However, individuals with a university level of education had enormous information regarding the destination, drug, and disease, which helped them to decide whether to follow or not follow our advice. In contrast to our results, Gagneux et al., 1996 [34], found no association between the adherence and the degree of education. Employment status also affected the degree of adherence in both groups, as adherence was insignificantly high among white collar workers in both groups. However, nonadherence was significantly higher among blue collar workers in both groups, which could be because white collar workers are usually highly educated (at least above the secondary level). However, blue collar workers usually do not complete their education level to a secondary level. Degree of adherence among domestic helpers usually is affected by the degree of adherence of their sponsors as they usually accompany their sponsors during their vacations so they usually follow their mode of adherence as well as the type of prophylaxis they got.

Travel for the purpose of leisure significantly affected the degree of adherence in both groups, which could be attributed to the fact that leisure travelers tended to go on safari and other travel-related adventures such as visiting wild life fields and forests and climbing mountains. They believed that these adventures are risky because they occur in open places; therefore, they likely tend to be more compliant than others. In organized travel, where travelers are on an organized trip, they are more likely to be adherent. Similar results were identified in the Dutch study in 1997 [26]. This could be explained because group travelers (organized tours) usually stimulate and encourage all participants to be compliant by social stimulation [26]. Another explanation is that organized tours are usually conducted by highly experienced tourist companies, and they obtain all of the health education materials that contain the risks of the travel destination and how they could be prevented. These companies disseminate this information to their travelers. Travel destinations in Africa significantly promoted adherence in both groups because most travelers to these areas are aware that malaria in African countries is highly endemic and is evenly distributed; therefore, the malaria risk for travelers is the highest in the world [9, 12], which encouraged the high adherence reported in this study. Additionally, travelers to African countries are usually exposed to travel-related hazards as they go on safari, visit open zoos, climb mountains, and live in camps and tents. They believe that such activities increase their risk of getting malaria because they occur in open places. To a lesser extent, travelers believe that the degree of health care in these countries is not high and this makes them more adherent. Also, most trips to African destinations were organized by travel agencies that ask every traveler to provide proof of malaria chemoprophylaxis as a prerequisite for getting an entrance visa. Similar results were reported by other studies [11, 20]. Age > 40 years and travel duration ≥ 5 weeks encouraged travelers to be more compliant, and similar results were reported in other studies [11, 12, 26].

Predictors of good adherence for both groups included five factors that differed in the order and strength for both groups. However, our results are very similar to those of the Dutch study [26]. This study provided valuable information for designing plans to increase adherence for those with a lower adherence rate and to strengthen adherence among those with higher rates of adherence.

5. Conclusion and Recommendations

Adherence with malaria chemoprophylaxis could be affected by many risk factors such as education, organized travel, leisure travel, and travel destination, as well as the duration of travel and the age of traveler. Therefore, adherence with malaria chemoprophylaxis should be improved in travelers to areas with high risks of malaria infection by designing health education programs that must be provided to those travelers in many occasions and periodically.

Travelers' health education programs should be designed with special emphasis on the need for a clear conveyance of the importance of continuing chemoprophylaxis.

Additionally, new methods of traveler education need to be developed and should be based on data from in-depth studies of travelers' motivations to take preventative measures.

Extra attention should be given to young, independent travelers and to those who have been found to show a low rate of adherence and may underestimate their risk of malaria on the basis of their thoughts and beliefs.

Conflict of Interests

The author declares that there is no conflict of interests regarding the publication of this paper.

References

[1] World Health Organization, *Fact Sheet Malaria*, World Health Organization, 2011, http://www.who.int/mediacentre/factsheets/fs094/en/.

[2] M. Henry, I. Diallo, J. Bordes et al., "Urban malaria in Dakar, Senegal: chemosusceptibility and genetic diversity of *Plasmodium falciparum* isolates," *The American Journal of Tropical Medicine and Hygiene*, vol. 75, no. 1, pp. 146–151, 2006.

[3] B. Pradines, P. Hovette, T. Fusai et al., "Prevalence of in vitro resistance to eleven standard or new antimalarial drugs among *Plasmodium falciparum* isolates from Pointe-Noire, Republic of the Congo," *Journal of Clinical Microbiology*, vol. 44, no. 7, pp. 2404–2408, 2006.

[4] R. H. Behrens and J. A. Roberts, "Is travel prophylaxis worth while? Economic appraisal of prophylactic measures against malaria, hepatitis A, and typhoid in travellers," *British Medical Journal*, vol. 309, no. 6959, pp. 918–922, 1994.

[5] H. O. Lobel, J. M. Roberts, B. Somaini, and R. Steffen, "Efficacy of malaria prophylaxis in American and Swiss travelers to Kenya," *The Journal of Infectious Diseases*, vol. 155, no. 6, pp. 1205–1209, 1987.

[6] T. W. Gyorkos, J. E. Svenson, J. D. MacLean, N. Mohamed, M. H. Remondin, and E. D. Franco, "Compliance with antimalarial chemoprophylaxis and the subsequent development of malaria: a matched case-control study," *The American Journal of Tropical Medicine and Hygiene*, vol. 53, no. 5, pp. 511–517, 1995.

[7] P. A. Phillips-Howard, A. Radalowicz, J. Mitchell, and D. J. Bradley, "Risk of malaria in British residents returning from malarious areas," *British Medical Journal*, vol. 300, no. 6723, pp. 499–503, 1990.

[8] R. H. Behrens and C. F. Curtis, "Malaria in travelers: epidemiology and prevention," *British Medical Bulletin*, vol. 49, no. 2, pp. 363–381, 1993.

[9] P. A. Phillips-Howard, M. Blaze, M. Hurn, and D. J. Bradley, "Malaria prophylaxis: survey of the response of British travellers to prophylactic advice," *British Medical Journal*, vol. 293, no. 6552, pp. 932–934, 1986.

[10] H. Kollaritsch and G. Wiedermann, "Compliance of Austrian tourists with prophylactic measures," *European Journal of Epidemiology*, vol. 8, no. 2, pp. 243–251, 1992.

[11] H. O. Lobel, P. A. Phillips-Howard, A. D. Brandling-Bennett et al., "Malaria incidence and prevention among European and North American travellers to Kenya," *Bulletin of the World Health Organization*, vol. 68, no. 2, pp. 209–215, 1990.

[12] R. Steffen, R. Heuser, R. Machler et al., "Malaria chemoprophylaxis among European tourists in Africa: use, adverse reactions and efficacy," *Bulletin of the World Health Organization*, vol. 68, pp. 313–322, 1990.

[13] Kuwait Demographics Profile 2014, http://www.state.gov/r/pa/ei/bgn/35876.htm.

[14] Centers for Disease Control and Prevention (CDC), *Malaria—Malaria and Travelers: Malaria Information and Prophylaxis, by Country*, Centers for Disease Control and Prevention, Atlanta, Ga, USA, 2015, http://www.cdc.gov/malaria/travelers/country_table/k.html.

[15] Ministry of Health, *Ports and Borders Health Division Statistics Book 2007–2010*, Public Health Department, Ministry of Health, Kuwait City, Kuwait, 2010.

[16] E. van den Enden, "Prevention and Treatment of Malaria," Illustrated lecture notes on Tropical Medicine, Edition 2004, Antwerp, Belgium, 2004, http://itg.author-e.eu/Generated/pubx/173/illustrated_lecture_notes_on_tropical_medicine.htm.

[17] F. A. Jacquerioz and A. M. Croft, *Drugs for Preventing Malaria in Travelers (Review)*, John Wiley & Sons, Cochrane Library, 2010, http://www.thecochranelibrary.com/userfiles/ccoch/file/CD006491.pdf.

[18] J. M. Bissonnette, "Adherence: a concept analysis," *Journal of Advanced Nursing*, vol. 63, no. 6, pp. 634–643, 2008.

[19] N. Senn, V. D'Acremont, P. Landry, and B. Genton, "Malaria chemoprophylaxis: what do the travelers choose, and how does pretravel consultation influence their final decision," *The American Journal of Tropical Medicine and Hygiene*, vol. 77, no. 6, pp. 1010–1014, 2007.

[20] WHO, *International Travel and Health Book 2012*, World Health Organization (WHO), Geneva, Switzerland, 2012.

[21] Kuwait Demographics Profile, 2014, http://www.indexmundi.com/kuwait/demographics_profile.html.

[22] The Demographic Profile of Kuwait, 2015, http://www.escwa.un.org/popin/members/kuwait.pdf.

[23] P. Meankaew, J. Kaewkungwal, A. Khamsiriwatchara, P. Khunthong, P. Singhasivanon, and W. Satimai, "Application of mobile-technology for disease and treatment monitoring of malaria in the 'Better Border Healthcare Programme'," *Malaria Journal*, vol. 9, article 237, 2010.

[24] P. Schlagenhauf, A. Tschopp, R. Johnson et al., "Tolerability of malaria chemoprophylaxis in non-immune travellers to sub-Saharan Africa: multicentre, randomised, double blind, four arm study," *British Medical Journal*, vol. 327, no. 7423, pp. 1078–1081, 2003.

[25] E. Petersen, T. Rønne, A. Rønn, I. Bygbjerg, and S. O. Larsen, "Reported side effects to chloroquine, chloroquine plus proguanil, and mefloquine as chemoprophylaxis against malaria in Danish travelers," *Journal of Travel Medicine*, vol. 7, no. 2, pp. 79–84, 2000.

[26] F. G. J. Cobelens and A. Leentvaar-Kuijpers, "Compliance with malaria chemoprophylaxis and preventative measures against mosquito bites among Dutch travellers," *Tropical Medicine and International Health*, vol. 2, no. 7, pp. 705–713, 1997.

[27] N. Resseguier, V. MacHault, L. Ollivier et al., "Determinants of compliance with malaria chemoprophylaxis among French soldiers during missions in inter-tropical Africa," *Malaria Journal*, vol. 9, article 41, 2010.

[28] D. Malvy, T. Pistone, A. Rezvani et al., "Risk of malaria among French adult travellers," *Travel Medicine and Infectious Disease*, vol. 4, no. 5, pp. 259–269, 2006.

[29] G. Ropers, M. D. R. van Beest Holle, O. Wichmann et al., "Determinants of malaria prophylaxis among German travelers to Kenya, Senegal, and Thailand," *Journal of Travel Medicine*, vol. 15, no. 3, pp. 162–171, 2008.

[30] H. O. Lobel, M. A. Baker, F. A. Gras et al., "Use of malaria prevention measures by North American and European travelers to East Africa," *Journal of Travel Medicine*, vol. 8, no. 4, pp. 167–172, 2001.

[31] S. Chatterjee, "Compliance of malaria chemoprophylaxis among travelers to India," *Journal of Travel Medicine*, vol. 6, no. 1, pp. 7–11, 1999.

[32] R. H. Behrens, R. B. Taylor, D. I. Pryce, and A. S. Low, "Chemoprophylaxis compliance in travelers with malaria," *Journal of Travel Medicine*, vol. 5, no. 2, pp. 92–94, 1998.

[33] P. Landry, D. Iorillo, R. Darioli, M. Burnier, and B. Genton, "Do travelers really take their mefloquine malaria chemoprophylaxis? Estimation of adherence by an electronic pillbox," *Journal of Travel Medicine*, vol. 13, no. 1, pp. 8–14, 2006.

[34] O. P. Gagneux, C. U. Blöchliger, M. Tanner, and C. F. Hatz, "Malaria and casual sex: what travelers know and how they behave," *Journal of Travel Medicine*, vol. 3, no. 1, pp. 14–21, 1996.

12

Molecular Characterization of *Leptospira* spp. in Environmental Samples from North-Eastern Malaysia Revealed a Pathogenic Strain, *Leptospira alstonii*

Muhammad Azharuddin Azali,[1] Chan Yean Yean,[2] Azian Harun,[2] Nurul Najian Aminuddin Baki,[2] and Nabilah Ismail[2]

[1] *School of Agriculture Science and Biotechnology, Faculty of Bioresources and Food Industry, Universiti Sultan Zainal Abidin, Tembila Campus, 22200 Besut, Terengganu, Malaysia*
[2] *Department of Medical Microbiology and Parasitology, School of Medical Sciences, Health Campus, Universiti Sains Malaysia, 16150 Kubang Kerian, Kelantan, Malaysia*

Correspondence should be addressed to Nabilah Ismail; drnabilah@usm.my

Academic Editor: Marcel Tanner

The presence of pathogenic *Leptospira* spp. in the environment poses threats to human health. The aim of this study was to detect and characterize *Leptospira* spp. from environmental samples. A total of 144 samples comprised of 72 soil and 72 water samples were collected from markets and recreational areas in a north-eastern state in Malaysia. Samples were cultured on Ellinghausen and McCullough modified by Johnson and Harris media. Leptospires were positive in 22.9% (n = 33) of the isolates. Based on partial sequences of 16S rRNA, a pathogenic leptospire, *Leptospira alstonii* (n = 1/33), was identified in 3% of the isolates followed by intermediate leptospire (*L. wolffii*, n = 1/33, and *L. licerasiae*, n = 7/33) and nonpathogenic leptospire, *L. meyeri* (n = 22/33) in 24.2% and 66.7%, respectively. This study demonstrates the presence of a clinically significant pathogenic *L. alstonii* in the environments which could pose health risks to the occupants and visitors.

1. Introduction

Leptospirosis is one of the most important zoonoses infecting both developing and developed countries in the world [1]. Traditionally, leptospirosis was classified as an occupational disease [2]. Later, leptospirosis was also associated with recreational activities through exposure to the contaminated soil or water [3–5]. An increasing number of people involved in outdoor activities have increased the chances of infection. Pets and rodents are the sources of infection in the housing areas. High density of rats in the markets poses potential threats to visitors and town service workers [6]. The expansion of housing areas also increases the opportunistic contact between humans and the infected wildlife. Environments are frequently associated with nonpathogenic leptospires. However, a novel pathogenic species, *L. kmetyi*, has been isolated from environmental samples in Malaysia [7].

Malaysia is a tropical country with high seasonal rainfall, warm temperatures, and wet and humid climate. These conditions lengthen the survival of leptospires in the environment. It is common that floods occur following heavy rainfall during monsoon season in the East Coast. The presence of leptospires in the environment during flooding may potentially cause an outbreak of leptospirosis. Kelantan which is located in the East Coast of Malaysia is among the affected states. The number of cases increased during flooding from on average 20 cases to 31 cases [8]. Many inhabitants in this state are also involved in agricultural activities which pose the highest risk as 50 cases were reported from the workers in this sector [8]. It was also reported that, in 2011, one death was recorded out of 276 cases [9]. Previously, one death was reported from a waterfall in Kelantan which is Jeram Pasu [10]. In order to identify the potential threats of leptospirosis in the environments, the present study aims to detect and characterize

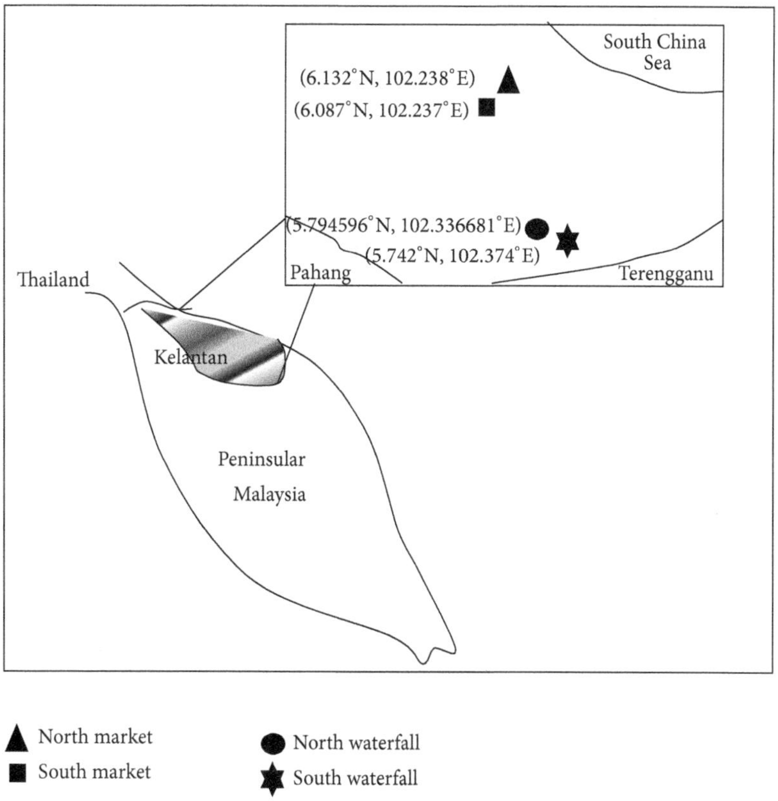

FIGURE 1: Location of sampling sites in north-eastern state of Malaysia.

Leptospira spp. isolated from the selected environments in Malaysia.

2. Material and Methods

2.1. Sampling Sites. Samplings were conducted from December 2012 to November 2013 at the selected recreational areas (waterfalls with spots of running and still water) and markets in the north-eastern state of Malaysia, Kelantan (Figure 1). Those sampling sites, which cover urban and rural areas of three districts, were selected based on previous reports of leptospirosis cases, rat infestations, and improper waste management.

2.2. Isolation of Leptospires

2.2.1. Sample Collection. Water samples in recreational areas were collected from shaded, suspected areas for the presence of animals and in-between rock areas. Water samples were collected about 1 foot below the water surface. Water samples were filtered through 0.2 μm Nalgene® Filter Unit and 40 mL of the samples were transferred into centrifuge tubes and then centrifuged at 4000 ×g, 27°C for 20 mins. Two mL of the samples were inoculated into 5 mL of liquid EMJH media with the addition of 5-fluorouracil (100 μg/mL). For soil samples, sampling locations were selected from wet and shaded areas, from garbage sites, and in the places where spoiled food was spotted. In sterile 50 mL falcon tubes, the soil samples were mixed with sterile water and shaken vigorously. The suspension was allowed to settle for 5–10 minutes before being filtered using 0.2 μm Nalgene® Filter Unit.

2.2.2. Culture of Leptospires. Several drops of the filtrates were inoculated into EMJH media supplemented with antimicrobial agents (5-fluorouracil, 100 μg/mL) and incubated at 30°C in a shaker incubator at 25 rpm to accelerate the growth of leptospires. The presence of leptospires was examined under dark-field microscopy using 20x and 40x magnification daily for 28 days. Leptospires can be distinguished by other spirochetes based on their characteristic thin helical structures with prominent hooked ends and motility.

2.2.3. Culture Purification. In an event of contamination, 1000 μL of contaminated cultures were transferred into fresh liquid EMJH media supplemented with sulfamethoxazole and trimethoprim (40/8 μg/mL), amphotericin B (5 μg/mL), and 5-fluorouracil (100 μg/mL) according to Chakraborty et al., with some modifications [14]. The concentration of trimethoprim was changed from 20 μg/mL to 8 μg/mL and fosfomycin was not added to the media. The cultures were examined under dark-field microscopy using 20x and 40x magnification daily for 28 days. If the contaminants were still present, the cultures were diluted in sterile distilled water using a serial dilution technique starting from dilutions 10^{-3}, 10^{-6}, 10^{-9}, and 10^{-12} and then transferred into solid EMJH media. The diluted culture was incubated for 3 weeks or until the leptospires colonies were observed on plates. Single,

Table 1: List of primers used.

Primer	Targeted genes	Annealing temperature (°C)	Product size	Sequences	Sources
G1	*secY*	55	285 bp	5′-CTGAATCGCTGTATAAAAGT 3′	[11]
G2				5′-GGAAAACAAATGGTCGGAAG 3′	
B64-I	*flaB*		563 bp	5′-CTGAATTCTCATCTCAACTC 3′	
B64-II				5′-GCAAAATCAGATGGACG AT 3′	
Pathogenic gene	*LipL32*	58	120 bp	5′-AGG TCT TTACAGAATTTCTTTCA 3′ 5′-TTACTTAGTCGCGTCAGAA 3′	This study
Sapro 1	*rrs*	55	240 bp	5′-AGAAATTTGTGCTAATACCGAATGT 3′	[12]
Sapro 2				5′-GGCGTCGCTGCTTCAGGCTTTCG 3′	
Bak2-F	16S rRNA	52	796 bp	5′-AGTTTGATCMTGGCTCAG 3′	[13]
Bak2-R				5′-GGACTACHAGGGTATCTAAT 3′	

isolated colonies were transferred from the plates into liquid media using sterile Pasteur pipettes. The cultures were examined under dark-field microscopy daily for 28 days.

2.3. Serological Characterization. The microscopic agglutination test (MAT) was performed using a set of hyperimmune rabbit antisera purchased from the Queensland Health Clinical and Statewide Services, Australia, including Autumnalis, Tarassovi, Pyrogenes, Javanica, Grippotyphosa, Copenhageni, Canicola, Ballum, Hardjoparjitno, Celledoni, Patoc, Djasiman, Icterohaemorrhagiae, Pomona, Australis, and Hebdomadis using the available method [15]. Cultures of 4 to 7 days of age were used as antigens. The turbidity of the cultures was adjusted to 0.5 McFarland. The plates were gently shaken to mix contents, covered to exclude debris and prevent evaporation, and incubated at 30°C for 2 hours. All of the isolates were screened for agglutination at titre ≥1 : 100 under dark-field microscope. Agglutination of at least 50% of the leptospires was considered as positive.

2.4. Molecular Characterization of the Isolates. DNA extraction was performed on isolates by using Qiagen DNeasy® Blood & Tissue Kit (Qiagen, USA) according to the manufacturer's protocols for Gram negative bacteria and stored at 20°C until use. A 20 μL-PCR reaction mixture containing 1x PCR buffer, 2.5 mM $MgCl_2$, 0.16 mM dNTP's premixed, 0.04 μM of each primer, and 0.75 units of Taq Polymerase was used in all PCR amplifications. Amplification was performed in MJ Research thermocycler with an initial denaturation at 94°C for 5 minutes, followed by 30 cycles of 94°C for 30 seconds, annealing for 30 seconds at Ta of the primers (Table 1), and extension at 72°C for 30 seconds. The cycles were then followed by the final extension at 72°C for 5 minutes. Primers G1/G2 and B64-I/B64-II were used to detect the *Leptospira* spp. Primer targeting virulence gene was used for the detection of *lipL32* gene. Bak2 primer pair, targeting 16SrRNA gene, was used for species identification. The primer sets Sapro 1 and Sapro 2 were used to detect the nonpathogenic leptospires. Amplified products were characterized by electrophoresis of 5 μL of each reaction on 1.5% agarose gel for 50 min at 90 V. The PCR product amplified by Bak2 primer pair was purified using QIAquick PCR Purification Kit (Qiagen, USA) and subsequently sequenced using Sanger sequencing kits and instruments supplied by Applied Biosystems®, US, performed by First Base Laboratories (Selangor, Malaysia). The DNA sequences were edited in BioEdit [16] and compared against the GenBank database using BLAST. The 16S rRNA gene partial sequences of all isolates were aligned with the 16S rRNA sequences of the type strains obtained from GenBank by using Multiple Sequence Comparison by Log-Expectation (MUSCLE) in MEGA 6 software [17]. The annotated sequences were submitted to the GenBank.

3. Results

3.1. Isolation of Leptospires. A total of 144 samples comprised of 72 water (markets, $n = 36$; recreational areas, $n = 36$) and 72 soil (markets, $n = 36$; recreational areas, $n = 36$) samples were collected. Out of those samples, 33 were positive for leptospires based on their characteristic morphology and motility. Among positive samples, 7 (5%) were water samples and 26 (18%) were soil samples. A total of 29 positive samples (water, $n = 7$; soil, $n = 22$) were collected from markets and only four positive samples (water, $n = 0$; soil, $n = 4$) were collected from recreational areas.

3.2. Serological Characterization. All of the leptospiral isolates in this study were not agglutinated with any of the reference hyperimmune sera used in MAT (Table 2). Hence, the isolates did not belong to any of the tested serogroups.

3.3. Molecular Characterization. Out of 33 isolates, 18 isolates were detected as *Leptospira* spp. using G1/G2 and B64-I/B64-II primers (Table 2). None of the isolates were found to contain the virulence gene. Molecular identification by 16S rRNA verified that, from 33 positive samples in this study, 31 isolates were identified as *Leptospira* spp. and two isolates were identified as leptospiral closest relatives, *Leptonema illini*. A pathogenic leptospire, *L. alstonii* (3%), was isolated from a soil sample in a market. Eight isolates (24.2%) were identified as intermediate pathogenic species comprised of seven *L. wolffii* and one *L. licerasiae*. A total of 22 isolates (66.7%) were identified as nonpathogenic leptospires, *L. meyeri*.

The phylogenetic tree constructed using the Neighbour-Joining method was illustrated in Figure 2. *Leptospira* spp.

TABLE 2: Results for molecular and serological tests.

Species (n = 33)	G1/G2; B64-I/B64-II (n)	SAPRO1/SAPRO2 (n)	Virulence gene (*LipL32*)	MAT
L. alstonii (n = 1)	1	1	—	—
L. wolffii (n = 7)	—	7	—	—
L. licerasiae (n = 1)	—	1	—	—
L. meyeri (n = 22)	17	22	—	—
Leptonema illini (n = 2)	—	2	—	—
Total (33)	18	33	0	0

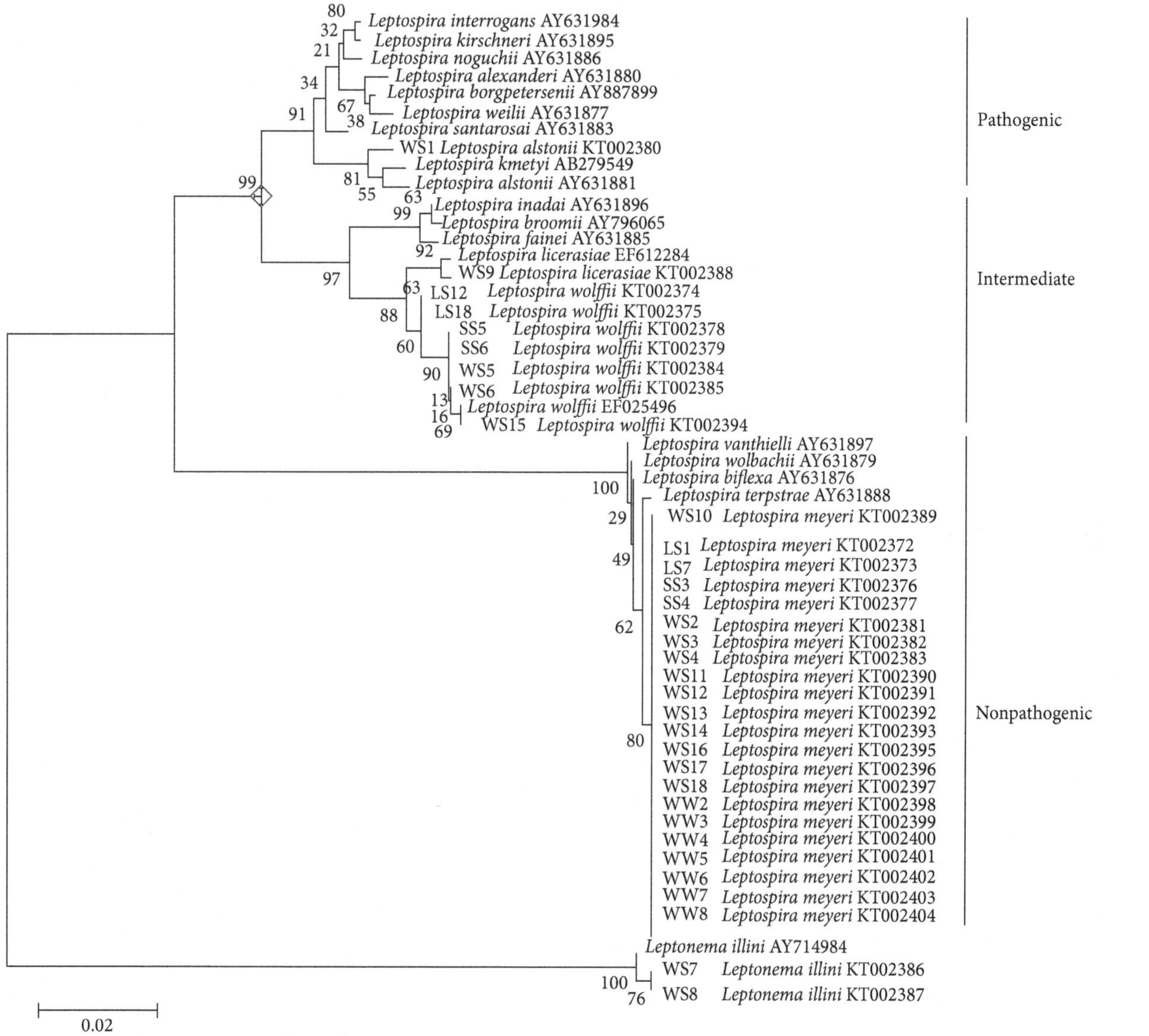

FIGURE 2: A phylogenetic tree generated by the Neighbour-Joining method using MEGA 6 based on 16S rRNA gene sequence of *Leptospira* isolates and the selected strains.

isolated in this study were clearly separated into three clades. Strain WS1 was discovered from soil samples included in the pathogenic clade. It was closely related to type strains of *L. alstonii* and *L. kmetyi*. LS12, LS18, SS5, SS6, WS5, WS6, WS9, and WS15 were grouped into intermediate pathogenic clade. LS1, LS7, SS4, WS1, WS2, WS3, WS4, WS10, WS11, WS12, WS13, WS14, WS16, WS17, WS18, WW2, WW3, WW4, WW5, WW6, WW7, and WW8 were grouped into nonpathogenic clade. These isolates were closely related to type strains of *L. meyeri* and *L. yanagawa*.

4. Discussion

Even though this is not the first study reporting the detection and characterization of leptospiral isolates from environmental samples, its isolation from recreational and market areas would give an impact to the community. Ganoza et al. reported that the prevalence of leptospires in water samples from markets was 67.9% [18]. In the present study, positive water samples from markets were found in 19.4% only. Leptospires may be unable to survive in the drainage water in this market. The water was found to contain detergent and appeared oily, most probably due to its close proximity to the nearby food stalls. It has been reported that 30 ppm of detergent (Ceepryn, Fixanol, and Sapamine) were lethal to leptospires in water in 5 minutes [19]. The prevalence of leptospires in water samples from recreational areas in Malaysia was 11.67% [20]. In the current study, a lower prevalence of 5.56% was noted, which could be due to the effect of inappropriate choice of sampling points. The chosen points may have not been exposed to the leptospiral contamination.

All isolates recovered in this study showed negative reactions to 16 reference hyperimmune sera tested in MAT. Similarly, negative results of MAT for environmental isolates were also reported from another study in which eight isolates from the selected urban sites in Malaysia were negative for a total of 25 hyperimmune sera tested [20]. The availability of the reference hyperimmune sera was very limited because none of local reference laboratories supplies the hyperimmune sera. Since the sera used in this study were procured overseas, the available panel of sera may not cover the circulating local serovar. A total of 37 serovars of *Leptospira* from 13 serogroups have been identified in Malaysia [21]. This highlights the importance of having locally produced hyperimmune sera available for local use.

In our study, G1/G2 and B64-I/B64-II primers detected 18 out of 33 isolates as *Leptospira* spp. However, 16S rRNA gene sequencing identified 31 out of 33 isolates as *Leptospira* spp. G1/G2 and B64-I/B64-II primers were not able to detect all strains of *Leptospira* spp. The occurrence of new strains of leptospires in humans, animals, and environment has increased the need for new primers that are more specific than G1/G2 and B64-I/B64-II. Leptospiral putative virulence gene, *LipL32*, rises as a new target for the detection of pathogenic leptospires though its role in virulence mechanisms remains unknown [22]. This is further complicated by the absence of this gene in pathogenic and intermediate leptospires isolated in this study. This gene was either absence or undetectable by PCR because in some cases the *LipL32* gene was not detectable in *L. licerasiae* by PCR but its product was detectable by both Southern blot hybridization and Western immunoblot [23]. In the previous study by Murgia et al., primer sets Sapro 1 and Sapro 2 were used to detect the saprophytic leptospires [11]. However, these primers were found to be unspecific [11] as pathogenic leptospire, *L. alstonii*, was amplified by this primer in this study.

In this study, a pathogenic species, *L. alstonii*, was isolated from a soil sample in market area. Our finding was in line with previous studies that also isolated *L. alstonii* from the environment [24]. Exposure to the soil in market areas which harboured pathogenic strains may explain the high seropositivity of leptospiral antibodies among garbage collectors and town cleaners in Kelantan [6]. *L. alstonii* was possibly harboured by frogs as it was initially isolated from frogs [25]. The isolation of leptospires from frogs specifically from kidney was reported as early as 1964 [26]. Several pathogenic serovars or serogroups such as bim, Australis, and Ballum have been isolated from frogs [27, 28]. However, inoculation of frogs with pathogenic serovars to establish experimental leptospirosis led to unsatisfactory results as leptospires were not recovered in their organs [29].

The intermediate species, *L. wolffii* and *L. licerasiae*, were isolated from markets and recreational areas. They are able to cause diseases in humans although less frequent [12]. The presence of pathogenic and intermediate species warrants adherence to precautions and preventive measures among the visitors to those areas. It was reported that Malaysians who were involved in recreational activities especially water related are 2.4 times more likely to acquire leptospirosis compared to those who were not involved in similar activities [30]. Leptospirosis was detected in wildlife in Malaysia including wild mammals-monkeys, bats, squirrels, and mongoose [31]. Those animals could be the reservoirs for leptospires in recreational areas located in remote areas.

A previous study reported high numbers of *L. meyeri* (88.1%) from environmental samples [24]. Our study also demonstrated the predominance of *L. meyeri* in Malaysia environment. Though this species was nonpathogenic, there is controversy surrounding *L. meyeri* pathogenicity status. *L. meyeri* serovar ranarum ICF which was previously considered as nonpathogenic was shown to be related to pathogenic strain suggesting that this species consisted of both pathogenic and nonpathogenic strains [32]. This strain was also amplified by sets of primers specific for pathogenic *Leptospira* and not the sets of primers specific for saprophytic strain [11]. This result is also supported by phylogenetic analysis in another study [13]. This disagreement demands a novel typing method of *Leptospira* spp. which covers not only pathogenic species but also intermediate and nonpathogenic strains to resolve the uncertainties in species' designation in the genus of *Leptospira*. The accurate species designation and classification are crucial because the presence of clinically imperative leptospires in the environment would not be overlooked.

Phylogenetic analysis of the studied isolates using 16S rRNA gene sequences concurred with the findings of previous report by Morey et al. in 2006 that the pathogenic, intermediate, and nonpathogenic species each formed one clade [33]. Intermediate groups were closely related to the pathogenic rather than nonpathogenic group. Isolates in the nonpathogenic group were closely related to both *L. meyeri* and *L. yanagawa*. It was reported that species within the nonpathogenic groups were separated by no more than 10 bp [33]. Using the 16S rRNA gene, *L. meyeri* recovered in this study were not separated. In order to demonstrate intraspecies genetic variations, the use of other gene loci is necessary, either singly or in combination. It was also suggested that a cut-off point of 1,000 base pairs (bp) was applied for leptospiral species identification [34]. The phylogenetic analysis of environmental isolates using 16S rRNA was also found to be better than using PFGE profiles.

5. Conclusion

The data presented in this study demonstrates the presence of a clinically significant pathogenic *L. alstonii* and the predominance of *L. meyeri* in the environment. The pathogenic strain was found to not contain one of the highly conserve putative leptospiral virulence genes. Early prevention is required to reduce the risks of infection amongst the population. Hence, continuous control and surveillance are essential in lowering the burden of the disease.

Competing Interests

The authors declare that they have no competing interests.

Acknowledgments

This study was supported in part by the KPI Fund, Universiti Sains Malaysia, Short Term Grant (304.PPSP.61311069) and RU Grant (1001.PPSP.812064).

References

[1] G. Pappas, P. Papadimitriou, V. Siozopoulou, L. Christou, and N. Akritidis, "The globalization of leptospirosis: worldwide incidence trends," *International Journal of Infectious Diseases*, vol. 12, no. 4, pp. 351–357, 2008.

[2] P. N. Levett, "Leptospirosis," *Clinical Microbiology Reviews*, vol. 14, no. 2, pp. 296–326, 2001.

[3] C. Radl, M. Müller, S. Revilla-Fernandez et al., "Outbreak of leptospirosis among triathlon participants in Langau, Austria, 2010," *Wiener Klinische Wochenschrift*, vol. 123, no. 23-24, pp. 751–755, 2011.

[4] S. Brockmann, I. Piechotowski, O. Bock-Hensley et al., "Outbreak of leptospirosis among triathlon participants in Germany, 2006," *BMC Infectious Diseases*, vol. 10, article 91, 2010.

[5] J. Morgan, S. L. Bornstein, A. M. Karpati et al., "Outbreak of leptospirosis among triathlon participants and community residents in Springfield, Illinois, 1998," *Clinical Infectious Diseases*, vol. 34, no. 12, pp. 1593–1599, 2002.

[6] M. N. Shafei, M. R. Sulong, N. A. Yaacob et al., "Seroprevalence of leptospirosis among town service workers in northeastern state of Malaysia," *International Journal of Collaborative Research on Internal Medicine & Public Health*, vol. 4, no. 4, pp. 395–403, 2012.

[7] A. T. Slack, S. Khairani-Bejo, M. L. Symonds et al., "*Leptospira kmetyi* sp. nov., isolated from an environmental source in Malaysia," *International Journal of Systematic and Evolutionary Microbiology*, vol. 59, no. 4, pp. 705–708, 2009.

[8] A. Hanim, "Penyakit kencing tikus meningkat," 2014, http://ww1.utusan.com.my/utusan/Timur/20140106/wt_02/Penyakit-kencing-tikus-meningkat.

[9] Bernama, "Six died from leptospirosis in Kelantan in first six months of 2013," 2015, http://www.mysinchew.com/node/87855.

[10] Kencing tikus: Air Terjun Jeram Pasu lengang, 2013, http://ww1.utusan.com.my/utusan/Timur/20131003/wt_03/Kencing-tikus-Air-Terjun-Jeram-Pasu-lengang.

[11] R. Murgia, N. Riquelme, G. Baranton, and M. Cinco, "Oligonucleotides specific for pathogenic and saprophytic leptospira occurring in water," *FEMS Microbiology Letters*, vol. 148, no. 1, pp. 27–34, 1997.

[12] J. N. Ricaldi, D. E. Fouts, J. D. Selengut et al., "Whole genome analysis of *Leptospira licerasiae* provides insight into leptospiral evolution and pathogenicity," *PLoS Neglected Tropical Diseases*, vol. 6, no. 10, Article ID e1853, 2012.

[13] J. V. Hookey, J. Bryden, and L. Gatehouse, "The use of 16S rDNA sequence analysis to investigate the phylogeny of Leptospiraceae and related spirochaetes," *Journal of General Microbiology*, vol. 139, no. 11, pp. 2585–2590, 1993.

[14] A. Chakraborty, S. Miyahara, S. Y. A. M. Villanueva, M. Saito, N. G. Gloriani, and S.-I. Yoshida, "A novel combination of selective agents for isolation of *Leptospira* species," *Microbiology and Immunology*, vol. 55, no. 7, pp. 494–501, 2011.

[15] J. R. Cole Jr., C. R. Sulzer, and A. R. Pursell, "Improved microtechnique for the leptospiral microscopic agglutination test," *Journal of Applied Microbiology*, vol. 25, no. 6, pp. 976–980, 1973.

[16] T. A. Hall, "BioEdit: a user-friendly biological sequence alignment editor and analysis program for Windows 95/98/NT," *Nucleic Acids Symposium Series*, no. 41, pp. 95–98, 1999.

[17] K. Tamura, G. Stecher, D. Peterson, A. Filipski, and S. Kumar, "MEGA6: molecular evolutionary genetics analysis version 6.0," *Molecular Biology and Evolution*, vol. 30, no. 12, pp. 2725–2729, 2013.

[18] C. A. Ganoza, M. A. Matthias, D. Collins-Richards et al., "Determining risk for severe leptospirosis by molecular analysis of environmental surface waters for pathogenic Leptospira," *PLoS Medicine*, vol. 3, no. 8, pp. 1329–1340, 2006.

[19] S. L. Chang, M. Buckingham, and M. P. Taylor, "Studies on *Leptospira Icterohaemorrhagiae*: IV. Survival in water and sewage: destruction in water by Halogen compounds, synthetic detergents, and heat," *Journal of Infectious Diseases*, vol. 82, no. 3, pp. 256–266, 1948.

[20] D. Benacer, P. Y. Who, S. N. M. Zain, F. Amran, and K. L. Thong, "Pathogenic and saprophytic *Leptospira* species in water and soils from selected urban sites in peninsular Malaysia," *Microbes and Environments*, vol. 28, no. 1, pp. 135–140, 2013.

[21] D. Benacer, S. N. Mohd Zain, F. Amran, R. L. Galloway, and K. L. Thong, "Isolation and molecular characterization of *Leptospira interrogans* and *Leptospira borgpetersenii* Isolates from the urban rat populations of Kuala Lumpur, Malaysia," *The American Journal of Tropical Medicine and Hygiene*, vol. 88, no. 4, pp. 704–709, 2013.

[22] A. Habarta, P. A. E. Abreu, N. Olivera et al., "Increased immunogenicity to LipL32 of *Leptospira interrogans* when expressed as a fusion protein with the cholera toxin B subunit," *Current Microbiology*, vol. 62, no. 2, pp. 526–531, 2011.

[23] M. A. Matthias, J. N. Ricaldi, M. Cespedes et al., "Human leptospirosis caused by a new, antigenically unique *Leptospira* associated with a *Rattus* species reservoir in the Peruvian Amazon," *PLoS Neglected Tropical Diseases*, vol. 2, no. 4, article e213, 2008.

[24] M. Saito, S. Y. A. M. Villanueva, A. Chakraborty et al., "Comparative analysis of Leptospira strains isolated from environmental soil and water in the Philippines and Japan," *Applied and Environmental Microbiology*, vol. 79, no. 2, pp. 601–609, 2013.

[25] L. Smythe, B. Adler, R. A. Hartskeerl, R. L. Galloway, C. Y. Turenne, and P. N. Levett, "Classification of *Leptospira*

genomospecies 1, 3, 4 and 5 as *Leptospira alstonii* sp. nov., *Leptospira vanthielii* sp. nov., *Leptospira terpstrae* sp. nov. and *Leptospira yanagawae* sp. nov., respectively," *International Journal of Systematic and Evolutionary Microbiology*, vol. 63, no. 5, pp. 1859–1862, 2013.

[26] S. L. Diesch, W. F. McCulloch, J. L. Braun, and H. C. Ellinghausen Jr., "Leptospires isolated from frog kidneys," *Nature*, vol. 209, no. 5026, pp. 939–940, 1966.

[27] C. O. R. Everard, D. G. Carrington, H. Korver, R. Burke, J. D. Everard, and C. Gravekamp, "Leptospires in the whistling frog (*Eleutherodactylus johnstonei*) on Barbados," *Journal of Tropical Medicine and Hygiene*, vol. 93, no. 2, pp. 140–145, 1990.

[28] C. Gravekamp, H. Korver, J. Montgomery et al., "Leptospires isolated from toads and frogs on the Island of Barbados," *Zentralblatt fur Bakteriologie*, vol. 275, no. 3, pp. 403–411, 1991.

[29] S. L. Diesch, W. F. McCulloch, and J. L. Braun, "Experimental leptospirosis in frogs," *Nature*, vol. 214, no. 5093, pp. 1139–1140, 1967.

[30] A. A. N. Rafizah, B. D. Aziah, Y. N. Azwany et al., "Risk factors of leptospirosis among febrile hospital admissions in northeastern Malaysia," *Preventive Medicine*, vol. 57, pp. S11–S13, 2013.

[31] S. Thayaparan, I. Robertson, F. Amraan, L. Su'ut, and M. T. Abdullah, "Serological prevalence of leptospiral infection in wildlife in Sarawak, Malaysia," *Borneo Journal of Resource Science and Technology*, vol. 2, no. 2, pp. 71–74, 2013.

[32] D. Postic, N. Riquelme-Sertour, F. Merien, P. Perolat, and G. Baranton, "Interest of partial 16S rDNA gene sequences to resolve heterogeneities between *Leptospira* collections: application to L. meyeri," *Research in Microbiology*, vol. 151, no. 5, pp. 333–341, 2000.

[33] R. E. Morey, R. L. Galloway, S. L. Bragg, A. G. Steigerwalt, L. W. Mayer, and P. N. Levett, "Species-specific identification of Leptospiraceae by 16S rRNA gene sequencing," *Journal of Clinical Microbiology*, vol. 44, no. 10, pp. 3510–3516, 2006.

[34] G. M. Cerqueira, A. J. A. McBride, A. Queiroz et al., "Monitoring Leptospira strain collections: the need for quality control," *American Journal of Tropical Medicine and Hygiene*, vol. 82, no. 1, pp. 83–87, 2010.

13

Perceptions about Eclampsia, Birth Preparedness, and Complications Readiness among Antenatal Clients Attending a Specialist Hospital in Kano, Nigeria

Umar Muhammad Lawan,[1] Idris Usman Takai,[2] and Hamza Ishaq[3]

[1]*Department of Community Medicine, Bayero University and Aminu Kano Teaching Hospital, Kano 700001, Nigeria*
[2]*Department of Obstetrics and Gynaecology, Bayero University and Aminu Kano Teaching Hospital, Kano 700001, Nigeria*
[3]*College of Health Sciences, Bayero University, Kano 700001, Nigeria*

Correspondence should be addressed to Umar Muhammad Lawan; drlawanumarus@yahoo.com

Academic Editor: Marcel Tanner

Background. Eclampsia is a reliable indicator of poor birth preparedness and complications readiness. We determined perceptions about eclampsia, birth preparedness, and complications readiness among antenatal clients in Kano, Nigeria. *Materials and Method.* A cross-sectional design was used to study 250 randomly selected antenatal clients. Data was analyzed using SPSS 16.0. *Result.* The mean age of the respondents was 26.1 ± 6.4 years. The majority perceived that eclampsia is preventable through good ANC (76.4%) and hospital delivery (70.8%). Overall, 66.8% had good perception about eclampsia. Having at least secondary school education and multigravidity were associated with good perception about eclampsia on multivariate analysis. About a third (39.6%) of the mothers was less prepared. On binary logistic regression, good perception about eclampsia and multigravidity were associated with being very prepared for birth. Up to 37.6% were not ready for complications. Half (50.4%) knew at least three danger signs of pregnancy, and 30.0% donated blood or identified suitable blood donor. On multivariate analysis, having at least secondary school education, being very prepared for birth, and multigravidity emerged as the only predictors of the respondents' readiness for complications. *Conclusion and Recommendations.* Health workers should emphasize the practicability of birth preparedness and complications readiness during ANC and in the communities, routinely review plans, and support clients meet-up challenging areas. The importance of girl-child education to at least secondary school should be buttressed.

1. Introduction

Eclampsia is a disturbance of the central nervous system in obstetric patient(s) characterised by seizure activity or coma with or without a prior history of hypertension in pregnancy, proteinuria, and/or oedema (preeclampsia) [1–3]. Eclampsia may occur during pregnancy, child birth, or as long as 3 weeks after birth.

Both preeclampsia and eclampsia account for significant maternal and fetal morbidity and mortality. Eclampsia alone accounts for approximately 50,000 maternal deaths worldwide annually [4]. Its reported incidence ranges from 1 in 100 to 1 in 3448 pregnancies globally [5]. Eclampsia is one of the leading causes of maternal mortality in Nigeria where as many as 545 maternal deaths per 100,000 live births occur annually [1, 2, 6]. The social burden of eclampsia is more marked in less developed nations especially in Africa where precipitating cultures and traditions like early marriage, short birth intervals, hot bath, and use of high osmolar potash gruel/drinks for immediate postpartum mothers prevail; maternal mortality is high and there is poor access to quality antenatal care and essential obstetric care services. Apart from the physical illness and psychological stress from the condition, victims and their families are often stigmatized and discriminated due to the prevailing perceptions that the condition runs in families, it is caused by evil spirits, it occurs as a punishment from God for bad deeds, or because it is perceivably associated with witches and wizards [7–9].

Scientifically, eclampsia is an indicator of poor birth preparedness and complication readiness [10]. Birth preparedness and complication readiness are a strategy designed to promote the timely use of skilled maternal and neonatal care especially during childbirth and on the premise that preparing for childbirth reduces delay in obtaining this care [6]. Birth and emergency preparedness plans should be discussed on first ANC visit, revised by subsequent visits, and finalized by 32nd week of gestation [11]. Birth plan/emergency preparedness plan encompasses the mothers' knowledge of danger signs; the desired place of birth; the birth attendant; and the location of the closest appropriate care facility. Other components of the plan include setting aside funds for birth-related and emergency expenses; a birth companion; support in looking after home and children while being away; transport to a health facility for the birth; transport in case of obstetric complication, and identification of compatible blood donors in case of emergency [6, 7, 12].

Empirical evidence suggests wrong perceptions about eclampsia in Nigeria and other parts of Africa [7–9], and mothers are often less prepared for deliveries or unexpected eventualities associated with pregnancy and child birth [1, 13–15]. This study was therefore to determine perceptions about eclampsia and level of birth preparedness and readiness to complications among antenatal clients attending a specialist hospital in Kano, Nigeria. We used the health belief model to conceptualize how the antenatal clients' perceptions of eclampsia as a proxy for obstetric emergencies influenced their planning for birth and emergencies. Findings from this study would be useful for clinicians, MNCH program managers, and researchers for designing ANC specific and community directed interventions aimed at reducing maternal mortality and morbidity in Nigeria and beyond.

2. Materials and Method

2.1. Setting. The study was conducted in Murtala Muhammad Specialist Hospital (MMSH) located within the ancient Kano city. The hospital serves the inhabitants of Kano state, surrounding states and people from neighboring Nigeria. MMSH has a bed capacity of about 250 and a monthly patients' turnover of about 18,000. About 1400 clients attend the facility for antenatal care each month.

2.2. Study Design, Subjects, and Sample Size. We used a cross-sectional design to study a random sample of 250 antenatal clients attending the ANC clinic in MMSH. The sample size was determined using an appropriate statistical formula for estimating minimum sample size for descriptive studies [16] and 13.4% proportion of women with good perception of eclampsia from a study conducted among major ethnic groups in Borno State, Nigeria [7]. The calculated sample size of 178 was inflated to 250 to compensate for incomplete responses and other contingencies.

2.3. Sampling. A systematic sampling technique was used for selection of the subjects based on the monthly clinic attendance of 1400 and using the ANC register. With a sampling interval of 6 (i.e., 1400/250), 1 in every 6 ANC clients was selected until the required sample size was met. The starting point for selection was determined by picking a random number from the clinic register between 1 and 6. Subsequent respondents were identified by adding the sampling interval to the preceding respondents' serial number on the ANC register until the required sample size was met.

2.4. Instrument and Method of Data Collection. Pretested semistructured interviewer-administered questionnaires were used for data collection. The questionnaire consisted of three sections that elicited the sociodemographic characteristics of the respondents, perception of the clients on causes/risk factors, prevention and management of eclampsia, and birth preparedness and complications readiness of the clients. The questionnaires were administered by four trained interviewers after obtaining informed consent from the mothers. Literate respondents indicated acceptance by signing the consent form, while nonliterate participants affixed their thumbprint. Permission and ethical clearance for the study were also sought and obtained from MMSH and Ethical Committee of Aminu Kano Teaching Hospital, respectively. Data was collected in August/September 2014.

2.5. Data Analysis. Data were analyzed using SPSS version 16.0 computer statistical software. Absolute numbers and simple percentages were used to summarize categorical variables, whereas quantitative variables were summarized using means and standard deviation. The clients' perceptions about eclampsia and birth preparedness and complications readiness were scored and graded using a scoring system adapted from a past study where each correct answer was given one point and wrong response was allocated no point [17]. Accrued points were subsequently graded in percentages. Out of the total of 17 points for perception, respondents that scored 10 to 17 points were adjudged to have "good perception," whereas those that scored 0 to 9 points had "poor perception," In the same vein out of a total of 8 points for preparedness, clients that scored 5 to 8 points were considered to be "very prepared" while those that scored 0 to 4 points were "less prepared." For complications readiness, clients that scored 4 to 7 points out of the total of 7 points were considered to be "ready" for complications whereas those that scored 0 to 3 points were "not ready."

The chi-square test and Fisher's exact probability test were used for bivariate analysis involving categorical variables, and binary logistic regression was used to determine factors that predict good perception of eclampsia, being very prepared for birth, and being ready for complications. A p value ≤ 0.05 was considered statistically significant.

3. Results

3.1. Sociodemographic Characteristics. The respondents' ages ranged from 15 to 40 years with a mean and standard deviation 26.1 ± 6.4 years. The majority of them were in the age bracket 20 to 24 years (29.6%), from Hausa and Fulani ethnic groups (219) (87.6%), married (242) (98.6%),

Table 1: Respondents' social and demographic characteristics.

Characteristic	Frequency (%) ($n = 250$)
Age (years)	
15–19	38 (15.2)
20–24	74 (29.6)
25–29	57 (22.8)
30–34	46 (18.4)
39-40	35 (14.0)
Education	
No education	20 (8.0)
Quranic only	75 (30.0)
Primary	80 (32.0)
Secondary	71 (28.0)
Postsecondary	4 (1.6)
Parity	
Primigravida	58 (23.2)
Multigravida	117 (46.8)
Grand multigravida	75 (30.0)
Ethnicity	
Hausa	179 (71.6)
Fulani	40 (16.0)
Yoruba	9 (3.6)
Igbo	6 (2.4)
Others	16 (6.4)
Marital status	
Married	242 (96.8)
Widowed	8 (3.2)
Occupations	
Unemployed	169 (67.6)
Petty trading	77 (30.8)
Civil service	2 (0.8)
Employed in private sector	2 (0.8)

Table 2: Assessment of the ANC clients' perception about eclampsia.

Parameters/indices	Frequency (%) ($n = 250$)
Believe it is possible to identify causes and risks of developing eclampsia††	189 (75.6)
Perceptions about the causes/risk factors of eclampsia†	
Preexisting hypertension	155 (62.0)
Poor prenatal care	111 (44.4)
Runs in families	35 (14.0)
Poor nutrition	46 (18.4)
Destiny	128 (51.2)
Evil spirits	47 (18.8)
Believe eclampsia is preventable††	210 (84.0)
Perceptions about ways of preventing eclampsia†	
Good antenatal care	191 (76.4)
Hospital delivery	177 (70.8)
Avoiding early marriage	28 (11.2)
Avoiding delivery at ≥35 years	9 (3.6)
Believe that eclampsia can be effectively managed††	195 (78.0)
Perceptions about the best source of treatment for eclampsia†	
Hospital	161 (64.4)
Spiritual/divine intervention	74 (29.6)
Hospital and divine/spiritual intervention	15 (6.0)
Grading of the ANC clients' perception about eclampsia	
Good (10–17)	167 (66.8)
Poor (0–9)	83 (33.2)

† refers to multiple responses: each of the responses given is out of the 250 sample.
†† refers to nonmultiple responses.

unemployed women (169) (67.6%), and with no secondary school level of education (175) (72.0%) as summarized in Table 1.

3.2. The ANC Clients' Perceptions about Eclampsia. The parameters used for assessing the ANC clients' perceptions about eclampsia are as summarized in Table 2. All the respondents had heard about eclampsia or seen some one with the condition. Up to three-quarters (75.6%) believed that it is possible to identify causes or risk factors of developing eclampsia in pregnancy. A significant proportion of them correctly perceived that preexisting hypertension and poor prenatal care are risk factors of the disease. Interestingly, however, some of the ANC clients wrongly perceived that eclampsia occur as a destiny from God (51.2%) or that it is inflicted upon the clients by evil spirits (18.8%). Commendably the majority of the clients perceived that eclampsia is preventable and that good antenatal care (76.4%) and hospital delivery (70.8%) are recognized preventive measures against the condition.

More than three-quarters of the clients (78.0%) perceived that eclampsia can be managed effectively. However, 29.6% and 6.0% claimed that it is best managed through spiritual means/seeking for divine intervention or through a combination of hospital care and divine intervention/spiritual, respectively.

Overall, when the respondents were cumulatively assessed on their perceptions about eclampsia, it was observed that 167 (66.8%) had good perceptions about the condition (Table 2). This study observed that age of the clients more than 24 years, Hausa/Fulani ethnicity, having at least secondary school level of education, and multigravidity were significantly associated with the clients' good perception about eclampsia. On binary logistic regression in a model consisting of these variables, having at least secondary school level of education and multigravidity emerged as the only

TABLE 3: Assesment of the ANC clients' Birth preparedness.

Parameters/indices	Frequency (%) (n = 250)
Can identify signs of normal labour	231 (92.4)
Agreed with spouse on place of delivery	198 (79.2)
Decided with spouse on how to get to place of delivery	183 (73.2)
Saved money for transport and delivery	211 (84.4)
Identified means of transport to desired place of delivery	141 (56.4)
Had made contingency plan on how to get to delivery place if identified means fails	118 (47.2)
Had obtained standing permission from spouse to get to place of delivery	96 (38.4)
Had made arrangement for companion(s) to place of delivery	194 (77.6)
Respondents' grading of Birth preparedness	
Very prepared (5–8)	171 (68.4)
Less prepared (0–4)	79 (39.6)

TABLE 4: Assessment of the ANC clients' complications readiness.

Parameters/indices	Frequency (%) (n = 250)
Knew at least 3 danger signs of pregnancy	126 (50.4)
Donated blood/identified suitable blood donor(s)	75 (30.0)
Saved money for transportation and delivery or in case of complication(s)	211 (84.4)
Obtained standing permission from spouse to go to hospital in case of labour or any complication(s)	96 (38.4)
Identified means of transportation to get to the hospital in case of labour or any complication(s)	141 (56.4)
Identified suitable person(s) to accompany them to hospital in case of labour or complication(s)	194 (77.6)
Had made contingency arrangement with a health worker in case of unexpected delivery at home	236 (94.4)
Grading of the ANC clients readiness to complications	
Ready (4–7)	156 (62.4)
Not ready (0–3)	94 (37.6)

client related factors associated with good perception about eclampsia (Table 5).

3.3. Birth Preparedness and Complications Readiness of the ANC Clients. We assessed the respondents' birth preparedness using nine (9) indices outlined in Table 3. Most of the respondents could identify correctly the signs of normal labour (92.4%) and had agreed with their spouses on choice of place of delivery (79.2%), how to get to the desired place of delivery in case of labour (73.2%), making arrangement for companion to hospital in case of labour (77.6%), and also saving some money for the purpose of transportation to the desired place of delivery, labour, and the accompanying expenses (84.4%). However, only half (56.4%) of the clients went ahead to identify the means of transportation to the hospital when labour starts or made a contingency arrangement on how to get to the place of delivery when the identified means of transportation fails (47.2%). Additionally only about a third (38.4%) of the clients had standing permission from their spouses on getting to the place of delivery when labour starts in their absence. Overall, when the clients were scored based on the preparedness indices, it was observed that about a third of them (79) (39.6%) were less prepared (Table 3). Being very prepared for birth was significantly associated with having good perception about eclampsia and multigravidity. On binary logistic regression, using a model consisting of the respondents' perception about eclampsia, multigravidity, and other important maternal factors including age, ethnicity, and educational status, good perception about eclampsia and multigravidity still emerged as the significant factors that were associated with being very prepared for birth (Table 5).

The ANC clients' readiness for complications was assessed using seven (7) indices outlined in Table 4. Except for the overlapping activities of preparation for normal delivery like saving money for delivery or arranging for companionship to hospital, the clients did not perform most of the indices used to assess their readiness for unexpected complications. Only about half of them (50.4%) knew at least three (3) danger signs of pregnancy, and less than one-third (30.0%) donated blood or identified suitable blood donor in case of emergency. Interestingly, most of the clients examined (94.4%) had made contingency arrangement with a health worker in case of unexpected delivery at home. This study also observed that more than one-third of the clients (37.6%) were not ready for unexpected events during pregnancy or at point of labour (Table 4). On bivariate analysis, clients' readiness for complications was found to be significantly associated with having good perception about eclampsia, being very prepared for birth, older age (age > 24 years), multigravidity, having at least secondary school level of education, and being from Hausa/Fulani ethnicity. When these variables were ran in multivariate analysis, having at least secondary school level of education, being very prepared for birth, and multigravidity emerged as the only predictors of the respondents' readiness for complications (Table 5).

4. Discussion

Antenatal care (ANC) is an important component of preventive care services and those health care providers offering this service can effectively lower and/or eliminate the risk of developing complications associated with pregnancy and delivery through antenatal health care talk (counseling) and possibly by the use of some forms of interventions.

TABLE 5: Factors associated with the ANC clients' perceptions about eclampsia, birth preparedness, and complications readiness.

Characteristic		Bi-variate		Binary logistic regression	
(A) Good perception about eclampsia	($n = 167$) Frequency (%)	Total	Statistical test (p value)	Z test (p value)	OR (95% C.I.)
Age >24 years	101 (60.5)	138	$\chi^2 = 5.67$ (0.017)	1.44 (0.149)	
Hausa/Fulani ethnicity	138 (82.6)	219	Fisher's (0.0002)	1.62 (0.106)	
Having at least secondary education	59 (35.3)	75	$\chi^2 = 6.80$ (0.0009)	2.57 (0.010)	3.06 (1.30, 7.16)
Multigravidity	136 (81.4)	192	$\chi^2 = 6.07$ (0.014)	2.20 (0.028)	2.67 (1.11, 6.37)
(B) Birth preparedness (very prepared)	($n = 171$) Frequency (%)	Total	Statistical test (p value)	Z test (p value)	OR (95% C.I.)
Having good perception about eclampsia	129 (75.4)	167	$\chi^2 = 18.21$ (0.0001)	3.17 (0.002)	2.86 (1.49, 5.49)
Age >24 years	101 (59.1)	138	$\chi^2 = 3.27$ (0.071)		
Hausa/Fulani ethnicity	146 (85.4)	219	Fisher's test (0.080)		
Having at least secondary education	59 (34.5)	75	$\chi^2 = 5.22$ (0.020)	1.67 (0.095)	
Multigravidity	139 (81.3)	192	$\chi^2 = 6.11$ (0.013)	2.18 (0.029)	2.41 (1.09, 5.29)
(C) Ready for complications	($n = 156$) Frequency (%)	Total	Statistical test (p value)	Z test (p value)	OR (95% C.I.)
Age >24 years	94 (60.3)	138	$\chi^2 = 4.29$ (0.038)	1.49 (0.137)	
Multigravidity	133 (85.3)	192	$\chi^2 = 16.65$ (0.0001)	4.03 (0.0001)	17.58 (4.36, 70.85)
Hausa/Fulani ethnicity	129 (82.7)	219	Fisher's test (0.001)	1.49 (0.137)	
Having at least secondary education	55 (35.3)	75	$\chi^2 = 5.46$ (0.020)	2.60 (0.009)	5.15 (1.50, 17.69)
Having good perception of eclampsia	117 (75.0)	167	$\chi^2 = 12.58$ (0.0001)	0.52 (0.606)	
Being very prepared for birth	144 (92.3)	171	$\chi^2 = 109.7$ (0.0001)	5.18 (0.0001)	314.87 (35.78, 2771.24)

4.1. Perceptions about Eclampsia. The major objective of antenatal care is to ensure optimal health outcomes for the mother and her baby. In our study, up to 76.4% of our respondents perceived that the risk of developing eclampsia can be prevented by good ANC as well as hospital delivery (70.8%). Eclampsia has been documented as one of the leading causes of maternal mortality in most Nigerian and other sources of the literature [1, 2, 4–9, 18, 19], and lack of awareness and/or utilization of maternal health care service are identified as leading risk factors for its occurrence [10, 18, 19]. According to Omotara [20], utilization of health care services in general is affected by awareness of the health care seekers. This is because women and their families lack understanding of the danger signs or gravity of the condition or because they do not know where to go to seek help in times of need. This invariably affects their abilities to make informed decision about seeking healthcare and as a result constrains them from exercising their reproductive rights. The average maternal mortality ratio for Kano state in northwestern region of Nigeria is 1600/100,000 live births [19]. This is almost 3 times higher than the national average of 545/100,000 live births [1, 2, 6, 18] and is one of the worst ratios in the world. The 70% wrong perception of eclampsia in our study further buttresses eclampsia as the leading cause of maternal mortality in our locality. This may not be unconnected with the level of higher education of the mothers as only 1.6% of them had postsecondary school education. This finding is particularly important because it reflects the need for improvements in the quality of maternal health care services received in our community. Furthermore, reports indicate that more than one-third of the population of Nigeria live in extreme poverty—defined by the World Bank as earnings of under $1 per day, while 9 out of 10 Nigerians live on less than $2 per day [21]. The zones in the northern part of the country where this study was carried out present the highest vulnerability, with highest proportion of the households experiencing chronic poverty [21]. This report is in keeping with the finding of this study in that majority of our respondents (67.6%) were not gainfully employed, and this may perhaps explain why more than one-third of them will seek spiritual and/or divine intervention in the management of eclampsia.

In our study, overall level of good perceptions regarding eclampsia was very high (66.8%) when compared with only 13.4% reported from a study conducted in Borno State, north-eastern part of the country [7]. This disparity may perhaps be associated with higher exposure of our respondents to maternal and child health issues, either from their educational attainment or from experiences surrounding their high parity. Our findings indicated that those respondents having at least secondary school level of education and multigravidity were more likely to have good perception about eclampsia than their counterparts. They may have perhaps accrued more experience from repeated child bearing and ANC exposures. The high level of good perception of eclampsia recorded in this study is quite commendable because it influenced their health seeking behavior [20]. This is corroborated by the fact that more than three-quarters of the clients studied perceived correctly that eclampsia can be prevented and managed effectively in the hospital.

4.2. Birth Preparedness and Complications Readiness. Birth preparedness is a fundamental component of antenatal care whose aim is to reduce unnecessary delays to seek emergency obstetric care in order to improve maternal and fetal outcomes [15]. Our respondents' performance on the indices used to assess birth preparedness was high, remarkable, and similar to a multicentre study conducted in Nigeria, where it was reported that awareness of the concept of birth preparedness was high [22]. Most of our respondents (92.4%) correctly identified the signs of labour and had agreed with their spouses on choice of place of delivery (79.2%). This is particularly commendable because being aware of when labour starts is a positive step towards activation of the birth preparedness and complication readiness plan. Past studies from parts of Africa and Asia reported lower levels of this stage of preparedness [14, 15, 23]. It is thus critical that all ANC attendees are well knowledgeable about signs of labour in order to gain easy access to skilled attendance at labour and delivery and to reduce and/or eliminate associated complications. Our study also observed that majority of our respondents had saved money for the purpose of transportation to their desired place of delivery. More than half had identified means of transportation to the hospital, and three-quarters had made arrangement for companionship. Similar levels of preparations were reported in previous studies [14, 15, 24]. Sadly, only about a third of our respondents had standing permission from their spouses on getting to the place of delivery when labour starts in their absence. This is not surprising because the majority of the clients studied (87.6%) were from the Hausa/Fulani ethnic group and predominantly Muslims among whom the practice of "purdah" which isolates the woman and encourages subjugation and overdependence on the man is common [18, 25]. In some cultures a woman cannot go to the hospital without the husband's prior permission; thus, even if she is pregnant or in labour and a complication arises, she may likely die at home if her husband is away [18, 25]. Some religions encourage fatalism by attributing every misfortune to the Almighty, thereby unnecessarily resigning themselves to fate rather than take positive steps to help themselves [18, 25].

Overall, up to 39.6% of the clients we examined were less prepared. This proportion is still lower than the 65% less prepared reported from a community-based study from Uganda [26] but slightly higher than the 28.3% reported from southern part of Nigeria [27]. This difference may be a result of sociocultural differences of the populations and perhaps the scale on which the key indices of birth preparedness were assessed.

We also observed that respondents' good perception about eclampsia and multigravidity was strong predictors of birth preparedness. This was similarly reported from Delhi [23] and other parts of Nigeria [27].

Except for the overlapping activities of preparations for normal delivery like saving money for delivery or arranging for companionship to hospital, our respondents did not perform well on most of the indices used to assess their readiness for unexpected complications. While most study participants (94.4%) viewed the occurrence of obstetric complications as a serious matter and noted the importance of saving funds in case of emergencies and had made contingency arrangement with a health worker in case of unexpected delivery at home, more than a third of them (37.6%) were not ready for unexpected events during pregnancy or at point of delivery. This clearly shows that despite high awareness of the need to have funds available, some of our respondents were not able to amass any savings. This is especially true in our locality with high level of poverty [21], where in most cases, poor patients and their families face serious challenges with mobilizing money in cases of emergencies.

Knowledge of the danger signs of obstetric complications is an essential step in recognition of complications and enables one to take appropriate action to access emergency care [10]. Only about half (50.4%) of our respondents knew at least three danger signs of pregnancy; this is in spite of the fact that up to 92.4% of them correctly identified the signs of normal labour. Our finding is commendable and higher than the 6.7% that knew three or more danger signs reported from a previous study from Asia [15]. Although less than one-third (30%) of our respondents donated blood or identified suitable blood donor in case of emergency, the finding is comparable to the 28.7% and 27.8% reported from parts of Asia [15, 23].

We also found that having at least secondary level of education ($p = 0.009$), being very prepared for birth ($p = 0.0001$), and multigravidity ($p = 0.0001$) emerged as the only predictors of the respondents' readiness for complications on multivariate analysis. This finding agrees with that of Hiluf and Fantahun from Ethiopia, where preparation for birth and its complication was found higher among literate mothers, women with parity range of 2 to 4, women with history of stillbirth, and those who were advised about birth preparedness during their antenatal care follow-up [28]. Similarly, a previous study from southeastern Nigeria reported that educational status and high parity of the respondents were the best predictors of awareness of the concept of birth preparedness and complication readiness [24]. Birth preparedness and complication readiness as components of focus antenatal care are an important concept that will significantly reverse the ugly trend of maternal and perinatal morbidity and mortality experienced in our community if strictly followed. Birth preparedness and complication readiness involve not only the pregnant woman, but also her family, community, and available health care providers and hence the need for collaborative efforts of this group of people for a robust, effective, and efficient health care delivery.

Based on the pertinent findings of our study, we recommend that health care workers should strengthen birth preparedness and complications readiness messages by emphasizing their practicability and reinforce this through repeated health education in hospitals during ANC and in the communities. They should routinely review progress made on both components of the plan on each ANC visits and support clients to meet challenging areas. The importance of girl-child education to at least secondary school level should be buttressed during these campaigns.

Conflict of Interests

The authors declare that there is no conflict of interests regarding the publication of this paper.

References

[1] E. A. A. Kuteyi, J. O. Kuku, I. C. Lateef, J. A. Ogudifpe, and B. M. A. Mogbeyteren, "Birth preparedness and complication readiness among pregnant women attending the three levels of health facilities in Ife central L.G. Nigeria," *Journal of Community Medicine and Primary Health Care*, vol. 23, no. 1, pp. 1–2, 2011.

[2] S. A. Starr, *Preventing the Tragedy of Maternal Deaths: A Report on the International Safe Motherhood Conference*, World Bank/WHO/UNFPA, Geneva, Switzerland, 1981, http://apps.who.int/medicinedocs/en/d/Jh2941e/.

[3] A. M. Richards, J. Moodlley, D. I. Graham, and M. R. R. Bullock, "Active management of the unconscious eclamptic patient," *BJOG: An International Journal of Obstetrics & Gynaecology*, vol. 93, no. 6, pp. 554–562, 1986.

[4] P. A. Long and J. N. Oats, "Preeclampsia in twin pregnancy, severity and pathogenesis," *Australian and New Zealand Journal of Obstetrics and Gynaecology*, vol. 27, no. 1, pp. 1–5, 1987.

[5] B. Moller and G. lindmark, "Eclampsia in Sweden, 1976–1980," *Acta Obstetricia et Gynecologica Scandinavica*, vol. 65, no. 4, pp. 307–314, 1986.

[6] JHIPEGO. Maternal and Neonatal Health (MNH) Program, *Birth Preparedness and Complication Readiness: Matrix of Shared Responsibilities*, MNH, 2001, http://www.jhpiego.org/files/bpcrmatrix.pdf.

[7] A. U. El-Nafaty and B. A. Omotara, "Perceived causes of eclampsia in four ethnic groups in Borno State, Nigeria," *African Journal of Reproductive Health*, vol. 2, no. 1, pp. 20–25, 1998.

[8] A. N. Adamu, K. A. Tunau, M. Hassan, and B. A. Ekele, "The perception of patients' relations on the cause of Eclampsia," *Gynecology & Obstetrics*, vol. 4, article 205, 2014.

[9] D. O. Akeju, M. Vidler, O. T. Oladapo et al., "Community perceptions of pre-eclampsia in Ogun State, Nigeria: a qualitative study," *Pregnancy Hypertens*, vol. 5, no. 1, pp. 101–102, 2015.

[10] JHPIEGO. Maternal and Neonatal Health, *Monitoring Birth Preparedness and Complication Readiness, Tools and Indicators for Maternal and Newborn Health*, Johns Hopkins, Bloomberg School of Public Health, Centre for International Communication Programs, 2004, http://www.jhpiego.org/.

[11] K. Barbara and P. Gomez, *Basic Maternal and Newborn Care: A Guide for Skilled Providers*, Jhpiego, Baltimore, Md, USA, 2004.

[12] R. A. McPherson, N. Khadka, J. M. Moore, and M. Sharma, "Are birth-preparedness programmes effective? Results from a field trial in Siraha District, Nepal," *Journal of Health, Population and Nutrition*, vol. 24, no. 4, pp. 479–488, 2006.

[13] Z. Iliyasu, I. S. Abubakar, H. S. Galadanci, and M. H. Aliyu, "Birth preparedness, complications readiness and fathers' participation in maternity care in northern Nigerian community," *African Journal of Reproductive Health*, vol. 14, no. 1, pp. 21–32, 2010.

[14] G. T. Debelew, M. F. Afework, and A. W. Yalew, "Factors affecting birth preparedness and complication readiness in Jimma Zone, Southwest Ethiopia: a multilevel analysis," *The Pan African Medical Journal*, vol. 19, article 272, 2014.

[15] S. M. Mutiso, Z. Qureshi, and J. Kinuthia, "Birth preparedness among antenatal clients," *East African Medical Journal*, vol. 85, no. 6, pp. 275–283, 2008.

[16] S. K. Lwanga and S. Lemeshow, *Sample Size Determination in Health Studies, a Practical Manual*, World Health Organization, Geneva, Switzerland, 1991, http://apps.who.int/iris/handle/10665/40062.

[17] U. Lawan, S. Abubakar, and M. Gambo, "HIV risk behaviors and knowledge of HIV/AIDS and its prevention among unmarried adolescents in Kano Metropolis, Northwestern Nigeria," *Journal of Behavioral Health*, vol. 1, no. 4, pp. 252–259, 2012.

[18] M. Bukar, V. Kunmanda, J. Moruppa, B. Ehalaiye, U. Takai, and D. Ndonya, "Maternal mortality at federal medical centre Yola, adamawa state: a five-year review," *Annals of Medical and Health Sciences Research*, vol. 3, no. 4, pp. 568–571, 2013.

[19] H. S. Galadanci, S. A. Idris, H. M. Sadauki, and I. A. Yakasai, "Programs and policies for reducing maternal mortality in Kano State, Nigeria: a review," *African Journal of Reproductive Health*, vol. 14, no. 3, pp. 31–36, 2010.

[20] B. A. Omotara, "Accesses, affordability and use of health services," in *Proceedings of the Scientific Session of the One Day Symposium Organized by the Nigerian Medical Associations*, Borno State Branch, Musa Usman Conference Centre, Maiduguri, Nigeria, January 1996.

[21] The World Bank, Nigeria Economic Report No. 1, 2013, http://www-wds.worldbank.org/external/default/WDSContentServer/WDSP/IB/2013/05/14/000333037_20130514101211/Rendered/PDF/776840WP0Niger0Box0342041B00PUBLIC0.pdf/.

[22] J. E. Ekabua, K. J. Ekabua, P. Odusolu, T. U. Agan, C. U. Iklaki, and A. J. Etokidem, "Awareness of birth preparedness and complication readiness in southeastern Nigeria," *ISRN Obstetrics and Gynecology*, vol. 2011, Article ID 560641, 6 pages, 2011.

[23] M. Hailu, A. Gebremariam, F. Alemseged, and K. Deribe, "Birth preparedness and complication readiness among pregnant women in Southern Ethiopia," *PLoS ONE*, vol. 6, no. 6, Article ID e21432, 2011.

[24] A. Acharya, R. Kaur, J. Prasuna, and N. Rasheed, "Making pregnancy safer-birth preparedness and complication readiness study among antenatal women attendees of a primary health center, delhi," *Indian Journal of Community Medicine*, vol. 40, no. 2, pp. 127–134, 2015.

[25] National Population Commission, *Nigeria Demographic and Health Survey (NDHS) 2013*, NPC and ICF International, Abuja, Nigeria, 2014.

[26] J. K. Kabakyenga, P.-O. Östergren, E. Turyakira, and K. O. Pettersson, "Knowledge of obstetric danger signs and birth preparedness practices among women in rural Uganda," *Reproductive Health*, vol. 8, article 33, 2011.

[27] A. A. Onayade, O. O. Akanbi, H. A. Okunola, C. F. Oyeniyi, O. O. Togun, and S. S. Sule, "Birth preparedness and emergency readiness plans of antenatal clinic attendees in Ile-ife, Nigeria," *The Nigerian Postgraduate Medical Journal*, vol. 17, no. 1, pp. 30–39, 2010.

[28] M. Hiluf and M. Fantahun, "Birth preparedness and complication readiness among women in Adigrat town, north Ethiopia," *Ethiopian Journal of Health Development*, vol. 22, no. 1, pp. 14–20, 2008.

Newer Classification System for Fissured Tongue: An Epidemiological Approach

Ramachandran Sudarshan,[1] G. Sree Vijayabala,[2] Y. Samata,[3] and A. Ravikiran[3]

[1] *Department of Oral Medicine and Radiology, Best Dental Science College and Hospital, Madurai 625104, India*
[2] *Department of Dentistry, ESIC Medical College and PGIMSR, Ashok Pillar Road, KK Nagar, Chennai 600078, India*
[3] *Department of Oral Medicine and Radiology, SIBAR Institute of Dental Sciences, Guntur 522509, India*

Correspondence should be addressed to Ramachandran Sudarshan; sudharshanram@yahoo.co.in

Academic Editor: Marcel Tanner

Introduction. Fissured tongue is a commonly encountered tongue disorder in dental practice. But there is a lack of data on different pattern, severity, and association of fissuring with various systemic disorders and other tongue anomalies. This study attempts to establish a classification system for fissured tongue and to know the correlation with the systemic health and other disorders of the tongue. *Materials and Methods.* A total of 1000 subjects between the age groups of 10 and 80 years were included in the study. Pattern of fissuring, allied systemic diseases, and related tongue anomalies were tabulated. *Results.* Out of 1000 subjects, 387 subjects presented with fissured tongue. Out of 387 subjects, hypertension was present in 57 cases, 18 subjects had diabetes, and 3 subjects had both hypertension and diabetes. Central longitudinal type was found to be the most common type of tongue fissuring. *Conclusion.* Fissured tongue has been found to be associated with certain systemic disease and further researches are required to know positive correlation. If a correlation exists, such disorders could be diagnosed earlier by identifying fissured tongue at an earlier age.

1. Introduction

In the medical philosophies, the tongue has been believed to be an indicator of health for several decades. Customarily, the tongue is known to be a mirror of the oral and general health. Hippocrates, Galen, and others considered the tongue as the barometer of health [1].

In the oral mucosal disorders, tongue lesions constitute substantial proportions. Variable range of prevalence rates has been reported in the different regions. This difference may get along with racial factors, gender and systemic disorders, and so forth [2].

Fissured tongue is an inherited disorder manifested with grooves that can vary in size and depth. A definite etiology does not exist but a polygenic mode of inheritance is postulated. It is an incidental finding diagnosed during the routine intraoral examination. Usually the fissured tongue is asymptomatic unless entrapment of debris within fissure occurs [3].

The rationale of this present study is a preliminary novel attempt to derive a classification for fissured tongue based on the pattern of fissuring, number of fissures on the tongue, and associated symptoms if any. Further correlation of these findings with the systemic health was also done to find out if any relevance exists.

2. Materials and Methods

The present study was conducted at the Department of Oral Medicine and Radiology, SIBAR Institute of Dental Sciences, Guntur. A total of 1000 consecutive patients among the age groups of 10 to 80 years were included in the study. All the patients were accessible at the hospital for regular checkup and dental treatment. The study was conducted from February 2012 to April 2012 by a single investigator as the fissured tongue is routinely noted as a common finding on intraoral examination [3]. Acquiescence to do the study was obtained from institutional review board and informed consent to take photographs was given by the study subjects. Only those patients who gave the informed consent participated

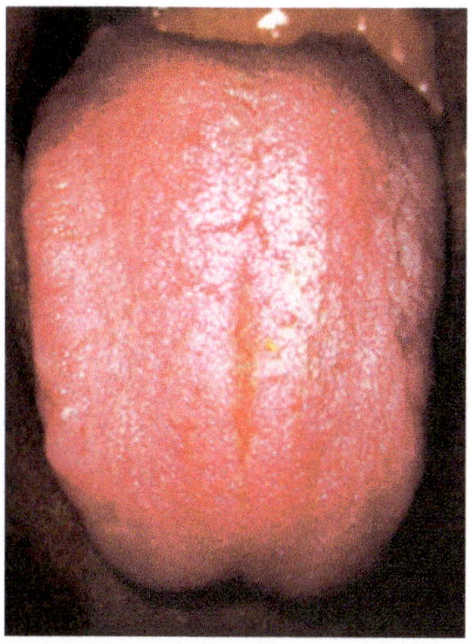

FIGURE 1: Central longitudinal and coated tongue.

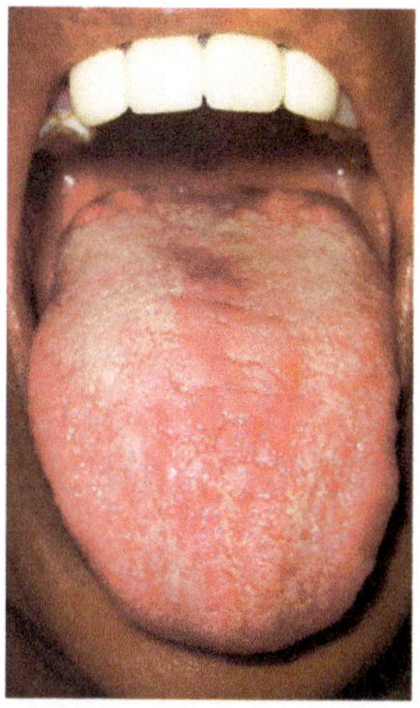

FIGURE 2: Central transverse type.

in the study. A detailed history regarding the demographic data, systemic health, and associated tongue symptoms was recorded. Medical history of the subjects was confirmed after evaluating their recent medical records. The subjects were seated on the dental chair and were examined using mouth mirror and straight probe and under illumination with dental chair light. Study subjects were asked to swish the mouth with sterile water before performing an intraoral examination of the tongue. The study subjects were asked to open the mouth and protrude the tongue as much as possible. The subjects were examined with sterile gloves and sterile gauze was used to hold the tip of the tongue to ease complete examination of the tongue. Clinical analysis regarding the pattern of fissuring of the tongue, number of fissures in tongue, and associated tongue anomalies was recorded. Statistical analysis was performed and a P value < 0.05 was considered to be statistically significant.

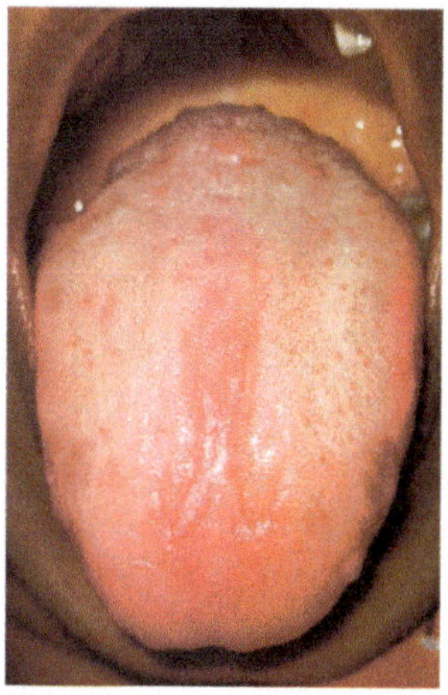

FIGURE 3: Lateral longitudinal type.

3. Results

Out of 387 subjects with fissured tongue, 235 (60.7%) were male subjects and 152 (39.3%) were female subjects.

Based on our observations, we have proposed a novel method of classification and classified fissured tongue as follows.

(1) Based on pattern of tongue fissures.

(a) Central longitudinal pattern in 196 (50.6%) subjects (Figure 1): vertical fissure running along the midline of the dorsal surface of the tongue.

(b) Central transverse pattern in 42 (10.9%) subjects (Figure 2): horizontal fissure/fissures crossing the midline.

(c) Lateral longitudinal pattern in 20 (5.2%) subjects (Figure 3): vertical fissure/fissures running laterally to the midline.

(d) Branching pattern in 68 (17.6%) subjects (Figure 4): transverse fissures extending from the central longitudinal fissure (branching tree appearance).

(e) Diffuse pattern in 61 (15.8%) cases (Figure 5): fissures diffusely distributed across the dorsal surface of the tongue.

(2) Based on number of tongue fissures.

(a) Mild: tongue fissures ranging from 1 to 3 in number.

(b) Moderate: tongue with more than 3 fissures.

(c) Severe: tongue with more than 10 fissures.

(3) Based on associated symptoms such as burning sensation and feeling of food lodgement.

(a) Without burning sensation.

(b) With burning sensation.

The predominantly observed fissuring pattern was the central longitudinal pattern (50.6%) and the least observed

TABLE 1: Correlation between patterning of fissuring and medical history.

Medical history	Pattern of fissuring										Total	
	Central longi.		Central trans.		Branching		Diffuse		Lateral longi.			
	N	%	*N*	%	*N*	%	*N*	%	*N*	%	*N*	%
Hypertension (HTN)	20	35.1	15	26.3	4	7.0	14	24.6	4	7.0	57	100.0
Diabetes Mellitus (DM)	2	11.1	2	11.1	7	38.9	7	38.9	0	0.0	18	100.0
Gastritis	4	44.4	0	0.0	3	33.3	2	22.2	0	0.0	9	100.0
Asthma	0	0.0	3	75.0	1	25.0	0	0.0	0	0.0	4	100.0
Trigeminal neuralgia	0	0.0	0	0.0	1	100.0	0	0.0	0	0.0	1	100.0
Syndrome associated	0	0.0	0	0.0	2	100.0	0	0.0	0	0.0	2	100.0
Epilepsy	0	0.0	0	0.0	0	0.0	1	100.0	0	0.0	1	100.0
HTN + DM	3	100.0	0	0.0	0	0.0	0	0.0	0	0.0	3	100.0
HTN + gastritis	2	100.0	0	0.0	0	0.0	0	0.0	0	0.0	2	100.0
Candidiasis + carcinoma	1	100.0	0	0.0	0	0.0	0	0.0	0	0.0	1	100.0
No medical history	164	56.7	22	7.6	50	17.3	37	12.8	16	5.5	289	100.0
Total	196	50.6	42	10.9	68	17.6	61	15.8	20	5.2	387	100.0

Fisher's Exact Test (<0.001).

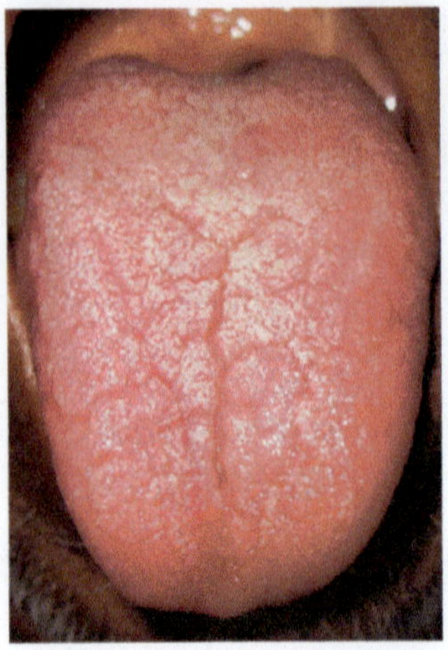

FIGURE 4: Branching type.

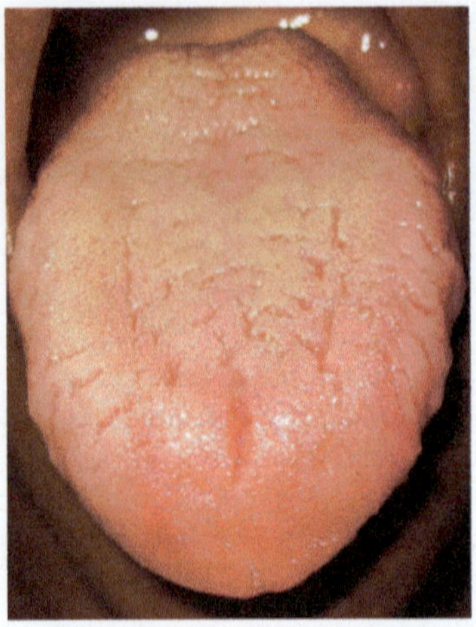

FIGURE 5: Diffuse type.

pattern was the lateral longitudinal pattern (5.2%). Fissuring pattern and number of fissures were correlated with gender (Pearson Chi-Square is 0.528) results depicted that out of 387 subjects 235 were males and 152 were females.

Pattern of fissuring and number of fissures were correlated and the results showed that the majority of mild cases were associated with central longitudinal pattern (76.9%) followed by central transverse (15.3%) and lateral longitudinal (7.8%) patterns. In moderate group of cases, the majority belonged to branching type (95.7%) followed by central transverse type (4.3%). In the severe group of cases, the majority were of diffuse type (96.8%) followed by branching type (3.2%) (Fisher's Exact Test < 0.001).

The majority of patients with fissured tongue were asymptomatic. Out of these 22 subjects, 6 (27.3%) subjects were in central longitudinal and diffuse types, 4 (18.2%) subjects were in central transverse and branching types, and 2 (9.1%) subjects were in lateral longitudinal type.

Pattern of fissuring in patients was correlated with their medical history. Out of 387 subjects with fissured tongue, 289 subjects were without any medical disorder and the remaining 98 subjects had associated systemic history (Table 1). Hypertension was present in 57 subjects, 18 subjects had diabetes, and 3 subjects had both hypertension and diabetes. Several other systemic disorders also coexisted with the occurrence of fissured tongue. In our observation it included asthma, gastritis, trigeminal neuralgia, epilepsy, candidiasis, carcinoma, and Down's syndrome. Several associated tongue disorders have also been observed in the subjects (Table 2).

4. Discussion

Fissured tongue is believed to be a normal variant in fewer than 10% of the population and perhaps genetically oriented.

TABLE 2: Correlation between pattern of fissuring and other tongue disorders.

Other tongue disorders	Pattern of fissuring										Total	
	Central longi.		Central trans.		Branching		Diffuse		Lateral longi.			
	N	%	N	%	N	%	N	%	N	%	N	%
No tongue disorders	188	53.4	37	10.5	63	17.9	48	13.6	16	4.5	352	100.0
Coated tongue	3	18.8	2	12.5	3	18.8	5	31.3	3	18.8	16	100.0
Oral submucous fibrosis	2	66.7	0	0.0	0	0.0	1	33.3	0	0.0	3	100.0
Depapillated tongue	1	33.3	2	66.7	0	0.0	0	0.0	0	0.0	3	100.0
Hairy tongue	0	0.0	0	0.0	0	0.0	1	100.0	0	0.0	1	100.0
Crenated tongue	0	0.0	0	0.0	1	50.0	0	0.0	1	50.0	2	100.0
Ankyloglossia	1	100.0	0	0.0	0	0.0	0	0.0	0	0.0	1	100.0
Lichen planus (reticular)	0	0.0	1	100.0	0	0.0	0	0.0	0	0.0	1	100.0
Geographic tongue	0	0.0	0	0.0	1	33.3	2	66.7	0	0.0	3	100.0
Erythema	1	100.0	0	0.0	0	0.0	0	0.0	0	0.0	1	100.0
Coated tongue + crenated tongue	0	0.0	0	0.0	0	0.0	1	100.0	0	0.0	1	100.0
Coated tongue + leukoplakia	0	0.0	0	0.0	0	0.0	1	100.0	0	0.0	1	100.0
Coated tongue + OSMF + depapillated tongue	0	0.0	0	0.0	0	0.0	1	100.0	0	0.0	1	100.0
Depapillated tongue + angular cheilitis	0	0.0	0	0.0	0	0.0	1	100.0	0	0.0	1	100.0
Total	196	50.6	42	10.9	68	17.6	61	15.8	20	5.2	387	100.0

Fisher's Exact Test (0.001).

The exact cause of fissured tongue is unidentified; nevertheless a polygenic mode of inheritance is alleged because the situation is seen clustering in families [4].

The asymptomatic fissured tongue is frequently perceived during intraoral examination as a subsidiary finding. Fissured tongue may be apparent at birth or become apparent during later stages with varying degree of depth from 2 to 6 mm [4, 5].

Gender based occurrence of fissured tongue was similar to a Libyan based adult population study that depicted that males were commonly affected [6]. But the findings were conflicting with the study conducted in Jordan that depicted that increased prevalence of fissured tongue in female subjects [2].

Fissured tongue has been discussed in the literature based on position as medial and lateral types. Several variations have been proposed in the presentation of grooves or furrows that are typically situated in the dorsolateral area of the tongue. The next pattern is a central fissure with several fissures branches at right angles from the central form. In the severe form, numerous fissures cover the entire dorsal surface dividing the tongue papillae into multiple separate "icelands" or lobules which correlates with our diffuse form of fissure patterning [7].

Burning sensation on the tongue may probably correlate with the systemic factors and poor oral hygiene. Local factors implicated in the etiology are ill fitting prosthesis, infection, parafunctional habits, allergic reaction, xerostomia and galvanism, and so forth [8]. Systemic factors concerned with burning sensation include medication, anemia, esophageal reflux, deficiency of vitamin B complex, zinc, iron, esophageal reflux, and psychological factors [9].

According to the literature, fissured tongue is usually asymptomatic. Few patients complain of mild pain. The circumstance is worsened by entrapment of food particles within the fissures and poor oral hygiene and nutrition [7].

A Hungarian epidemiological survey depicted that fissured tongue was coexistent with diabetes mellitus followed by hypertension [10]. But in our study, most of the systemically debilitated patients had hypertension followed by diabetes. Most of the hypertensive patients had central longitudinal pattern of fissuring which was found to be the common type in patients without any medical history. Reports suggest that an association exists between geographic tongue and fissured tongue [11, 12]. Contradicting to the previous reported studies, coated tongue was found to be more associated with fissured tongue rather than geographic tongue which was similar to the observation of the Jordanian study [2]. Fissured tongue was found to be associated with certain syndromes like Melkersson-Rosenthal syndrome, Coffin-Lowry syndrome, Fraser's Syndrome, Down's syndrome, Oral-Facial-Digital Syndrome Type I, Mohr Syndrome, Pierre Robin Syndrome, Maroteaux-Lamy Syndrome, ECC syndrome, and even Sjögren syndrome [13, 14].

5. Conclusion

This study portrays the newer classification for fissured tongue, its pattern, frequencies of pattern, associated symptoms, and coexisting systemic disorders. The association of fissured tongue with several systemic disorders has to be extensively studied in a larger population to validate its specific relation with systemic illness. Genetic preponderance of fissured tongue should also be extensively investigated. Further, if this genetic preponderance is substantiated in multicentre trials, fissured tongue diagnosed in early stages of life might be supportive of earlier diagnosis of systemic disorders.

Conflict of Interests

The authors declare that there is no conflict of interests regarding the publication of this paper.

References

[1] F. Mojarrad and P. B. Vaziri, "Prevalence of tongue anomalies in Hamadan, Iran," *Iranian Journal of Public Health*, vol. 37, no. 2, pp. 101–105, 2008.

[2] A.-M. Darwazeh and A.-A. Almelaih, "Tongue lesions in a Jordanian population. Prevalence, symptoms, subject's knowledge and treatment provided," *Medicina Oral, Patologia Oral y Cirugia Bucal*, vol. 16, no. 6, pp. e745–e749, 2011.

[3] M. Goswami, A. Verma, and M. Verma, "Benign migratory glossitis with fissured tongue," *Journal of Indian Society of Pedodontics and Preventive Dentistry*, vol. 30, no. 2, pp. 173–175, 2012.

[4] B. S. Kumar, G. Anil, J. Jayarajan, and A. Skaria, "Prevalence of fissured tongue occurring alone and in association with syndromes—a cross sectional study," *Kerala Dental Journal*, vol. 34, no. 1, pp. 26–28, 2011.

[5] S. A. Fuoad and P. Prasad, "Fissured tongue in psoriatic patient—a case report," *Research and Reviews: Journal of Dental Sciences*, vol. 2, no. 1, pp. 1–4, 2014.

[6] S. M. Byahatti and M. S. H. Ingafou, "The prevalence of tongue lesions in libyan adult patients," *Journal of Clinical and Experimental Dentistry*, vol. 2, no. 4, pp. e163–e168, 2010.

[7] M. Rathee, A. Hooda, and A. Kumar, "Fissured tongue: a case report and review of literature," *The Internet Journal of Nutrition and Wellness*, vol. 10, no. 1, 2010.

[8] P. López-Jornet, F. Camacho-Alonso, P. Andujar-Mateos, M. Sánchez-Siles, and F. Gómez-García, "Burning mouth syndrome: update," *Medicina Oral, Patologia Oral y Cirugia Bucal*, vol. 15, no. 4, pp. e562–e568, 2010.

[9] A. Aggarwal and S. R. Panat, "Burning mouth syndrome: a diagnostic and therapeutic dilemma," *Journal of Clinical and Experimental Dentistry*, vol. 4, no. 3, pp. e180–e185, 2012.

[10] T. Vörös-Balog, C. Dombi, N. Vincze, and J. Bánóczy, "Epidemiologic survey of tongue lesions and analysis of the etiologic factors involved," *Fogorvosi Szemle*, vol. 92, no. 5, pp. 157–163, 1999.

[11] J. Jahanbani, L. Sandvik, T. Lyberg, and E. Ahlfors, "Evaluation of oral mucosal lesions in 598 referred iranian patients," *The Open Dentistry Journal*, vol. 3, no. 1, pp. 42–47, 2009.

[12] H. Ebrahimi, S. Pourshahidi, A. A. Tadbir, and S. B. Shyan, "The relationship between geographic tongue and stress," *Iranian Red Crescent Medical Journal*, vol. 12, no. 3, pp. 313–315, 2010.

[13] R. Sharma, P. Narang, Y. G. Reddy, and A. K. Sharma, "A triad of developmental anomalies-an unusual case," *Journal of Clinical and Diagnostic Research*, vol. 7, no. 6, pp. 1264–1265, 2013.

[14] A. R. Shikhman, "The connection between gluten intolerance and Sjogren's syndrome," *Journal of Gluten Sensitivity*, pp. 22–23, 2011.

15

Short-Course Induction Treatment with Intrathecal Amphotericin B Lipid Emulsion for HIV Infected Patients with Cryptococcal Meningitis

Gerardo Alvarez-Uria,[1] Manoranjan Midde,[1] Raghavakalyan Pakam,[1] Pradeep Sukumar Yalla,[1] Praveen Kumar Naik,[1] and Raghuprakash Reddy[2]

[1]*Department of Infectious Diseases, RDT Bathalapalli Hospital, Kadiri Road, Bathalapalli 515661, India*
[2]*Department of Microbiology, RDT Bathalapalli Hospital, Kadiri Road, Bathalapalli 515661, India*

Correspondence should be addressed to Gerardo Alvarez-Uria; gerardouria@gmail.com

Academic Editor: Marcel Tanner

Cryptococcal meningitis (CM) is a common cause of death among HIV infected patients in developing countries, especially in sub-Saharan Africa. In this observational HIV cohort study in a resource-limited setting in India, we compared the standard two-week intravenous amphotericin B deoxycholate (AmBd) (Regimen I) with one week of intravenous AmBd along with daily therapeutic lumbar punctures and intrathecal AmB lipid emulsion (Regimen II) during the intensive phase of CM treatment. 78 patients received Regimen I and 45 patients received Regimen II. After adjustment for baseline characteristics (gender, age, altered mental status or seizures at presentation, CD4 cell count, white blood cells, cerebrospinal fluid white cells, and haemoglobin), the use of Regimen II was associated with a significant relative risk reduction in mortality (adjusted hazard ratio 0.4, 95% confidence interval, 0.22–0.76) and 26.7% absolute risk reduction (95% confidence interval, 9.9–43.5) at 12 weeks. The use of Regimen II resulted in lower costs of drugs and hospital admission days. Since the study is observational in nature, we should be cautious about our results. However, the good tolerability of intrathecal administration of AmB lipid emulsion and the clinically important mortality reduction observed with the short-course induction treatment warrant further research, ideally through a randomized clinical trial.

1. Introduction

Cryptococcal meningitis (CM) is a common opportunistic infection in HIV infected patients with severe immunosuppression. In middle- and low-income countries, the mortality of CM ranges from 55% to 70% [1, 2]. In sub-Saharan Africa, CM accounts for 10–20% of deaths among HIV infected patients [1]. Globally, it is estimated that approximately 957,900 cases of CM occur each year, resulting in 624,700 deaths [1].

The World Health Organization (WHO) recommends two-week induction treatment with amphotericin B deoxycholate (AmBd) and flucytosine or fluconazole, followed by eight-week consolidation treatment with oral fluconazole [3]. However, a two-week treatment with AmBd is not feasible for many resource-poor settings because it is frequently associated with nephrotoxicity and requires a prolonged admission in a health-care facility with frequent monitoring of the renal function and electrolytes [4]. The nephrotoxicity of AmBd occurs mainly during the second week of therapy, and severe renal toxicity is rare when the treatment is shortened to seven days or less [5–7].

Previous studies have shown strong correlation between the rate of fungal clearance in cerebrospinal fluid (CSF) and survival in CM. AmB has a strong fungicidal activity against *Cryptococcus*, but AmBd and lipid formulations of AmB have poor penetration into CSF [8, 9]. To achieve higher concentration in CSF, intrathecal administration of AmB has been used for the treatment of CM in China, and observational studies suggest that it could be associated with improved survival [10]. However, AmBd has a direct irritant effect, and intrathecal administration of AmBd might be poorly tolerated because of inflammation of the meninges and nerve roots [11, 12]. Previous studies in humans and animals indicate that intrathecal administration of lipid formulations of AmB is better tolerated than AmBd [13–15]. Furthermore, data from a murine model suggest that the combination of intravenous antifungal agents with intrathecal administration of liposomal AmB could be beneficial in terms of survival and reduction of fungal load in CSF [16, 17].

The aim of this study was to compare the standard two-week intravenous therapy with an induction regimen including one week of intravenous AmBd and intrathecal AmB lipid emulsion (AmBle), both regimens accompanied by oral fluconazole for two weeks, in patients from a prospective HIV cohort study in India.

2. Methods

2.1. Setting. The Vicente Ferrer HIV Cohort Study (VFHCS) is a prospective cohort study of HIV infected patients who have attended the Rural Development Trust Hospital in Bathalapalli, Anantapur District, AP, India. The VFHCS is registered at ClinicalTrials.gov (number NCT02454569). The hospital belongs to a nongovernmental organization and provides medical care to HIV infected people free of charge. In our setting, 72% of the population live in rural areas [18], and the HIV epidemic is largely driven by heterosexual transmission and it is characterized by low CD4 cell counts at presentation, poor socioeconomic conditions, and high levels of illiteracy [19–21].

2.2. Definitions and Design. All HIV infected patients from the VFHCS database diagnosed with CM from 1 October 2010 to 31 January 2015 were included. Patients who did not complete four weeks of follow-up since the initiation of CM treatment were excluded. There were no other exclusion criteria. The diagnosis of CM was based on the presence of *Cryptococcus* antigens in CSF by latex agglutination [2]. Fungal burden in CSF was not measured. Altered mental status was defined in patients with confusion, disorientation, coma, or low consciousness.

2.3. Treatment. All patients were admitted to the hospital. As in most low- and middle-income countries, flucytosine is not available in India, so fluconazole was used during the induction phase.

Before 15 June 2013, patients were treated with the standard two-week induction treatment with intravenous AmBd 0.7–1 mg/kg and oral fluconazole 1200 mg once daily followed by 600 mg once daily for eight weeks (consolidation phase) and 200 mg once daily thereafter (maintenance phase) [3]. Owing to the lack of disposable manometers, CSF opening pressure was not measured. Therapeutic lumbar punctures with removal of at least 20 mL of CSF (typically 30–40 mL) were performed on alternate days during the first six days of induction therapy, and according to the apparent opening pressure (rapid flow of CSF through the lumbar puncture needle) and patient's symptoms, such as blurred vision, headache, or altered mental status.

The procedure for therapeutic lumbar punctures and the treatment used during the consolidation and the maintenance phases were identical in both groups.

After 15 June 2013, patients received intravenous AmBd 0.7 mg/kg once daily for seven days, intrathecal AmBle 2.5 mg (Amphomul, Bharat Serums and Vaccines, India) once daily for seven days [22, 23], and oral fluconazole 600 mg twice daily for 14 days. Lumbar punctures were performed daily and, after removing at least 20 mL of CSF (typically 30–40 mL), a solution of 0.5 mL (2.5 mg) of AmBle in four mL of 10% dextrose was inoculated slowly into the subarachnoid space. After removing the lumbar puncture needle, patients were asked to lay flat on the bed for one hour. To assess toxicity, patients were asked daily about symptoms related to the local irritating effect of AmB such as lumbar pain, leg pain, vomiting, or retention of urine or stools after the intrathecal administration of AmBle.

AmBle was presented in a vial of 50 mg/10 mL emulsion, so only one vial was used for each patient with CM. The cost of each vial was 1,080 Indian rupees (around 17 USD in March 2015). While the total cost of drugs used in the two-week standard AmB treatment was 3,465 Indian rupees (around 55 USD in March 2015), the total cost of the one-week short-intrathecal AmB treatment was 2,932 Indian rupees (around 47 USD in March 2015).

Patients from both groups received one litre of normal saline solution with 20 mmol of potassium chloride before each infusion of intravenous AmBd [3], and patients not taking antiretroviral therapy (ART) were recommended to initiate ART after four weeks of the initiation of CM treatment. There were no changes in the availability of ART during the two periods of the study.

2.4. Statistical Analysis. Statistical analysis was performed using Stata Statistical Software (Stata Corporation, Release 12.1; College Station, Texas, USA). Time-to-event methods were used. Time was measured from treatment initiation to death. Patients who did not die during the first 12 weeks of treatment were censored at week 12 or at their latest visit date, whatever occurred first. Univariate and multivariate analyses were performed with Cox regression proportional hazard models. The proportional hazard assumption was assessed performing log-log survival curves based on Schoenfeld residuals [24]. In a sensitivity analysis, we also performed a multivariate analysis using flexible parametric survival analysis with three degrees of freedom [25]. The selection of variables included in the multivariate analyses was based on the results of a large cohort study investigating determinants of mortality of HIV-associated cryptococcal meningitis and the availability of data in our cohort [26]. The study was approved by the Ethics Committee of the Rural Development Trust Hospital.

3. Results

3.1. Study Population. During the study period, 126 patients were treated from CM. Two patients who received the standard AmB regimen and one patient who received the

TABLE 1: Baseline characteristics by treatment group.

	Value	Standard Rx (n = 78)	Short i.t. Rx (n = 45)	P value
Gender	Male	53 (67.95)	35 (77.78)	0.245
	Female	25 (32.05)	10 (22.22)	
Abnormal mental status or seizures	No	51 (65.38)	36 (80)	0.086
	Yes	27 (34.62)	9 (20)	
On antiretroviral therapy	No	39 (50)	20 (44.44)	0.552
	Yes	39 (50)	25 (55.56)	
CD4 cell count (cells/μL)	0–25	20 (25.64)	10 (22.22)	0.753
	26–50	18 (23.08)	12 (26.67)	
	51–100	11 (14.1)	9 (20)	
	>100	29 (37.18)	14 (31.11)	
Age, mean (SD)	Years	36.72 (9.25)	38.29 (9.13)	0.362
White blood cells, mean (SD)	Cells/nL	6.24 (4.74)	6.42 (5.71)	0.862
Hemoglobin, mean (SD)	g/dL	9.18 (2.49)	9.43 (1.9)	0.538
CSF white cells, median (IQR)	Cells/mL	17 (6–76)	16 (4–40)	0.52

CSF: cerebrospinal fluid; IQR: interquartile range; i.t.: intrathecal; Rx: treatment.
Data are presented as number (%) unless otherwise indicated. Standard Rx: two-week intravenous amphotericin B deoxycholate (AmBd). Short i.t. Rx: one week of intravenous AmBd and intrathecal AmB lipid emulsion. P values were calculated using Chi^2 test for categorical variables and t-test (not assuming equal variances) for continuous variables.

short-intrathecal AmB regimen did not complete four weeks of follow-up and were excluded. 123 patients were included in the final analysis, 78 patients in the standard AmB regimen group, and 45 patients in the short-intrathecal AmB regimen group. Baseline characteristics and between group differences are described in Table 1. We did not find significant differences between groups, although the proportion of patients with altered mental status or seizures was higher in the standard AmB regimen group (34.6% versus 22%, P value = 0.086). Of those not on ART at the time of starting CM treatment, the median time from CM treatment to initiation of ART was 35 days (interquartile range: 29–51) in the standard AmB regimen group and 36 days (interquartile range: 26–48) in the short-intrathecal AmB regimen group.

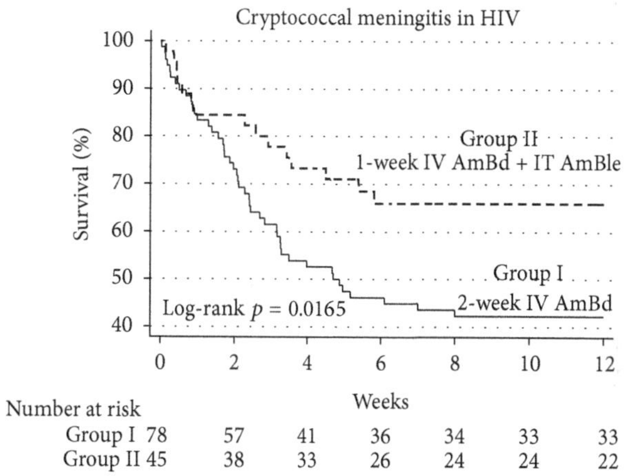

FIGURE 1: Kaplan-Meier survival estimates by treatment group. IV AmBd, intravenous amphotericin B deoxycholate. IT AmBle, intrathecal amphotericin B lipid emulsion.

3.2. Mortality. Sixty patients died during the study period, 45 in standard AmB group, and 15 in the short-intrathecal group. Kaplan-Meier survival estimates by treatment group are shown in Figure 1. Compared with patients who received the standard AmB regimen, patients in the short-intrathecal AmB regimen group had significant lower mortality (P = 0.0165). Univariate and multivariate analyses of factors associated with mortality are described in Table 2. Compared with the standard AmB regimen, patients who received the short-intrathecal AmB regimen had a significant lower risk of death in univariate (hazard ratio (HR) 0.5, 95% confidence interval [CI], 0.28–0.89, P = 0.019) and multivariate analyses (adjusted HR 0.4, 95% CI, 0.22–0.76, P = 0.005). We also performed a multivariate analysis using flexible parametric survival methods, showing similar results (adjusted HR 0.4, 95% CI, 0.21–0.75, P = 0.004). Adjusted risk differences and numbers needed to treat are shown in Figure 2. The use of the short-intrathecal AmB regimen was associated with a 26.7% absolute risk reduction (95% CI, 9.9–43.5) in mortality at 12 weeks.

3.3. Tolerability of Intrathecal AmBle. Intrathecal administration of AmBle was well tolerated. We did not observe drug adverse reactions described in previous studies using intrathecal AmBd such as lumbar pain, leg pain, vomiting, prostration, or altered mental status [11, 12]. Of 45 patients in the short-intrathecal AmB regimen group, only one patient developed acute urinary retention, which resolved after one day.

4. Discussion

In this observational cohort study in a resource-limited setting, the use of a short-course intravenous AmBd regimen along with intrathecal AmBle was well tolerated and was associated with a clinically important reduction in mortality

TABLE 2: Univariate and multivariate analysis of factors associated with mortality using Cox proportional hazard methods.

	Hazard ratio	Adjusted hazard ratio
Female	0.794 (0.442–1.424)	0.800 (0.431–1.484)
AMS or seizures	2.337* (1.394–3.918)	1.716 (0.982–2.998)
CD4 count (cells/mcl)		
0–25	1 (reference)	1 (reference)
26–50	1.115 (0.551–2.255)	0.875 (0.405–1.892)
51–100	0.903 (0.395–2.064)	1.116 (0.476–2.614)
>100	1.020 (0.522–1.993)	0.970 (0.487–1.934)
On ART	0.896 (0.54–1.486)	1.012 (0.588–1.739)
Age (years)	1.015 (0.989–1.043)	1.013 (0.985–1.042)
WBC (cells/nL)	1.097* (1.054–1.143)	1.147* (1.092–1.204)
Haemoglobin (g/dL)	0.922 (0.820–1.036)	0.860* (0.758–0.976)
CSF WC (cells/mL)	0.995* (0.991–0.999)	0.995* (0.992–0.999)
Treatment		
Standard	1 (reference)	1 (reference)
Short i.t. course	0.496* (0.276–0.890)	0.403* (0.215–0.756)

*P value < 0.05. AMS: altered mental status; ART: antiretroviral therapy; CSF WC: cerebrospinal fluid white cells; i.t.: intrathecal; Rx: treatment; WBC: white blood cells.

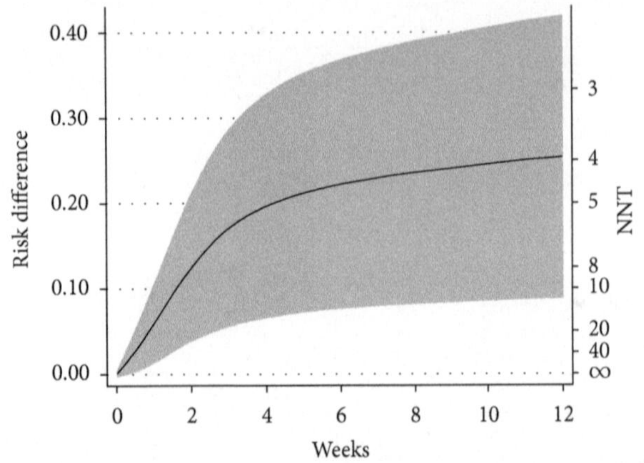

FIGURE 2: Adjusted risk difference and number needed to treat using flexible parametric survival methods. NNT: number needed to treat.

compared with the standard of care in low- and middle-income countries.

The WHO recommends two weeks of intravenous AmBd and flucytosine or fluconazole during the intensive phase of CM treatment. However, this regimen is impractical in resource-poor settings because of the cost of medicines and hospital care [4]. Therefore, fluconazole monotherapy is the treatment most commonly used in low- and middle-income countries, albeit its lower efficacy compared with AmB regimens [4]. The short-intrathecal AmB regimen was associated not only with an increased survival but also with a lower cost in terms of days of hospitalization and drugs. In addition, one week of intravenous AmBd could be given safely without laboratory monitoring, as long as hydration and potassium supplements are provided [7, 27].

Unlike previous experiences with intrathecal AmBd [11, 12], intrathecal AmBle was very well tolerated, and only one patient developed a transient urinary retention. This is in accordance with the case reports of patients receiving other lipid forms of AmB intrathecally and with the results from animal models [13–15, 17]. To our knowledge, this is one of the first studies investigating the effectivity of a lipid form of AmB administered intrathecally in CM. A previous study performed in mice showed that combination therapy including intrathecal liposomal AmB and fluconazole was able to reduce mortality compared with intravenous liposomal AmB monotherapy [16]. Moreover, mice treated with intrathecal liposomal AmB had minimal inflammatory signs in the meninges [16, 17].

In developed countries, disposable manometers are used to control the intracranial pressure [28]. In our study, we did not measure the intracranial pressure of patients with CM. However, this reflects the situation in most resource-limited settings, where disposable manometers are rarely used due to cost, unavailability, and safety issues. A study performed in South Africa and Uganda suggests that therapeutic lumbar punctures can have a dramatic effect on survival of CM regardless of the initial intracranial pressure [29]. Although at least four therapeutic lumbar punctures were performed in the standard AmB regimen group, the mortality reduction seen with the short-intrathecal AmB regimen could be related to the fact that patients in this group undertook more therapeutic lumbar punctures. We speculate that the combination of therapeutic lumbar punctures and intrathecal administration of AmBle might have achieved a more rapid clearance of the fungal load in CSF. However, new studies are needed to confirm these hypotheses.

In some African countries, refusal of lumbar punctures is common due to the belief among patients and relatives that the procedure can cause death [30]. However, in our setting, lumbar puncture refusal was rare, and patients frequently referred to improvement of their symptoms after the procedure. In our experience, the fact that "spinal taps" were used as means of administrating antifungal medication in a "difficult-to-reach" space helped improve the acceptability of therapeutic lumbar punctures among patients and doctors. New studies are needed to evaluate the acceptability of frequent lumbar punctures in settings with higher HIV prevalence in the general population such as sub-Saharan Africa.

The study has some limitations. Given the observational nature of the study, we must be cautious about the survival benefits of the new short-course induction regimen. This was an observational study using routine clinical data in a resource-poor setting. The selection of treatment was not randomized and the two regimens compared in this study were given at different periods of time, so it is possible that our results could be influenced by unknown confounders not included in the multivariate analysis. In addition, we did not measure the CSF opening pressure or surrogates for fungal burden in CSF such as quantitative cultures or *Cryptococcus* antigen titres, which are important predictors of mortality

[26]. On the other hand, unlike clinical trials, no patient was excluded because of the severity of the disease, so our results could be generalized to other resource-poor setting where patients are diagnosed with CM at advanced stages [31].

5. Conclusions

The study demonstrates that intrathecal administration of AmBle is well tolerated. In addition, the short induction therapy with intravenous AmBd along with daily therapeutic lumbar punctures and intrathecal AmBle achieved a clinically important reduction in mortality compared with the standard of care in low- and middle-income countries. Being an observational study, we must be cautious about the survival benefits of the new regimen. Still, the mortality of CM in resource-poor setting is unacceptably high, and our findings deserve further research.

Conflict of Interests

The authors declare that they have no competing interests.

References

[1] B. J. Park, K. A. Wannemuehler, B. J. Marston, N. Govender, P. G. Pappas, and T. M. Chiller, "Estimation of the current global burden of cryptococcal meningitis among persons living with HIV/AIDS," *AIDS*, vol. 23, no. 4, pp. 525–530, 2009.

[2] D. J. Sloan and V. Parris, "Cryptococcal meningitis: epidemiology and therapeutic options," *Clinical Epidemiology*, vol. 6, no. 1, pp. 169–182, 2014.

[3] World Health Organization, "Diagnosis, prevention and management of cryptococcal disease in HIV-infected adults, adolescents and children," December 2011, http://www.who.int/hiv/pub/cryptococcal_disease2011/en/.

[4] R. Rajasingham, M. A. Rolfes, K. E. Birkenkamp, D. B. Meya, and D. R. Boulware, "Cryptococcal meningitis treatment strategies in resource-limited settings: a cost-effectiveness analysis," *PLoS Medicine*, vol. 9, no. 9, Article ID e1001316, 2012.

[5] T. Bicanic, R. Wood, G. Meintjes et al., "High-dose amphotericin B with flucytosine for the treatment of cryptococcal meningitis in HIV-infected patients: a randomized trial," *Clinical Infectious Diseases*, vol. 47, no. 1, pp. 123–130, 2008.

[6] T. Bicanic, G. Meintjes, R. Wood et al., "Fungal burden, early fungicidal activity, and outcome in cryptococcal meningitis in antiretroviral-naive or antiretroviral-experienced patients treated with amphotericin B or fluconazole," *Clinical Infectious Diseases*, vol. 45, no. 1, pp. 76–80, 2007.

[7] A. T. Jackson, J. C. Nussbaum, J. Phulusa et al., "A phase II randomized controlled trial adding oral flucytosine to high-dose fluconazole, with short-course amphotericin B, for cryptococcal meningitis," *AIDS*, vol. 26, no. 11, pp. 1363–1370, 2012.

[8] V. Strenger, A. Meinitzer, J. Donnerer et al., "Amphotericin B transfer to CSF following intravenous administration of liposomal amphotericin B," *Journal of Antimicrobial Chemotherapy*, vol. 69, no. 9, pp. 2522–2526, 2014.

[9] S. Kethireddy and D. Andes, "CNS pharmacokinetics of antifungal agents," *Expert Opinion on Drug Metabolism and Toxicology*, vol. 3, no. 4, pp. 573–581, 2007.

[10] W. Fang, Z. Fa, and W. Liao, "Epidemiology of *Cryptococcus* and cryptococcosis in China," *Fungal Genetics and Biology*, vol. 78, pp. 7–15, 2015.

[11] C. Yuchong, C. Jianghan, W. Hai, and G. Julin, "Lumbar puncture drainage with intrathecal injection of amphotericin B for control of cryptococcal meningitis," *Mycoses*, vol. 54, no. 4, pp. e248–e251, 2011.

[12] J. N. Galgiani, N. M. Ampel, J. E. Blair et al., "Coccidioidomycosis," *Clinical Infectious Diseases*, vol. 41, no. 9, pp. 1217–1223, 2005.

[13] K. V. Clemons, R. A. Sobel, P. L. Williams, and D. A. Stevens, "Comparative toxicities and pharmacokinetics of intrathecal lipid (amphotericin B colloidal dispersion) and conventional deoxycholate formulations of amphotericin B in rabbits," *Antimicrobial Agents and Chemotherapy*, vol. 45, no. 2, pp. 612–615, 2001.

[14] B. Mete, N. Saltoglu, E. Vanli et al., "Simultaneous cryptococcal and tuberculous meningitis in a patient with systemic lupus erythematosus," *Journal of Microbiology, Immunology and Infection*, 2013.

[15] B. L. Grannan, V. Yanamadala, A. S. Venteicher, B. P. Walcott, and J. C. Barr, "Use of external ventriculostomy and intrathecal anti-fungal treatment in cerebral mucormycotic abscess," *Journal of Clinical Neuroscience*, vol. 21, no. 10, pp. 1819–1821, 2014.

[16] J. Capilla, A. Flavia, E. Mayayo, and J. Guarro, "Efficacy of intrathecal liposomal amphotericin B plus oral posaconazole in the treatment of acute meningeal cryptococcosis in a murine model," *International Journal of Antimicrobial Agents*, vol. 42, no. 3, pp. 282–283, 2013.

[17] A. F. Gazzoni, J. Capilla, E. Mayayo, and J. Guarro, "Efficacy of intrathecal administration of liposomal amphotericin B combined with voriconazole in a murine model of cryptococcal meningitis," *International Journal of Antimicrobial Agents*, vol. 39, no. 3, pp. 223–227, 2012.

[18] *Office of the Registrar General & Census Commissioner*, Census of India, New Delhi, India, 2011.

[19] G. Alvarez-Uria, M. Midde, R. Pakam, and P. K. Naik, "Gender differences, routes of transmission, socio-demographic characteristics and prevalence of HIV related infections of adults and children in an HIV cohort from a rural district of India," *Infectious Disease Reports*, vol. 4, no. 1, article e19, 2012.

[20] G. Alvarez-Uria, R. Pakam, M. Midde, and P. K. Naik, "Entry, retention, and virological suppression in an HIV cohort study in India: description of the cascade of care and implications for reducing HIV-related mortality in low- and middle-income countries," *Interdisciplinary Perspectives on Infectious Diseases*, vol. 2013, Article ID 384805, 8 pages, 2013.

[21] G. Alvarez-Uria, P. K. Naik, R. Pakam, L. Bachu, and M. Midde, "Natural history and factors associated with early and delayed mortality in HIV-infected patients treated of tuberculosis under directly observed treatment short-course strategy: a prospective cohort study in India," *Interdisciplinary Perspectives on Infectious Diseases*, vol. 2012, Article ID 502012, 9 pages, 2012.

[22] S. Sundar, K. Pandey, C. P. Thakur et al., "Efficacy and safety of amphotericin B emulsion versus liposomal formulation in Indian patients with visceral leishmaniasis: a randomized, open-label study," *PLoS Neglected Tropical Diseases*, vol. 8, no. 9, article e3169, 2014.

[23] S. Sundar, J. Chakravarty, D. Agarwal, A. Shah, N. Agrawal, and M. Rai, "Safety of a pre-formulated amphotericin B lipid emulsion for the treatment of Indian Kala-azar," *Tropical Medicine & International Health*, vol. 13, no. 9, pp. 1208–1212, 2008.

[24] D. G. Kleinbaum and M. Klein, *Survival Analysis, a Self-Learning Text*, Springer, 2nd edition, 2005.

[25] P. Royston and P. C. Lambert, *Flexible Parametric Survival Analysis Using Stata: Beyond the Cox Model*, StataCorp, 2011, https://ideas.repec.org/b/tsj/spbook/fpsaus.html.

[26] J. N. Jarvis, T. Bicanic, A. Loyse et al., "Determinants of mortality in a combined cohort of 501 patients with HIV-associated cryptococcal meningitis: implications for improving outcomes," *Clinical Infectious Diseases*, vol. 58, no. 5, pp. 736–745, 2014.

[27] C. K. Muzoora, T. Kabanda, G. Ortu et al., "Short course amphotericin B with high dose fluconazole for HIV-associated cryptococcal meningitis," *Journal of Infection*, vol. 64, no. 1, pp. 76–81, 2012.

[28] J. R. Perfect, W. E. Dismukes, F. Dromer et al., "Clinical practice guidelines for the management of cryptococcal disease: 2010 update by the infectious diseases society of America," *Clinical Infectious Diseases*, vol. 50, no. 3, pp. 291–322, 2010.

[29] M. A. Rolfes, K. H. Hullsiek, J. Rhein et al., "The effect of therapeutic lumbar punctures on acute mortality from cryptococcal meningitis," *Clinical Infectious Diseases*, vol. 59, no. 11, pp. 1607–1614, 2014.

[30] K. T. Thakur, K. Mateyo, L. Hachaambwa et al., "Lumbar puncture refusal in sub-Saharan Africa: a call for further understanding and intervention," *Neurology*, vol. 84, no. 19, pp. 1988–1990, 2015.

[31] A. Kambugu, D. B. Meya, J. Rhein et al., "Outcomes of cryptococcal meningitis in Uganda before and after the availability of highly active antiretroviral therapy," *Clinical Infectious Diseases*, vol. 46, no. 11, pp. 1694–1701, 2008.

16

Voluntary Counseling and Testing for HIV in Rural Area of Democratic Republic of the Congo: Knowledge, Attitude, and Practice Survey among Service Users

Mida Kautako-Kiambi,[1] Mathilde B. Ekila,[2] Smith Kama-Lemba,[1] Roger Wumba,[3] and Michel N. Aloni[4]

[1] *Centre de Santé de Référence et Maternité de la Cité de Mbanza-Ngungu, Mbanza-Ngungu, Bas-Congo, Democratic Republic of the Congo*
[2] *Division of Infectious Diseases, Department of Internal Medicine, University Hospital of Kinshasa, School of Medicine, University of Kinshasa, Kinshasa, Democratic Republic of the Congo*
[3] *Department of Tropical Medicine, University Hospital of Kinshasa, Faculty of Medicine, University of Kinshasa, Kinshasa, Democratic Republic of the Congo*
[4] *Division of Hemato-Oncology and Nephrology, Department of Pediatrics, University Hospital of Kinshasa, School of Medicine, University of Kinshasa, Kinshasa, Democratic Republic of the Congo*

Correspondence should be addressed to Mida Kautako-Kiambi; midakk@yahoo.fr

Academic Editor: Shyam Sundar

Aims. To determine the prevalence of HIV, the level of sexual risk for HIV, and determinants of VCT attendance among adult population living in a rural area. *Methods.* A cross-sectional study was conducted in Mbanza-Ngungu, Democratic Republic of the Congo. An anonymous questionnaire was designed to extract relevant data. *Results.* In our cohort, 69% were respondents of more than 24 years of age and the single marital status was most represented (64.1%). A high proportion of respondents (90.6%) visited VCT service for requiring information (good acceptability). Positive test for HIV was reported in 9.4% of respondents. In this cohort, 49.6% of respondents had declared themselves to never use condom. In binary analysis, there was association between positive HIV test and age ($p = 0.04$) and religions ($p = 0.02$). In this cohort, it was observed that positive HIV test was significantly associated with confidentiality ($p = 0.02$). However, there was no association between positive HIV test and condom use ($p = 0.25$), knowledge of VCT ($p = 0.81$), service requested ($p = 0.20$), and previous HIV test ($p = 0.68$). *Conclusions.* Preventive information for AIDS should be recommended in the population living in rural zone.

1. Introduction

Since 80s, HIV/AIDS infection remains one of the most devastating diseases worldwide. Approximately 33 million people are living with HIV and among them 97% are living in developing countries. Developing countries account for 97% of the HIV cases reported in the world. Sub-Saharan Africa is the first region of the world affected by the disease [1].

PNUD-DRC in 2009 report states that the prevalence of AIDS is around 4% and approximately 1,034,086 infected people (more than 15 years of age) are affected by the disease in the Democratic Republic of the Congo (DRC) [2]. It is be estimated that 80% of people who tested positive for HIV were in later stages and many infected individuals ignore their HIV status [3].

The situation requires measures to be strengthened, including public Voluntary Counseling and Testing (VCT) which is an entry point for prevention, education, care, and support for HIV infected individuals [4, 5]. However, rare published studies focused on persons who access these services in this country [6].

We therefore conducted a cross-sectional study in Mbanza-Ngungu, a semirural area located in the western part of the DRC. The objectives of this study were to determine the prevalence of HIV, the level of sexual risk for HIV, and determinants of VCT attendance among adult population living in this area. This piece of information will give the whole view of patients and may serve to rule out general public health in our midst.

2. Materials and Methods

2.1. Ethical Approval. Pending the installation of an ethical committee in the province of Bas-Congo of the DRC and the central health zone of Mbanza-Ngungu hospitals, the study was assessed and approved by the Provincial Health Officer (the highest ranked medical authority in the Oriental Province) and the Director's Board of Nsona-Nkulu Hospital and Maternity of Mbanza-Ngungu city. The aim and the procedures of the study were explained to the respondents. A written informed consent signed by participants was obtained before their inclusion. The respondents were informed that they could withdraw anytime without further obligation. Confidentiality of data was maintained.

2.2. Study Design. This cross-sectional study was conducted between January 2011 and July 2011 in Mbanza-Ngungu, Democratic Republic of the Congo. In this area, the HIV prevalence was estimated to be around 1.1% in the adult population between 15 and 49 years of age and from 3.3% to 4.9% for pregnant women [2]. Mbanza-Ngungu is a semirural territory in Bas-Congo Province in the western part of the Democratic Republic of the Congo; it has a population of nearly 100,000 people.

2.3. Study Population. The study included all individuals who visited the VCT services. Pregnant women were excluded from the study. The responders were classified in two categories of age: group 1 (≤24 years of age) and group 2 (>24 years of age).

This study was conducted in two VCT services located in health facilities in Mbanza-Ngungu, namely, Nsona-Nkulu hospital and Maternity of Mbanza-Ngungu city. They were selected for the study because they offered information, education, and management for the population of the city.

2.4. Data Collection. The respondents were selected and included in this study using a simple random sampling method. An anonymous questionnaire was designed to extract relevant data from the case records. The questionnaire was prepared in French and translated in Kikongo (the predominant language in Mbanza-Ngungu). The questionnaire was pretested in 20 respondents not selected for the study.

The respondents selected for the study had completed an anonymous questionnaire. The structured questionnaire is self-administered. The structured questionnaire contained of a total of questions addressing three axes: (i) demographic data (age, gender); (ii) prevention behavior for HIV/AIDS; (iii) knowledge and attitude.

Table 1: Sociodemographics and characteristics of the 234 study participants.

Variables	Frequency	Percent
Gender		
Male	117	50
Female	117	50
Age (years)		
≤24	73	31.2
>24	161	68.8
Education		
Primary	141	60.3
Secondary	84	35.9
Tertiary	9	3.8
Occupation		
Unemployed	55	23.5
Employed	124	53.0
Students	55	23.5
Marital status		
Single/widowed/divorced/separated	150	64.1
Married/cohabitation	84	35.9
Religion		
Christianity	182	77.8
Kimbanguism	14	6.0
Islam	5	2.1
Without religion	17	8.3
Animist	16	6.8

2.5. Data Analysis. Data from the returned questionnaires were stored confidentially and were manually entered into a microcomputer using Microsoft Office Excel 2010. After data cleaning (control for quality and coherence), they were exported on SPSS 19.0 for statistical analysis. Descriptive analyses were used to get mean for quantitative variables and proportion for all the qualitative variables. The confidence interval at 95% was calculated. Chi2 tests, Fisher's exact tests, and Student's t-tests were used for comparisons between variables. For identification of factors associated with the use of VCT services, we performed a binary logistics analysis. Differences were considered significant when $p < 0.05$.

3. Results

3.1. Sample Characteristics. A total of 234 respondents gave informed consent from 247 received during the period of the study. The participation rate was 95%. These data were used for analysis.

Sociodemographics and general characteristics of the respondents are presented in Table 1. The proportion of males and females visitors was similar. In our cohort, 161 (69%) were respondents more than 24 years of age (Table 1). Only 4% of respondents achieved the tertiary education level. Regarding the occupation, 53% of the respondents were categorized as employed. The respondents with single marital status were most represented (64.1%). The majority (77.8%) of

Table 2: Knowledge, attitude, and behavioral variables frequency (%).

Variables	Frequency (%)
Source of information	
Media (TV, radio, journal, etc.)	28 (12)
Health service, health care worker	110 (47)
Vicinity (sexual partner, family, friend, etc.)	68 (29.1)
Church	5 (2.1)
Other	23 (9.8)
Purpose of visit	
New sexual partner or marriage	22 (8.4)
Simple curiosity	94 (40.2)
Risk sexual relation	7 (3)
Sickness	31 (13.2)
Death from HIV in the family	11 (4.7)
Being oriented by VCT client or health agent	9 (3.8)
Rape	6 (2.6)
Retesting (after a first test)	41 (17.5)
Other	13 (5.7)
Service requested during visit	
Information	22 (9.4)
VCT	10 (4.3)
Information and VCT	202 (86.3)
HIV testing expected result by subjects	
Negative	112 (48.1)
Positive	5 (2.1)
Do not know	116 (49.8)
HIV testing result	
Negative	199 (85)
Positive	22 (9.4)
Undetermined	13 (5.6)
Previous HIV testing	
No	100 (42.7)
Yes	134 (57.3)
Sexual relation 3 months before VCT	
Yes	128 (54.7)
No	106 (45.3)
Use of condom	
Never	116 (49.6)
Sometimes	116 (49.6)
Always	2 (0.8)
Confidence of HIV test (if positive) with	
No body	37 (15.8)
Sexual partner	110 (47)
A family member	47 (20.1)
Pastor/priest	4 (1.7)
Other	36 (15.4)

VCT: Voluntary Counseling and Testing.

the respondents were Christians. Other details are reported in Table 1.

3.2. Knowledge and Attitude. Knowledge and attitude of respondents are summarized in Table 2. Forty-seven percent of the respondents know VCT service. The three main sources of VCT information are health agents, the vicinity, and the media. Other details are reported in Table 2.

The most common reasons of the visits were the curiosity, HIV retesting, and the context of another disease. Other reasons are summarized in Table 2. Only 8.4% of the visits were due to counseling before marriage or a new relationship. A high proportion of respondents (90.6%) visit VCT service for requiring information (*good acceptability*). Two percent of respondents had supposed that they were infected and expected a positive HIV test. Positive test for HIV was reported in 22 (9.4%) respondents and 13 (5.6%) had an undetermined result. A total of 134 (57.3%) respondents were screened for HIV infection in the past. A minority (0.8%) of them had confirmed using condom during each suspected sexual relation. In contrast, 116 respondents (49.6%) had declared themselves to never use condom. Among them 65 (56%) were single. Forty-seven percent of responders agree to inform their sexual partner if the HIV test was positive. Other details are shown in Table 2.

Frequencies of positive test for HIV in 234 responders according sociodemographic characteristics are summarized in Table 3.

Table 3: HIV positive tests in 234 study participants according sociodemographics and characteristics.

Variables	Frequency	Percent
Gender		
Male	10/117	8.6
Female	12/117	10.3
Age (years)		
≤24	2/73	2.7
>24	20/161	12.4
Education		
Primary	14/141	9.9
Secondary	7/84	8.3
Tertiary	1/9	11.1
Job category		
Unemployed	6/55	10.9
Employed	15/121	12.4
Students	1/55	1.8
Marital status		
Single/widowed/divorced/separated	13/150	8.7
Married/cohabitation	9/84	10.7
Religion		
Christians	13/182	71.4
Kimbanguism	1/14	7.1
Muslim	1/5	20.0
Without religion	1/17	5.9
Animist	6/16	37.5

3.3. Binary Analysis. The results of the bivariate analysis between positive HIV testing and sociodemographic characteristics of respondents are shown in Table 4. There was no association between positive result for HIV test and gender ($p = 0.47$), education level ($p = 0.64$), job category ($p = 0.93$), and marital status ($p = 0.98$). However, there was

Table 4: HIV testing result from VCT versus sociodemographic variables.

Variables	Coefficient	p value	OR [95% CI]
Age	1.65	0.04	5.2 [1.1–24.7]
Education level	0.23	0.64	1.3 [0.5–3.3]
Job category	0.06	0.93	1.0 [0.3–4.1]
Religion	−1.27	0.02	0.3 [0.1–0.8]
Gender	−0.34	0.47	0.7 [0.3–1.8]
Marital status	0.01	0.98	1.0 [0.4–2.8]

VCT: Voluntary Counseling and Testing.

Table 5: HIV testing result from VCT versus attitude and behavioral variables.

Variables	Coefficient	p value	OR [95% CI]
Condom use	−0.56	0.25	0.6 [0.2–1.5]
Confidentiality	−1.1	0.02	0.3 [0.1–0.8]
VCT service knowledge	−0.12	0.81	0.9 [0.3–2.2]
Service requested	1.38	0.20	4.0 [0.5–33.6]
Previous HIV test	0.20	0.68	1.2 [0.5–3.1]

VCT: Voluntary Counseling and Testing.

association between positive HIV test and age ($p = 0.04$) and religions ($p = 0.02$).

Table 5 shows the association between positive HIV test and behaviors and attitude of the study population. In this cohort, it was observed that positive HIV test was significantly associated with confidentiality ($p = 0.02$). However, there was no association between positive HIV test and condom use ($p = 0.25$), knowledge of VCT ($p = 0.81$), service requested ($p = 0.20$), and previous HIV test ($p = 0.68$).

4. Discussion

To our knowledge, the present study is one of the first attempts to describe characteristics and attitude about HIV/AIDS in individuals attending VCT in a rural area of Central Africa. VCT serves as an entry point and represents one of the strategies adopted by the international community to control HIV explosion [4].

In this study, the HIV prevalence was 9.4%. This trend is higher than those observed in previous studies in another part of the province of Bas-Congo where the prevalence varies between 1.1% and 5.7% [7]. This difference can be explained by the target population in this study. This prevalence is probably increased in some high-risk specific groups attending the VCTs.

In Mbanza-Ngungu, the greater proportion of respondents with increased risk of HIV infection was individuals aged more than 24 years. Different studies reported similar results in the DRC [3, 8–10].

Educational level was not found to be a significant factor affecting the result of HIV test. Previous studies show that education level is a major determinant for HIV testing and counseling [9, 11, 12]. This situation could be explained by the underrepresentation of responders with high level education in a rural area in the context of the DRC.

In this cohort, job category was not found as a significant risk factor for positive HIV test. This result is not in accordance with those published in 2011 by the multisectorial program against HIV/AIDS of the DRC. This situation is probably due to underrepresentation of group with high risk of HIV infection (sex professionals, truck drivers, and female soldiers) in our cohort [13–15].

Christianity is found to be a significantly protective factor against HIV infection, in our cohort. A recent study in Tanzania found that religious beliefs have a significant influence on HIV-related stigma [16]. In Congolese rural area, Christianity coexists with several African traditional religions and sociocultural beliefs. By their convictions, African traditional religions could constitute a barrier for HIV disclosure and an obstacle for prevention strategies. However, recent studies in other provinces of DRC showed that Catholic (relative to non-Catholic Christian) religious affiliation was associated with an increased risk of HIV [10].

In our cohort, the positive HIV test was predominant in females. The female preponderance noted in this cohort was comparable with previous studies in Africa [3, 17].

In our cohort, there was no association between positive HIV test and marital status. This observation has been confirmed by subsequent studies [10]. However, in rural area in Kenya, married women were 4.8 times more likely to be HIV positive than those never married [18]. Similar observation was recently reported in Mozambique [19]. Efforts need to be strengthened to make couples aware of HIV spread and disclosure.

This study reveals that respondents with single marital status visited more VCT service than the couples. The low frequency of responders in couple might be related to the false idea that marital partnerships prevent from HIV in African culture [20, 21].

Our results show that respondents that are willing to disclose their status to a confidant had probably a negative HIV test. This suggests that they knew they are in good health and more of them (69%) have HIV testing in the past. It is important to note that 16% of respondents did not wish to disclose their HIV status and 51% of them have a sexual partner. These findings are comparable with previous studies in Africa [22, 23].

Sex with occasional partners was considered as risky sexual behaviors. The use of condom remains an effective preventing factor of HIV sexual transmission [24, 25]. In our cohort, only 0.8% of respondents have declared regularly using condom and approximately 50% of them use condom occasionally. Similar observations have been previously reported in other categories of population living in the DRC [26–28].

5. Conclusion

VCT is an entry point for HIV prevention and therapeutic support. This study shows the need to strengthen information on AIDS prevention in rural areas in the DRC.

Preventive information on AIDS should be recommended in the population living in rural zone, an area at high risk, to contract HIV/AIDS. However, HIV/AIDS control requires a comprehensive approach, including the leaders and community education.

Conflict of Interests

The authors declare that there is no conflict of interests.

Acknowledgments

The authors thank all patients who participated in this study. They thank all their colleagues involved in the collection of samples and all the nurses of VCT service of Mbanza-Ngungu for the support given for the present study.

References

[1] Joint United Nations Programme on HIV/AIDS (UNAIDS), *Global Report: UNAIDS Report on the Global AIDS Epidemic*, WHO Library Cataloguing-in-Publication Data, 2010.

[2] PNUD-RDC, *Pauvreté et conditions de vie des ménages dans le Bas-Congo*, 2009.

[3] M. Kautako-Kiambi, M. Aloni-Ntetani, P. Pululu et al., "Socio-demographic, biological and clinical profile of patients living with HIV during screening in a voluntary counselling and screening centre in a rural area of Mbanza-Ngungu, Democratic Republic of Congo, in 2006–2011," *Bulletin de la Société de Pathologie Exotique*, vol. 106, no. 3, pp. 180–183, 2013.

[4] World Health Organization, *Global HIV/AIDS Response—Epidemic Update and Health Sector Progress Towards Universal Access—Progress Report*, World Health Organization, Geneva, Switzerland, 2011, http://www.who.int/hiv/pub/progress_report2011/summary_en.pdf.

[5] J. Ditekemena, R. Matendo, O. Koole et al., "Male partner voluntary counselling and testing associated with the antenatal services in Kinshasa, Democratic Republic of Congo: a randomized controlled trial," *International Journal of STD and AIDS*, vol. 22, no. 3, pp. 165–170, 2011.

[6] P. Kayembe, N. Kyloka, M. Mulwakila, and K. Mashinda, *Inventaire et évaluation des travaux de recherche menés en RDC sur le VIH/SIDA de 2005 à 2010*, PNMLS-RDC, 2011.

[7] Comité DSRP Provincial, *Document provincial de stratégie de réduction de la pauvreté*, Province du Bas-Congo, 2007.

[8] DRC, *Epidemiological fact sheet on HIV and AIDS*, UNAIDS, WHO, Geneva, Switzerland, 2008.

[9] J. T. Bertrand, L. F. Brown, M. Kinzonzi, M. Mansilu, and B. Djunghu, "AIDS knowledge in three sites in Bas-Zaire," *AIDS Education and Prevention*, vol. 4, no. 3, pp. 251–266, 1992.

[10] M. Hawkes, E. S. Şivasivugha, S. K. Ngigi, C. K. Masumbuko, J. Brophy, and Z. T. Kibendelwa, "HIV and religion in the Congo: a mixed-methods study," *Current HIV Research*, vol. 11, no. 3, pp. 246–253, 2013.

[11] EDS-RDC, 2007, http://www.measuredhs.com/pubs/pdf/SR141/SR141.pdf.

[12] A. K. Ziraba, N. J. Madise, J. K. Kimani et al., "Determinants for HIV testing and counselling in Nairobi urban informal settlements," *BMC Public Health*, vol. 11, article 663, 2011.

[13] International HIV/AIDS Alliance, *The Cost Efficiency of HIV Prevention for Vulnerable and Most-at-Risk Populations and the Reality of Funding. What's Preventing Prevention Campaign Briefing 2*, International HIV/AIDS Alliance, Hove, UK, 2010.

[14] *Rapport d'activité sur la riposte au VIH/SIDA*, PNMLS, 2012.

[15] J. C. Omba Kalonda, "Sexual violence in the Democratic Republic of Congo: impact on public health?" *Medecine Tropicale*, vol. 68, no. 6, pp. 576–578, 2008.

[16] J. Zou, Y. Yamanaka, M. John, M. Watt, J. Ostermann, and N. Thielman, "Religion and HIV in Tanzania: influence of religious beliefs on HIV stigma, disclosure, and treatment attitudes," *BMC Public Health*, vol. 9, article 75, 2009.

[17] R. W. Ryder, V. Batter, N. Kaseka et al., "Effect of HIV-1 infection on tuberculosis and fertility in a large workforce in Kinshasa, Democratic Republic of the Congo," *AIDS Patient Care and STDs*, vol. 14, no. 6, pp. 297–304, 2000.

[18] J. Negin, J. Wariero, P. Mutuo, S. Jan, and P. Pronyk, "Feasibility, acceptability and cost of home-based HIV testing in rural Kenya," *Tropical Medicine and International Health*, vol. 14, no. 8, pp. 849–855, 2009.

[19] S. Agha, "Factors associated with HIV testing and condom use in Mozambique: implications for programs," *Reproductive Health*, vol. 9, article 20, 2012.

[20] D. G. Willms, M.-I. Arratia, and P. Makondesa, "Can interfaith research partnerships develop new paradigms for condom use and HIV prevention? The implementation of conceptual events in Malawi results in a 'spiritualised condom'," *Sexually Transmitted Infections*, vol. 87, no. 7, pp. 611–615, 2011.

[21] M. S. Steele, E. Bukusi, C. R. Cohen, B. A. Shell-Duncan, and K. K. Holmes, "The ABCs of HIV prevention in men: associations with HIV risk and protective behaviors," *Journal of Acquired Immune Deficiency Syndromes*, vol. 43, no. 5, pp. 571–576, 2006.

[22] H. T. Gebrekristos, M. N. Lurie, N. Mthethwa, and Q. A. Karim, "Disclosure of HIV status: experiences of patients enrolled in an integrated TB and HAART pilot programme in South Africa," *African Journal of AIDS Research*, vol. 8, no. 1, pp. 1–6, 2009.

[23] A. Desclaux, S. Boye, and B. Taverne, "The social relegation of widows living with HIV in the time of ART in Senegal," *Bulletin de la Société de Pathologie Exotique*, vol. 107, no. 4, pp. 273–278, 2014.

[24] P. Pitché, K. Gbetoglo, B. Saka et al., "HIV prevalence and behavioral studies in female sex workers in Togo: a decline in the prevalence between 2005 and 2011," *Pan African Medical Journal*, vol. 15, article 62, 2013.

[25] M.-C. Boily, M. Pickles, C. M. Lowndes et al., "Positive impact of a large-scale HIV prevention programme among female sex workers and clients in South India," *AIDS*, vol. 27, no. 9, pp. 1449–1460, 2013.

[26] P. K. Kayembe, M. A. Mapatano, A. B. Fatuma et al., "Knowledge of HIV, sexual behavior and correlates of risky sex among street children in Kinshasa, Democratic Republic of Congo," *East African Journal of Public Health*, vol. 5, no. 3, pp. 186–192, 2008.

[27] N. R. Ngatu, R. Hirota, M. Eitoku et al., "Perception of the risk of sexual transmission of HIV among Congolese and Japanese university students," *Environmental Health and Preventive Medicine*, vol. 17, no. 2, pp. 139–146, 2012.

[28] M. Ntumbanzondo, R. Dubrow, L. M. Niccolai, K. Mwandagalirwa, and M. H. Merson, "Unprotected intercourse for extra money among commercial sex workers in Kinshasa, Democratic Republic of Congo," *AIDS Care*, vol. 18, no. 7, pp. 777–785, 2006.

17

Antibacterial Action of Curcumin against *Staphylococcus aureus*

Sin-Yeang Teow,[1] Kitson Liew,[2] Syed A. Ali,[3] Alan Soo-Beng Khoo,[2,4] and Suat-Cheng Peh[1,5]

[1] *Sunway Institute for Healthcare Development (SIHD), Sunway University, 47500 Bandar Sunway, Selangor Darul Ehsan, Malaysia*
[2] *Molecular Pathology Unit, Cancer Research Centre (CaRC), Institute for Medical Research (IMR), 50588 Jalan Pahang, Kuala Lumpur, Malaysia*
[3] *Advanced Medical and Dental Institute (AMDI), Universiti Sains Malaysia (USM), 13200 Kepala Batas, Pulau Pinang, Malaysia*
[4] *Institute for Research, Development and Innovation, International Medical University (IMU), 57000 Bukit Jalil, Kuala Lumpur, Malaysia*
[5] *Anatomical Pathology Department, Sunway Medical Centre, 47500 Bandar Sunway, Selangor Darul Ehsan, Malaysia*

Correspondence should be addressed to Sin-Yeang Teow; ronaldt@sunway.edu.my

Academic Editor: Sukla Biswas

Curcumin, the major constituent of *Curcuma longa* L. (Zingiberaceae family) or turmeric, commonly used for cooking in Asian cuisine, is known to possess a broad range of pharmacological properties at relatively nontoxic doses. Curcumin is found to be effective against *Staphylococcus aureus* (*S. aureus*). As demonstrated by *in vitro* experiment, curcumin exerts even more potent effects when used in combination with various other antibacterial agents. Hence, curcumin which is a natural product derived from plant is believed to have profound medicinal benefits and could be potentially developed into a naturally derived antibiotic in the future. However, there are several noteworthy challenges in the development of curcumin as a medicine. *S. aureus* infections, particularly those caused by the multidrug-resistant strains, have emerged as a global health issue and urgent action is needed. This review focuses on the antibacterial activities of curcumin against both methicillin-sensitive *S. aureus* (MSSA) and methicillin-resistant *S. aureus* (MRSA). We also attempt to highlight the potential challenges in the effort of developing curcumin into a therapeutic antibacterial agent.

1. Introduction

Curcumin or diferuloylmethane is the major phytochemical of *Curcuma longa* L. (Zingiberaceae family), which is commonly known as turmeric. Curcumin is the polyphenolic compound that gives the yellow colour of the herb. Turmeric is mainly cultivated in tropical and subtropical regions and is mainly produced by India. Traditionally, it has been used to flavour food, dye cloths, and treat various human ailments [1]. Curcumin is extracted from turmeric by solvent extraction (preferably with ethanol) through various methods (e.g., Soxhlet, ultrasonic, microwave, and supercritical carbon dioxide) followed by purification via column chromatography [2, 3]. Ever since the identification of curcumin as the main constituent of turmeric, multiple pharmacological activities of curcumin that include antimicrobial, antidiabetic, anti-inflammatory, anticancer, and antioxidant have been reported [4–6]. More excitingly, when combined with other drugs, curcumin has been found to enhance the effects of antibacterial [7–9], antifungal [10, 11], anticancer [12, 13], and antioxidant [14, 15] activities.

Curcumin usually exhibits low to no toxicity at the active doses. A systematic review from the MEDLINE computerized database (1966 to 2002) has shown that curcumin is safe when consumed up to 8 g each day consecutively for 3 months in a phase I human trial that involved 25 subjects [16]. Similarly, the dose of 8 g per day was safe when used in combination with gemcitabine that showed marked therapeutic effects in pancreatic cancer patients [17, 18]. Interestingly, curcumin is also able to reverse the Aflatoxin B1-induced toxicity and iron-overloaded liver toxicity in rats [19–21]. Despite being extensively studied, the exact mechanism(s) of curcumin's multiple biological and pharmacological activities remains to be explored. Based on the available literature, there are two hypotheses describing the poly-pharmacological effects of curcumin. First, curcumin is known to act on multiple targets [4, 5, 22–24], hence having diverse roles in regulating various cellular processes. Secondly, products resulting from the curcumin degradation have been shown to be highly diverse depending on the chemical or biochemical reactions involved [25–27]. Most of these products are stable and function differently that may lead to the multiple effects.

The most studied activity of the curcumin in the past 10 years is the anticancer effects [28]. However, the first paper describing the biological action of curcumin was its antibacterial activity against various bacteria: *S. aureus*, *Trichophyton gypseum*, *Salmonella paratyphi*, and *Mycobacterium tuberculosis* [29]. To date, studies on the antibacterial activity of curcumin that indicate inhibition properties of a wide range of bacteria are increasingly documented [6, 23, 30]. Recent publications have also reported that curcumin is active against a plethora of drug-resistant bacterial strains [8, 9, 31, 32]. *S. aureus* infection is a major problem in many developing countries, especially in hospitals where the MRSA spreading is difficult to control [33]. Over the years, the multidrug-resistant *S. aureus* infection has increased the global morbidity and mortality [34, 35]. Due to the difficulty in treating the infection, it has consequently imposed an elevating burden on healthcare resources [36–38]. Cumulative findings in recent years have shown that curcumin is active against both MSSA and MRSA [8, 9, 30, 32, 39, 40]. In view of the need for a more efficacious and safe therapeutic modality towards the drug-resistant *S. aureus*, we discuss the reported antibacterial activities of curcumin against *S. aureus* and its potentials and limitations to be developed into a potent antibiotic.

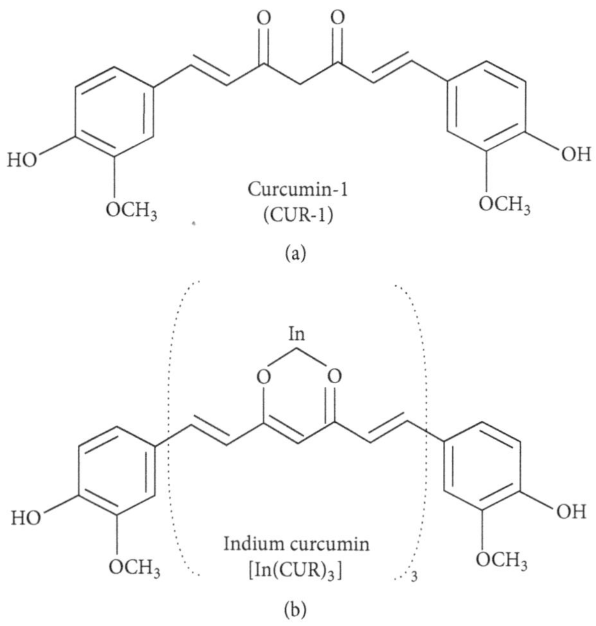

FIGURE 1: Chemical structures of antibacterial curcumin analogues against *S. aureus*. Upper panel shows the structure of curcumin-1 [30, 41] while the lower panel shows the metal complexes of curcumin, indium curcumin [42, 43]. The chemical structures above were drawn using a free online tool, ChemWriter (http://chemwriter.com/).

2. Curcumin-Mediated Inhibition of *S. aureus*

Curcumin inhibits the growth of both Gram-positive and Gram-negative bacteria [6, 23, 30]. *S. aureus* is one of the Gram-positive strains that is susceptible to curcumin-mediated inhibition. *S. aureus* is a pathogen that causes various infections including infective endocarditis (IE), bacteremia, skin and soft tissue, osteoarticular, and pleuropulmonary infections [33]. Over the years, *S. aureus* has evolved and developed multiple strategies to evade human immune system and to resist antibiotics treatment. This has given rise to the evolution of MRSA, and the emergence of healthcare-associated (HA) and community-associated (CA) MRSA has caused a major problem to the human society [45, 46]. In this section, we discuss the past and current works that show the curcumin-mediated killings of MSSA and MRSA (summarized in Table 1).

Mun et al. [9] showed that the minimal inhibitory concentrations (MICs) of curcumin against 10 strains of *S. aureus* (including 2 ATCC MSSA and MRSA standard strains, 4 MRSA clinical isolates, and 4 MRSA from culture collection) ranged from 125 to 250 μg/mL while a study by Wang et al. [40] showed the MIC of 256 μg/mL against MSSA. Using a broth microdilution assay, our group [8] also showed that 250 μg/mL curcumin was required to kill the two ATCC MSSA (#25923) and MRSA (#43300) strains. However, another study demonstrated that the MICs against the ATCC standard MSSA and MRSA were 219 and 217 μg/mL, respectively, that are slightly lower than the former study [47]. Recently, Kali et al. [48] showed the mean curcumin MIC of 126.9 μg/mL against 15 Gram-positive bacterial isolates including thirteen *S. aureus* and two *Enterococcus faecalis*. Nonetheless, this study is not used for comparison in Table 1 because the obtained MIC might not be representative for curcumin's effect against *S. aureus* as the study was carried out in combination with *Enterococcus faecalis*.

A more potent inhibition was achieved when curcumin-1 (CUR-1), a major component of commercial preparations of curcumin (purity > 98%), was used against *S. aureus*. The chemical structure of curcumin-1 is shown in Figure 1. Tyagi et al. [30] showed that the curcumin-1 was active against MSSA at concentration of as low as 25 μM (equivalent to 9.21 μg/mL), as it killed 50% of the bacteria after 2 hr incubation. The activity was time- and dose-dependent, and 100% killing was achieved at 50 μM (equivalent to 18.42 μg/mL) after 2 hr exposure [30]. In contrast, Sasidharan et al. [41] showed that the same compound had a MIC of 250 μg/mL against *S. aureus*, which is comparable to the native curcumin [8, 9]. In an *in vivo* mouse model, administration of 100 mg/kg curcumin was shown to protect the mice infected with both MSSA and MRSA from pneumonia by targeting the α-hemolysin (Hla) protein of *S. aureus* [40]. In summary, the curcumin MICs against *S. aureus* ranged from 18.42 to 256 μg/mL (refer to Table 1). The variation could be due to

TABLE 1: Antibacterial activity of curcumin against *S. aureus*.

Compound (solvent)	MIC (μg/mL)	*S. aureus* strain	Test method	Reference
Curcumin (DMSO) Indium curcumin (DMSO)	187.5 93.8	MSSA (ATCC 25923)	Broth macrodilution	[42]
Curcumin (DMSO)	125–250	MSSA (ATCC 25923) MRSA (ATCC 33591) MRSA (4 Clinical isolates) MRSA (4 from CCARM)#	Broth microdilution	[9]
Curcumin-1 (DMSO)	250	MSSA (MTCC 902)*	Broth microdilution	[41]
Curcumin (DMF)	250	MSSA (ATCC 25923) MRSA (ATCC 43300) MSSA (1 Clinical isolates) MSSA (10 Env. isolates)	Broth microdilution	[8]
Curcumin-1 (DMSO)	18.42	MSSA (ATCC 29213)	Colony counting method	[30]
Curcumin (ethanol)	219 217	MSSA (ATCC 29213) MRSA (ATCC 43300)	Broth macrodilution	[47]
Curcumin (ethanol)	125	MSSA (ATCC 25923)	Broth macrodilution	[49]
Curcumin (DMSO)	256	MSSA (USA 300) MSSA (8325-4)	Broth microdilution	[40]

#CCARM: culture collection of antimicrobial resistant microbes.
*Purchased from Microbial Type Culture Collection Centre (MTCC), IMTECH, Chandigarh, India.
Env.: environmental.

(i) strain difference (i.e., MRSA versus MSSA); (ii) source of bacterial strains (i.e., ATCC standard strains versus clinical isolates); (iii) type of antibacterial assay (i.e., disk diffusion versus broth microdilution); and (iv) type of curcumin and its solvent (i.e., commercial compound versus in-house purified compound). Overall, the cumulative findings showed that there is no difference of MICs against MSSA and MRSA, suggesting that the sensitivity towards curcumin treatment is not altered by the multidrug resistance machinery in *S. aureus*.

There have been several explanations on how curcumin acts and kills the bacteria which are illustrated in Figure 2. Rai et al. [44] have demonstrated that curcumin interacts with FtsZ (prokaryotic homologue of eukaryotic cytoskeletal protein tubulin) *in vitro* and inhibits the assembly of FtsZ protofilaments in *Bacillus subtilis* 168. Although it has not been examined directly on *S. aureus*, it is believed that inhibiting the assembly dynamics of FtsZ is one of the main mechanisms of curcumin in inhibiting bacterial cell proliferation. FtsZ is also believed to be a novel target for the development of antibacterial drugs against *S. aureus*. [63, 64]. Mun et al. [32] showed that the antibacterial action of curcumin against both MSSA and MRSA was markedly enhanced when used in combination with ATPase inhibitors and mild detergents that compromise ATP-binding cassette (ABC) transporters and cytoplasmic membrane integrity, respectively. The same study has also shown that curcumin binds to peptidoglycan (PGN), and the increasing concentrations of PGN block the curcumin antibacterial activity. Tyagi et al. [30] also showed that curcumin-1 inhibited *S. aureus* growth by perturbing the bacterial membrane integrity. In this study, the bacterial membrane of *S. aureus* was examined using two fluorescent probes: propidium iodide and calcein. The membrane leakage upon exposure to curcumin was also evaluated by fluorescence and scanning electron microscopies. Although existing evidence suggests that curcumin inhibits *S. aureus* mainly by damaging the bacterial membrane, further investigation is required to identify additional bacterial target proteins besides FtsZ and PGN. This is important not only to enhance the understanding of the curcumin interaction with its target proteins, but also to further improve the activity of curcumin against *S. aureus*, particularly the MRSA strains. Similar studies should also be performed on the curcumin derivatives such as curcumin-1 (curcumin with highest purity >98%) and indium curcumin (metal complex with curcumin) which have shown more potent antibacterial effects than the native curcumin. The chemical structures of curcumin-1 and indium curcumin are shown in Figure 1.

3. Synergism of Curcumin with Antibiotics against *S. aureus*

In addition to showing potent antibacterial activity when used alone, curcumin also exerts marked activity against *S. aureus* when used at subinhibitory dose in combination with various other antibiotics [8, 9, 31, 32]. These findings are interesting since curcumin is naturally derived from turmeric, which is one of the major ingredients of Asian cuisine [1, 23]. Of note, crude turmeric extracts have previously shown marked antibacterial activities against *S. aureus* [6, 65, 66]. This section discusses the synergistic antibacterial activity of curcumin with antibiotics against MSSA and MRSA. Table 2 summarizes studies that demonstrated the synergism of antibiotics-curcumin. In this table, we include the information of curcumin type, solvent, and concentration, type of bacteria-killing assay, and *S. aureus* strains for comparison.

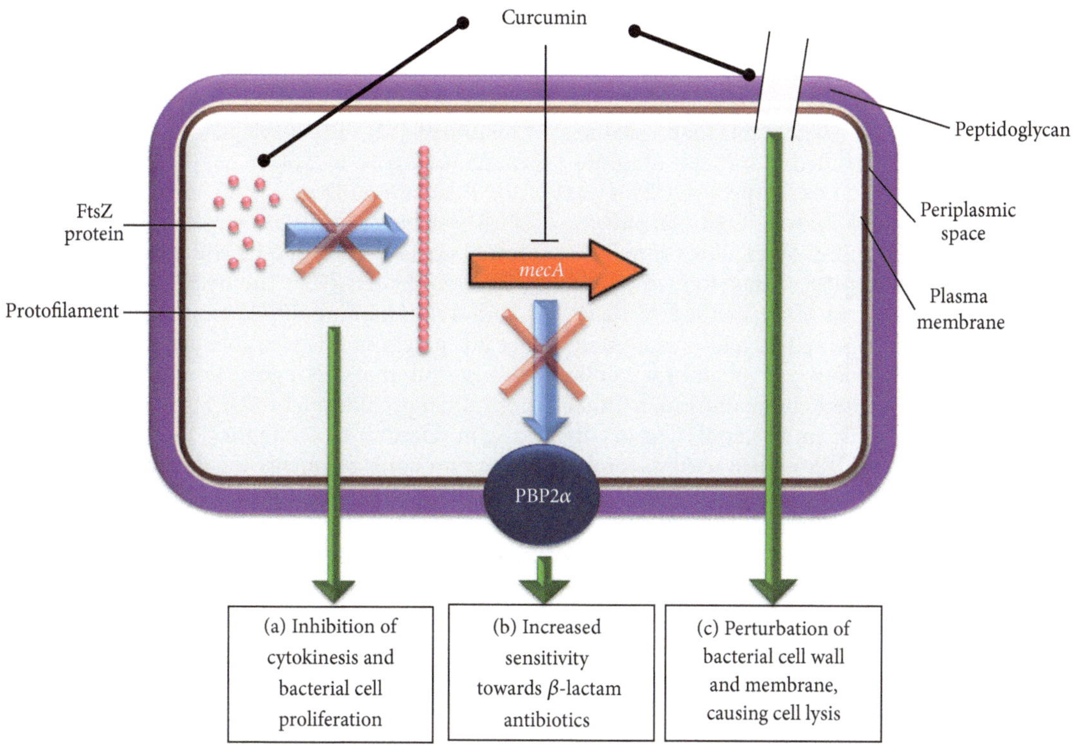

FIGURE 2: The potential mechanisms underlying the antibacterial effect of curcumin against *S. aureus*. Circle-shaped arrow indicates binding whereas blocked arrow represents inhibition. (a) Curcumin may bind into FtsZ proteins, thereby inhibiting the assembly of FtsZ protofilaments. This, in turn, suppresses the formation of Z-ring leading to inhibition of cytokinesis and bacterial proliferation [44]. (b) In the case of MRSA, curcumin could inhibit the *mecA* gene transcription, causing reduced expression of PBP2α proteins. As a result, MRSA can be sensitized towards the antibacterial action of β-lactam antibiotics such as Penicillin and Methicillin [32]. (c) The binding between curcumin and peptidoglycan on *S. aureus* cell wall could trigger damage on the cell wall and membrane, leading to cell lysis of *S. aureus* [30, 32].

TABLE 2: Synergism of curcumin against *S. aureus*.

Compound (solvent)	Subinhibitory concentration	Antibiotics	*S. aureus* strain	Test method	Reference
Curcumin (not reported)	500 μg/disc	Cefixime Cephotaxime Vancomycin Tetracycline	MSSA (1 clinical isolate)	Disk diffusion	[31]
Curcumin (DMSO)	Checkerboard (various serial dilutions)	Oxacillin Ampicillin Ciprofloxacin Norfloxacin	MSSA (ATCC 25923) MRSA (ATCC 33591) MRSA (1 clinical isolate)	Broth microdilution	[9]
Curcumin-1 (DMSO)	Checkerboard (various serial dilutions)	Cefaclor Cefodizime Cefotaxime	MSSA (MTCC 902)*	Broth microdilution	[41]
Curcumin (DMF)	25 μg/mL	Gentamicin Amikacin Ciprofloxacin	MSSA (ATCC 25923) MRSA (ATCC 43300) MSSA (1 clinical isolate) MSSA (10 environ. isolates)	Disk diffusion & broth microdilution	[8]
Curcumin (DMSO)	32 μg/mL	Penicillin Erythromycin Ciprofloxacin	MSSA (ATCC 25923) MSSA (13 clinical isolates)	Disk diffusion	[48]

*Purchased from Microbial Type Culture Collection Centre (MTCC), IMTECH, Chandigarh, India.

The first study that reported the synergism of curcumin against *S. aureus* was seven years ago by Moghaddam et al. [31]. Using a disk diffusion method, Moghaddam et al. [31] showed that 500 μg/disc of curcumin exerted synergistic antibacterial effect on the MSSA when used in combination with four antibiotics. Combination with cefotaxime, cefixime, tetracycline, and vancomycin resulted in increase of inhibition zone of 52.6, 24.9, 26.5, and 24.4%, respectively. This was then followed by Mun et al. [9] study in 2013 that showed curcumin's synergism with Oxacillin, Ampicillin, Ciprofloxacin, and Norfloxacin against the MRSA. This study employed checkerboard broth microdilution assay method to determine the synergistic activity. This method allows more standardised testing and is less laborious and suitable for studies with multiple concentrations of test compounds [67]. Other studies also showed the synergistic antibacterial effect of curcumin against both MSSA and MRSA when used in combination with antibiotics such as Cefaclor, Cefodizime, Cefotaxime, Gentamicin, Amikacin, Penicillin, and Erythromycin (refer to Table 2). Based on reported findings, the curcumin synergism in combination with antibiotics appears to be relatively nonspecific. Antibiotics classes that have shown synergism with curcumin include β-lactams, Cephalosporins, Aminoglycosides, Glycopeptides, Tetracyclines, and Fluoroquinolones. This might due to the multitargeting action of curcumin or their undetermined breakdown products as pointed out in the previous section. More studies are needed to evaluate the mechanism of curcumin synergism based on the different classes of antibiotics. In addition to antibacterial action, curcumin also reverses the drug resistance when used in combination with other anticancer agents such as cisplatin, 5-fluorouracil, oxaliplatin, and doxorubicin in multiple types of cancer cells including breast [68], colon [69], head and neck [70], and ovary [71]. The curcumin may have acted on the target or pathway related to the development of drug resistance, hence restoring the killing effect of the drugs [72, 73]. This may be one of the mechanisms on how curcumin enhances the effect of antibacterial drugs, especially when they are targeting *S. aureus*-infected human cells.

In recent years, MRSA infection has emerged as a serious infection due to its multidrug resistance (MDR) especially in the hospital setting [74]. The MRSA infection may spread rapidly especially when the disease is not well controlled. Curcumin exhibits potent activity against MRSA, not only when used alone, but also in combination with other antibiotics. In an effort to understand the curcumin's anti-MRSA effect, Mun et al. [32] showed that the Tris and Triton X-100 inhibited the bacterial growth to 63% and 59%, respectively, when used together with curcumin. This suggests that bacterial membrane permeability is partly responsible in regulating the antibacterial efficacy of curcumin against MRSA. The same group has also shown that ATPase inhibitors (DCCD and NaN_3) which block the ATP-binding cassette (ABC) enhanced the MRSA killing when used together with curcumin. The importance of membrane permeability/integrity in curcumin effect was also confirmed when the increase of peptidoglycan (PGN) concentration successively blocked the curcumin antibacterial activity [32]. These findings suggest that any drug or inhibitor that primarily acts on the bacterial membrane has higher chance of showing enhanced activity when used together with curcumin. It is also noteworthy that the expression of Penicillin-binding protein 2α (PBP2α), a protein responsible in conferring resistance towards β-lactam antibiotics, was downregulated in MRSA upon curcumin treatment [32]. This protein which is encoded by *MecA*, a nonnative gene in MRSA has significantly reduced affinity for β-lactam antibiotics such as Methicillin and Penicillin. Cell-wall biosynthesis, the target of β-lactam, could therefore carry on in MRSA despite the presence of potent doses of these antibiotics [75]. The detailed mode of action of curcumin in inhibiting PBP2α expression in MRSA is not clear at this juncture. It is plausible that curcumin may act on the transcription of *MecA* gene, thereby blocking the expression of PBP2α protein (Figure 2).

In addition to antibiotics, there are evidences showing that curcumin augments the activity of other natural compounds against MSSA and MRSA. Balan et al. [76] demonstrated that combination of curcumin and whey proteins markedly inhibited *S. aureus* growth *in vitro*. Sharma et al. [77] have also previously reported the combination effect of curcumin with several phytochemicals such as cinnamaldehyde, ellagic acid, and eugenol against *Staphylococcus epidermidis* (*S. epidermidis*), which is closely related to *S. aureus*. The combination activities as such against *S. aureus* remain to be investigated. Indeed, there have been many studies showing the potent antibacterial action of other natural compounds against *S. aureus* such as thymoquinone [78], rhein [79], emodin [80], silibinin [81], osthol [82], tannic acid [83], and epigallocatechin gallate [84]. These findings warrant the potential use of abovementioned compounds in combination with curcumin against *S. aureus*.

4. The Challenges of Using Curcumin as Antibiotic

Cumulative findings suggest that curcumin has broad-spectrum antibacterial activities and has synergistic effects with other antibiotics in combination therapies *in vitro* [1, 6, 85]. Curcumin has also shown potent antibacterial action in the mouse model [40]. Nonetheless, the curcumin antibacterial activity has never been evaluated in clinical trials with an aim of using it as a future antibiotic. In this section, we discuss the underlying challenges from the clinical perspectives in developing curcumin into a potential antibiotic.

While curcumin is known to possess the pharmacological activities at relatively low doses, several studies have evidenced some cytotoxicity of curcumin [50–54, 86]. The first study that demonstrated the curcumin toxicity was by Goodpasture and Arrighi [50]. They showed that turmeric resulted in an induction of chromosome aberrations in tested cell lines starting from 10 μg/mL. Other studies have also shown the toxic effects of curcumin mainly on the DNA damage and chromosome aberrations [51–53]. While DNA alteration is the starting point of carcinogenesis, the use of curcumin under abovementioned conditions might be an issue. In other words, curcumin treatment may cause cancers even though the anticancer action of curcumin is well documented. In 1993, a study has concluded that turmeric oleoresin (turmeric extract containing 79–85% of curcumin) has carcinogenic property in rats and mice [54]. Mice taking 0.2 mg/kg body weight of curcumin daily average were found to have carcinomas in their small intestines. Curcumin has also shown to promote lung cancer in another study [55]. The tumour-promoting activity of curcumin has been linked to the induction of reactive oxygen species (ROS) production such as superoxide anion and hydrogen peroxide [87–89].

As curcumin is an active iron chelator, it may potentially affect systemic iron metabolism especially those who have suboptimal iron status [56]. Furthermore, curcumin has been reported to block the enzymes that metabolize drugs such as cytochrome P450s [57, 58]. This may lead to the accumulation of nonmetabolized drugs in blood and result in undesired toxicity. In human, nonetheless, the side effects of curcumin have been relatively mild. A human trial has shown that curcumin ranging from 0.9 to 3.6 g per day up to 4 months only caused some adverse effects that included nausea, diarrhea, and increased serum alkaline phosphatase and lactate dehydrogenase [90]. In 2010, Balaji and Chempakam [91] have predicted a few toxigenic and potent compounds from turmeric using a cost-effective cheminformatics approach. This method can be adopted to select the effective but nontoxic curcumin or its derivatives for further biological studies. However, the selected compound has to be evaluated in a long-term study at its active dose against *S. aureus* in order to confirm the safety of using curcumin as a potential antibiotic.

Curcumin is usually extracted from turmeric plant mainly by solvent extraction followed by column-based purification [2, 3]. Curcumin is sparingly soluble in water (<0.1 mg/mL) and is mainly dissolved in organic solvents such as DMSO, DMF, or ethanol (Tables 1 and 2). This may be the major concern when it is administered into human system as human plasma is composed of 92% of water. The water-insoluble nature may affect curcumin bioavailability and hence affect its pharmacological potential [26, 27, 61]. To this end, several methods have been developed in recent years to circumvent the poor solubility and stability of curcumin, thereby maximizing its pharmacological or biological actions. For example, it has been reported that the use of heat could enhance the curcumin solubility [59, 60]. Kurien et al. [59] have reported the improved water solubility of curcumin from 0.6 to 7.4 μg/mL, without displaying heat-mediated destruction of the chemical structure. Development of curcumin bioconjugates has also shown to be an effective method of enhancing the curcumin solubility. For instances, conjugation of curcumin with hyaluronic acid formed micelles in aqueous phase at physiological pH and appeared to be nontoxic [92]. Dey and Sreenivasan have also conjugated curcumin with alginate, a natural polysaccharide product, in order to increase its stability and bioavailability [93]. Other macromolecules that could serve as carrier systems for curcumin include beta-casein [94], chitosan/Tween 20 [95], emulsomes [96], sodium caseinate [97], and albumin [98, 99]. The development of curcumin nanoformulations has been extensively reviewed in light of its anticancer action [100–102]. While increasing number of curcumin nanoformulation is being introduced into the therapeutic field, it is important to ensure that the bioconjugates or nanoformulations do not diminish the antibacterial effects of curcumin at the expense of improved bioavailability in order to develop them into effective antibiotics in the future.

Table 3: Challenges of curcumin use in clinical setting.

Challenge	References
Cytotoxicity	
DNA damage and chromosome aberrations	[50–53]
Carcinogenesis	
Promote tumour formation *in vivo*	[54, 55]
Iron chelation	
Alter systemic iron metabolism	[56]
Enzyme inhibition	
Inhibit drug-metabolizing enzymes	[57, 58]
Solubility	
Hydrophobic nature does not support water solubility	[59, 60]
Bioavailability	
Degradation by plasma protease and nonspecific protein binding	[26, 27, 61, 62]

In addition to potential toxicity, poor solubility, and low bioavailability, curcumin encounters multiple challenges when it is administered either through oral or intravenous route due to the nature of body system [26, 59, 61, 62]. A large amount of curcumin may get degraded in the presence of detoxifying and metabolic enzymes, or it may bind to the circulatory proteins such as albumin which may potentially reduce its activity. Contradictorily, there have been evidences showing that degraded products from curcumin are responsible of its pharmacological activities [26, 27]. Furthermore, it has been shown that albumin-bound curcumin exerted similar level of activity compared to the DMSO-dissolved curcumin in serum [103]. Of note, the curcumin degradation and binding with physiological proteins have not been evaluated in light of the curcumin antibacterial action. Whether or not these factors would affect the activity of curcumin, further investigations are required. Notably, development of the curcumin bioconjugates, nanoformulations, or derivatives could be the key to overcome the challenges mentioned above (summarized in Table 3). The development of modified curcumin has been recently reviewed [62, 100, 101].

5. Conclusion

Curcumin has shown potent antibacterial activity and other pharmacological actions in the past 50 years. Curcumin has been marketed globally as a health supplement mainly for its antioxidant and anti-inflammatory properties. In addition, it also has high potential to be developed into an antibiotic against *S. aureus* and other bacterial strains in the future. However, the challenges mentioned in the preceding sections should be taken into consideration to open the door for the development of more biologically active curcumin derivatives. To the best of our understanding, this is the first review that compares and summarizes the curcumin antibacterial activity against *S. aureus*. More investigation is required in order to better understand the broad action of curcumin prior to develop this compound or its derivatives into a potential antibiotic.

Competing Interests

The authors declared that there are no competing interests.

Acknowledgments

The authors would like to thank the Director General of Health Malaysia for permission to publish this study and the Director of the Institute for Medical Research for her support.

References

[1] A. Goel, A. B. Kunnumakkara, and B. B. Aggarwal, "Curcumin as 'Curecumin': from kitchen to clinic," *Biochemical Pharmacology*, vol. 75, no. 4, pp. 787–809, 2008.

[2] M. Li, M. O. Ngadi, and Y. Ma, "Optimisation of pulsed ultrasonic and microwave-assisted extraction for curcuminoids by response surface methodology and kinetic study," *Food Chemistry*, vol. 165, pp. 29–34, 2014.

[3] K. I. Priyadarsini, "The chemistry of curcumin: from extraction to therapeutic agent," *Molecules*, vol. 19, no. 12, pp. 20091–20112, 2014.

[4] S. C. Gupta, S. Prasad, J. H. Kim et al., "Multitargeting by curcumin as revealed by molecular interaction studies," *Natural Product Reports*, vol. 28, no. 12, pp. 1937–1955, 2011.

[5] R. K. Maheshwari, A. K. Singh, J. Gaddipati, and R. C. Srimal, "Multiple biological activities of curcumin: a short review," *Life Sciences*, vol. 78, no. 18, pp. 2081–2087, 2006.

[6] S. Z. Moghadamtousi, H. A. Kadir, P. Hassandarvish, H. Tajik, S. Abubakar, and K. Zandi, "A review on antibacterial, antiviral, and antifungal activity of curcumin," *BioMed Research International*, vol. 2014, Article ID 186864, 12 pages, 2014.

[7] S. Bansal and S. Chhibber, "Curcumin alone and in combination with augmentin protects against pulmonary inflammation and acute lung injury generated during *Klebsiella pneumoniae* B5055-induced lung infection in BALB/c mice," *Journal of Medical Microbiology*, vol. 59, no. 4, pp. 429–437, 2010.

[8] S.-Y. Teow and S. A. Ali, "Synergistic antibacterial activity of curcumin with antibiotics against *Staphylococcus aureus*," *Pakistan Journal of Pharmaceutical Sciences*, vol. 28, no. 6, pp. 2109–2114, 2015.

[9] S.-H. Mun, D.-K. Joung, Y.-S. Kim et al., "Synergistic antibacterial effect of curcumin against methicillin-resistant *Staphylococcus aureus*," *Phytomedicine*, vol. 20, no. 8-9, pp. 714–718, 2013.

[10] A. S. Garcia-Gomes, J. A. R. Curvelo, R. M. A. Soares, and A. Ferreira-Pereira, "Curcumin acts synergistically with fluconazole to sensitize a clinical isolate of *Candida albicans* showing a MDR phenotype," *Medical Mycology*, vol. 50, no. 1, pp. 26–32, 2012.

[11] M. Sharma, R. Manoharlal, A. S. Negi, and R. Prasad, "Synergistic anticandidal activity of pure polyphenol curcumin i in combination with azoles and polyenes generates reactive oxygen species leading to apoptosis," *FEMS Yeast Research*, vol. 10, no. 5, pp. 570–578, 2010.

[12] B. B. Patel and A. P. N. Majumdar, "Synergistic role of curcumin with current therapeutics in colorectal cancer: minireview," *Nutrition and Cancer*, vol. 61, no. 6, pp. 842–846, 2009.

[13] A. O. Boztas, O. Karakuzu, G. Galante et al., "Synergistic interaction of paclitaxel and curcumin with cyclodextrin polymer complexation in human cancer cells," *Molecular Pharmaceutics*, vol. 10, no. 7, pp. 2676–2683, 2013.

[14] N. Aftab and A. Vieira, "Antioxidant activities of curcumin and combinations of this curcuminoid with other phytochemicals," *Phytotherapy Research*, vol. 24, no. 4, pp. 500–502, 2010.

[15] O. Naksuriya and S. Okonogi, "Comparison and combination effects on antioxidant power of curcumin with gallic acid, ascorbic acid, and xanthone," *Drug Discoveries and Therapeutics*, vol. 9, no. 2, pp. 136–141, 2015.

[16] N. Chainani-Wu, "Safety and anti-inflammatory activity of curcumin: a component of tumeric (*Curcuma longa*)," *Journal of Alternative and Complementary Medicine*, vol. 9, no. 1, pp. 161–168, 2003.

[17] M. Kanai, K. Yoshimura, M. Asada et al., "A phase I/II study of gemcitabine-based chemotherapy plus curcumin for patients with gemcitabine-resistant pancreatic cancer," *Cancer Chemotherapy and Pharmacology*, vol. 68, no. 1, pp. 157–164, 2011.

[18] N. Dhillon, B. B. Aggarwal, R. A. Newman et al., "Phase II trial of curcumin in patients with advanced pancreatic cancer," *Clinical Cancer Research*, vol. 14, no. 14, pp. 4491–4499, 2008.

[19] S. Poapolathep, K. Imsilp, K. Machii, S. Kumagai, and A. Poapolathep, "The effects of curcumin on aflatoxin B1- induced toxicity in rats," *Biocontrol Science*, vol. 20, no. 3, pp. 171–177, 2015.

[20] D. J. Messner, G. Sivam, and K. V. Kowdley, "Curcumin reduces the toxic effects of iron loading in rat liver epithelial cells," *Liver International*, vol. 29, no. 1, pp. 63–72, 2009.

[21] F. A. Badria, A. S. Ibrahim, A. F. Badria, and A. A. Elmarakby, "Curcumin attenuates iron accumulation and oxidative stress in the liver and spleen of chronic iron-overloaded rats," *PLoS ONE*, vol. 10, no. 7, Article ID e0134156, 2015.

[22] M.-H. Teiten, S. Eifes, M. Dicato, and M. Diederich, "Curcumin-the paradigm of a multi-target natural compound with applications in cancer prevention and treatment," *Toxins*, vol. 2, no. 1, pp. 128–162, 2010.

[23] S. C. Gupta, S. Patchva, W. Koh, and B. B. Aggarwal, "Discovery of curcumin, a component of golden spice, and its miraculous biological activities," *Clinical and Experimental Pharmacology and Physiology*, vol. 39, no. 3, pp. 283–299, 2012.

[24] H. Zhou, C. S. Beevers, and S. Huang, "The targets of curcumin," *Current Drug Targets*, vol. 12, no. 3, pp. 332–347, 2011.

[25] C. Schneider, O. N. Gordon, R. L. Edwards, and P. B. Luis, "Degradation of curcumin: from mechanism to biological implications," *Journal of Agricultural and Food Chemistry*, vol. 63, no. 35, pp. 7606–7614, 2015.

[26] L. Shen and H.-F. Ji, "The pharmacology of curcumin: Is it the degradation products?" *Trends in Molecular Medicine*, vol. 18, no. 3, pp. 138–144, 2012.

[27] L. Shen, C.-C. Liu, C.-Y. An, and H.-F. Ji, "How does curcumin work with poor bioavailability? Clues from experimental and theoretical studies," *Scientific Reports*, vol. 6, Article ID 20872, 2016.

[28] D. Ghosh, D. Bagchi, and T. Konishi, *Clinical Aspects of Functional Foods and Nutraceuticals*, CRC Press/Taylor and Francis Group, 2014.

[29] E. Schraufstätter and H. Bernt, "Antibacterial action of curcumin and related compounds," *Nature*, vol. 164, no. 4167, pp. 456–457, 1949.

[30] P. Tyagi, M. Singh, H. Kumari, A. Kumari, and K. Mukhopadhyay, "Bactericidal activity of curcumin I is associated with damaging of bacterial membrane," *PLoS ONE*, vol. 10, no. 3, Article ID e0121313, 2015.

[31] K. Moghaddam, M. Iranshahi, M. Yazdi, and A. Shahverdi, "The combination effect of curcumin with different antibiotics against Staphylococcus aureus," *International Journal of Green Pharmacy*, vol. 3, no. 2, pp. 141–143, 2009.

[32] S.-H. Mun, S.-B. Kim, R. Kong et al., "Curcumin reverse methicillin resistance in *Staphylococcus aureus*," *Molecules*, vol. 19, no. 11, pp. 18283–18295, 2014.

[33] S. Y. C. Tong, J. S. Davis, E. Eichenberger, T. L. Holland, and V. G. Fowler, "*Staphylococcus aureus* infections: epidemiology, pathophysiology, clinical manifestations, and management," *Clinical Microbiology Reviews*, vol. 28, no. 3, pp. 603–661, 2015.

[34] H. W. Boucher and G. R. Corey, "Epidemiology of methicillin-resistant *Staphylococcus aureus*," *Clinical Infectious Diseases*, vol. 46, supplement 5, pp. S344–S349, 2008.

[35] E. Klein, D. L. Smith, and R. Laxminarayan, "Hospitalizations and deaths caused by methicillin-resistant *Staphylococcus aureus*, United States, 1999-2005," *Emerging Infectious Diseases*, vol. 13, no. 12, pp. 1840–1846, 2007.

[36] B. Tarai, P. Das, and D. Kumar, "Recurrent challenges for clinicians: emergence of methicillin-resistant *Staphylococcus aureus*, vancomycin resistance, and current treatment options," *Journal of Laboratory Physicians*, vol. 5, no. 2, pp. 71–78, 2013.

[37] C. L. Ventola, "The antibiotic resistance crisis—part 1: causes and threats," *Pharmacy and Therapeutics*, vol. 40, no. 4, pp. 277–283, 2015.

[38] R. V. Rasmussen, V. G. Fowler Jr., R. Skov, and N. E. Bruun, "Future challenges and treatment of *Staphylococcus aureus* bacteremia with emphasis on MRSA," *Future Microbiology*, vol. 6, no. 1, pp. 43–56, 2011.

[39] A. P. D. Ribeiro, A. C. Pavarina, L. N. Dovigo et al., "Phototoxic effect of curcumin on methicillin-resistant *Staphylococcus aureus* and L929 fibroblasts," *Lasers in Medical Science*, vol. 28, no. 2, pp. 391–398, 2013.

[40] J. Wang, X. Zhou, W. Li, X. Deng, Y. Deng, and X. Niu, "Curcumin protects mice from *Staphylococcus aureus* pneumonia by interfering with the self-assembly process of α-hemolysin," *Scientific Reports*, vol. 6, Article ID 28254, 2016.

[41] N. K. Sasidharan, S. R. Sreekala, J. Jacob, and B. Nambisan, "*In vitro* synergistic effect of curcumin in combination with third generation cephalosporins against bacteria associated with infectious diarrhea," *BioMed Research International*, vol. 2014, Article ID 561456, 8 pages, 2014.

[42] S. Tajbakhsh, K. Mohammadi, I. Deilami et al., "Antibacterial activity of indium curcumin and indium diacetylcurcumin," *African Journal of Biotechnology*, vol. 7, no. 21, pp. 3832–3835, 2008.

[43] K. Mohammadi, K. H. Thompson, B. O. Patrick et al., "Synthesis and characterization of dual function vanadyl, gallium and indium curcumin complexes for medicinal applications," *Journal of Inorganic Biochemistry*, vol. 99, no. 11, pp. 2217–2225, 2005.

[44] D. Rai, J. K. Singh, N. Roy, and D. Panda, "Curcumin inhibits FtsZ assembly: an attractive mechanism for its antibacterial activity," *Biochemical Journal*, vol. 410, no. 1, pp. 147–155, 2008.

[45] G. Y. Liu, "Molecular pathogenesis of *Staphylococcus aureus* infection," *Pediatric Research*, vol. 65, no. 5, part 2, pp. 71R–77R, 2009.

[46] L. G. Miller and S. L. Kaplan, "*Staphylococcus aureus*: a community pathogen," *Infectious Disease Clinics of North America*, vol. 23, no. 1, pp. 35–52, 2009.

[47] H. Gunes, D. Gulen, R. Mutlu, A. Gumus, T. Tas, and A. E. Topkaya, "Antibacterial effects of curcumin: an *in vitro* minimum inhibitory concentration study," *Toxicology and Industrial Health*, vol. 32, no. 2, pp. 246–250, 2016.

[48] A. Kali, D. Bhuvaneshwar, P. V. Charles, and K. Seetha, "Antibacterial synergy of curcumin with antibiotics against biofilm producing clinical bacterial isolates," *Journal of Basic and Clinical Pharmacy*, vol. 7, no. 3, pp. 93–96, 2016.

[49] S. Sandikci Altunatmaz, F. Yilmaz Aksu, G. Issa, B. Basaran Kahraman, D. Dulger Altiner, and S. Buyukunal, "Antimicrobial effects of curcumin against *L. monocytogenes, S. aureus, S. Typhimurium* and *E. coli* O157 : H7 pathogens in minced meat," *Veterinární Medicína*, vol. 61, no. 5, pp. 256–262, 2016.

[50] C. E. Goodpasture and F. E. Arrighi, "Effects of food seasonings on the cell cycle and chromosome morphology of mammalian cells in vitro with special reference to turmeric," *Food and Cosmetics Toxicology*, vol. 14, no. 1, pp. 9–14, 1976.

[51] J. Cao, L. Jia, H.-M. Zhou, Y. Liu, and L.-F. Zhong, "Mitochondrial and nuclear DNA damage induced by curcumin in human hepatoma G2 cells," *Toxicological Sciences*, vol. 91, no. 2, pp. 476–483, 2006.

[52] P. Urbina-Cano, L. Bobadilla-Morales, M. A. Ramírez-Herrera et al., "DNA damage in mouse lymphocytes exposed to curcumin and copper," *Journal of Applied Genetics*, vol. 47, no. 4, pp. 377–382, 2006.

[53] R. D. Verschoyle, W. P. Steward, and A. J. Gescher, "Putative cancer chemopreventive agents of dietary origin-how safe are they?" *Nutrition and Cancer*, vol. 59, no. 2, pp. 152–162, 2007.

[54] National Toxicology Program, "NTP toxicology and carcinogenesis studies of turmeric oleoresin (CAS No. 8024-37-1) (major component 79%-85% curcumin, CAS No. 458-37-7) in F344/N rats and B6C3F1 mice (feed studies)," *National Toxicology Program Technical Report Series*, vol. 427, pp. 1–275, 1993.

[55] S. T. Dance-Barnes, N. D. Kock, J. E. Moore et al., "Lung tumor promotion by curcumin," *Carcinogenesis*, vol. 30, no. 6, pp. 1016–1023, 2009.

[56] Y. Jiao, J. Wilkinson IV, X. Di et al., "Curcumin, a cancer chemopreventive and chemotherapeutic agent, is a biologically active iron chelator," *Blood*, vol. 113, no. 2, pp. 462–469, 2009.

[57] R. Appiah-Opong, J. N. M. Commandeur, B. van Vugt-Lussenburg, and N. P. E. Vermeulen, "Inhibition of human recombinant cytochrome P450s by curcumin and curcumin decomposition products," *Toxicology*, vol. 235, no. 1-2, pp. 83–91, 2007.

[58] R. Thapliyal and G. B. Maru, "Inhibition of cytochrome P450 isozymes by curcumins *in vitro* and *in vivo*," *Food and Chemical Toxicology*, vol. 39, no. 6, pp. 541–547, 2001.

[59] B. T. Kurien, A. Singh, H. Matsumoto, and R. H. Scofield, "Improving the solubility and pharmacological efficacy of curcumin by heat treatment," *Assay and Drug Development Technologies*, vol. 5, no. 4, pp. 567–576, 2007.

[60] B. T. Kurien and R. H. Scofield, "Heat-solubilized curcumin should be considered in clinical trials for increasing bioavailability," *Clinical Cancer Research*, vol. 15, no. 2, p. 747, 2009.

[61] P. Anand, A. B. Kunnumakkara, R. A. Newman, and B. B. Aggarwal, "Bioavailability of curcumin: problems and promises," *Molecular Pharmaceutics*, vol. 4, no. 6, pp. 807–818, 2007.

[62] S. Prasad, A. K. Tyagi, and B. B. Aggarwal, "Recent developments in delivery, bioavailability, absorption and metabolism

of curcumin: the golden pigment from golden spice," *Cancer Research and Treatment*, vol. 46, no. 1, pp. 2–18, 2014.

[63] T. Matsui, J. Yamane, N. Mogi et al., "Structural reorganization of the bacterial cell-division protein FtsZ from *Staphylococcus aureus*," *Acta Crystallographica Section D: Biological Crystallography*, vol. 68, no. 9, pp. 1175–1188, 2012.

[64] P. Singh and D. Panda, "FtsZ inhibition: a promising approach for anti-staphylococcal therapy," *Drug News and Perspectives*, vol. 23, no. 5, pp. 295–304, 2010.

[65] P. Gul and J. Bakht, "Antimicrobial activity of turmeric extract and its potential use in food industry," *Journal of Food Science and Technology*, vol. 52, no. 4, pp. 2272–2279, 2015.

[66] A. Gupta, S. Mahajan, and R. Sharma, "Evaluation of antimicrobial activity of *Curcuma longa* rhizome extract against *Staphylococcus aureus*," *Biotechnology Reports*, vol. 6, pp. 51–55, 2015.

[67] J. E. Foweraker, C. R. Laughton, D. F. Brown, and D. Bilton, "Comparison of methods to test antibiotic combinations against heterogeneous populations of multiresistant *Pseudomonas aeruginosa* from patients with acute infective exacerbations in cystic fibrosis," *Antimicrobial Agents and Chemotherapy*, vol. 53, no. 11, pp. 4809–4815, 2009.

[68] G. S. Sen, S. Mohanty, D. M. S. Hossain et al., "Curcumin enhances the efficacy of chemotherapy by tailoring p65NFκB-p300 cross-talk in favor of p53-p300 in breast cancer," *The Journal of Biological Chemistry*, vol. 286, no. 49, pp. 42232–42247, 2011.

[69] V. Ruiz de Porras, S. Bystrup, A. Martínez-Cardús et al., "Curcumin mediates oxaliplatin-acquired resistance reversion in colorectal cancer cell lines through modulation of CXC-Chemokine/NF-κB signalling pathway," *Scientific Reports*, vol. 6, article 24675, 2016.

[70] B. Sivanantham, S. Sethuraman, and U. M. Krishnan, "Combinatorial effects of curcumin with an anti-neoplastic agent on head and neck squamous cell carcinoma through the regulation of EGFR-ERK1/2 and apoptotic signaling pathways," *ACS Combinatorial Science*, vol. 18, no. 1, pp. 22–35, 2016.

[71] H. Wahl, L. Tan, K. Griffith, M. Choi, and J. R. Liu, "Curcumin enhances Apo2L/TRAIL-induced apoptosis in chemoresistant ovarian cancer cells," *Gynecologic Oncology*, vol. 105, no. 1, pp. 104–112, 2007.

[72] S. Saha, A. Adhikary, P. Bhattacharyya, T. Das, and G. Sa, "Death by design: where curcumin sensitizes drug-resistant tumours," *Anticancer Research*, vol. 32, no. 7, pp. 2567–2584, 2012.

[73] T. Nabekura, "Overcoming multidrug resistance in human cancer cells by natural compounds," *Toxins*, vol. 2, no. 6, pp. 1207–1224, 2010.

[74] R. Köck, K. Becker, B. Cookson et al., "Methicillin-resistant *Staphylococcus aureus* (MRSA): burden of disease and control challenges in Europe," *Euro Surveillance*, vol. 15, no. 41, Article ID 19688, 2010.

[75] S. J. Peacock and G. K. Paterson, "Mechanisms of methicillin resistance in *Staphylococcus aureus*," *Annual Review of Biochemistry*, vol. 84, pp. 577–601, 2015.

[76] P. Balan, G. Mal, S. Das, and H. Singh, "Synergistic and additive antimicrobial activities of curcumin, Manuka honey and whey proteins," *Journal of Food Biochemistry*, vol. 40, no. 5, pp. 647–654, 2016.

[77] G. Sharma, K. Raturi, S. Dang, S. Gupta, and R. Gabrani, "Combinatorial antimicrobial effect of curcumin with selected phytochemicals on *Staphylococcus epidermidis*," *Journal of Asian Natural Products Research*, vol. 16, no. 5, pp. 535–541, 2014.

[78] K. Chaieb, B. Kouidhi, H. Jrah, K. Mahdouani, and A. Bakhrouf, "Antibacterial activity of Thymoquinone, an active principle of *Nigella sativa* and its potency to prevent bacterial biofilm formation," *BMC Complementary and Alternative Medicine*, vol. 11, article 29, 2011.

[79] D.-K. Joung, H. Joung, D.-W. Yang et al., "Synergistic effect of rhein in combination with ampicillin or oxacillin against methicillin-resistant Staphylococcus aureus," *Experimental and Therapeutic Medicine*, vol. 3, no. 4, pp. 608–612, 2012.

[80] Y.-S. Lee, O.-H. Kang, J.-G. Choi et al., "Synergistic effect of emodin in combination with ampicillin or oxacillin against methicillin-resistant *Staphylococcus aureus*," *Pharmaceutical Biology*, vol. 48, no. 11, pp. 1285–1290, 2010.

[81] H.-K. Kang, H.-Y. Kim, and J.-D. Cha, "Synergistic effects between silibinin and antibiotics on methicillin-resistant *Staphylococcus aureus* isolated from clinical specimens," *Biotechnology Journal*, vol. 6, no. 11, pp. 1397–1408, 2011.

[82] P. Joshi, S. Singh, A. Wani et al., "Osthol and curcumin as inhibitors of human Pgp and multidrug efflux pumps of *Staphylococcus aureus*: reversing the resistance against frontline antibacterial drugs," *MedChemComm*, vol. 5, no. 10, pp. 1540–1547, 2014.

[83] H. Akiyama, K. Fujii, O. Yamasaki, T. Oono, and K. Iwatsuki, "Antibacterial action of several tannins against *Staphylococcus aureus*," *Journal of Antimicrobial Chemotherapy*, vol. 48, no. 4, pp. 487–491, 2001.

[84] W.-H. Zhao, Z.-Q. Hu, S. Okubo, Y. Hara, and T. Shimamura, "Mechanism of synergy between epigallocatechin gallate and β-lactams against methicillin-resistant *Staphylococcus aureus*," *Antimicrobial Agents and Chemotherapy*, vol. 45, no. 6, pp. 1737–1742, 2001.

[85] S. C. Gupta, S. Patchva, and B. B. Aggarwal, "Therapeutic roles of curcumin: lessons learned from clinical trials," *AAPS Journal*, vol. 15, no. 1, pp. 195–218, 2013.

[86] E. Burgos-Morón, J. M. Calderón-Montaño, J. Salvador, A. Robles, and M. López-Lázaro, "The dark side of curcumin," *International Journal of Cancer*, vol. 126, no. 7, pp. 1771–1775, 2010.

[87] S. J. McNally, E. M. Harrison, J. A. Ross, O. J. Garden, and S. J. Wigmore, "Curcumin induces heme oxygenase 1 through generation of reactive oxygen species, p38 activation and phosphatase inhibition," *International Journal of Molecular Medicine*, vol. 19, no. 1, pp. 165–172, 2007.

[88] J. Kang, J. Chen, Y. Shi, J. Jia, and Y. Zhang, "Curcumin-induced histone hypoacetylation: the role of reactive oxygen species," *Biochemical Pharmacology*, vol. 69, no. 8, pp. 1205–1213, 2005.

[89] T. Atsumi, S. Fujisawa, and K. Tonosaki, "Relationship between intracellular ROS production and membrane mobility in curcumin- and tetrahydrocurcumin-treated human gingival fibroblasts and human submandibular gland carcinoma cells," *Oral Diseases*, vol. 11, no. 4, pp. 236–242, 2005.

[90] R. A. Sharma, S. A. Euden, S. L. Platton et al., "Phase I clinical trial of oral curcumin: biomarkers of systemic activity and compliance," *Clinical Cancer Research*, vol. 10, no. 20, pp. 6847–6854, 2004.

[91] S. Balaji and B. Chempakam, "Toxicity prediction of compounds from turmeric (*Curcuma longa* L)," *Food and Chemical Toxicology*, vol. 48, no. 10, pp. 2951–2959, 2010.

[92] S. Manju and K. Sreenivasan, "Conjugation of curcumin onto hyaluronic acid enhances its aqueous solubility and stability," *Journal of Colloid and Interface Science*, vol. 359, no. 1, pp. 318–325, 2011.

[93] S. Dey and K. Sreenivasan, "Conjugation of curcumin onto alginate enhances aqueous solubility and stability of curcumin," *Carbohydrate Polymers*, vol. 99, pp. 499–507, 2014.

[94] M. Esmaili, S. M. Ghaffari, Z. Moosavi-Movahedi et al., "Beta casein-micelle as a nano vehicle for solubility enhancement of curcumin; food industry application," *LWT—Food Science and Technology*, vol. 44, no. 10, pp. 2166–2172, 2011.

[95] M. G. O'Toole, R. M. Henderson, P. A. Soucy et al., "Curcumin encapsulation in submicrometer spray-dried chitosan/Tween 20 particles," *Biomacromolecules*, vol. 13, no. 8, pp. 2309–2314, 2012.

[96] M. H. Ucisik, S. Küpcü, B. Schuster, and U. B. Sleytr, "Characterization of CurcuEmulsomes: nanoformulation for enhanced solubility and delivery of curcumin," *Journal of Nanobiotechnology*, vol. 11, no. 1, article 37, 2013.

[97] K. Pan, Q. Zhong, and S. J. Baek, "Enhanced dispersibility and bioactivity of curcumin by encapsulation in casein nanocapsules," *Journal of Agricultural and Food Chemistry*, vol. 61, no. 25, pp. 6036–6043, 2013.

[98] C. Thomas, L. S. Pillai, and L. Krishnan, "Evaluation of albuminated curcumin as soluble drug form to control growth of cancer cells *in vitro*," *Journal of Cancer Therapy*, vol. 5, no. 7, pp. 723–734, 2014.

[99] T. H. Kim, H. H. Jiang, Y. S. Youn et al., "Preparation and characterization of water-soluble albumin-bound curcumin nanoparticles with improved antitumor activity," *International Journal of Pharmaceutics*, vol. 403, no. 1-2, pp. 285–291, 2011.

[100] M. M. Yallapu, M. Jaggi, and S. C. Chauhan, "Curcumin nanoformulations: a future nanomedicine for cancer," *Drug Discovery Today*, vol. 17, no. 1-2, pp. 71–80, 2012.

[101] M. M. Yallapu, M. Jaggi, and S. C. Chauhan, "Curcumin nanomedicine: a road to cancer therapeutics," *Current Pharmaceutical Design*, vol. 19, no. 11, pp. 1994–2010, 2013.

[102] N. Ghalandarlaki, A. M. Alizadeh, and S. Ashkani-Esfahani, "Nanotechnology-applied curcumin for different diseases therapy," *BioMed Research International*, vol. 2014, Article ID 394264, 23 pages, 2014.

[103] W. W. Quitschke, "Differential solubility of curcuminoids in serum and albumin solutions: implications for analytical and therapeutic applications," *BMC Biotechnology*, vol. 8, article 84, 2008.

18

Clinical Profile and Visual Outcome of Ocular Bartonellosis in Malaysia

Chai Lee Tan,[1] Lai Chan Fhun,[1,2] Evelyn Li Min Tai,[1]
Nor Hasnida Abdul Gani,[3] Julieana Muhammed,[1] Tengku Norina Tuan Jaafar,[3]
Liza Sharmini Ahmad Tajudin,[1] and Wan-Hazabbah Wan Hitam[1]

[1]*Department of Ophthalmology, School of Medical Sciences, Universiti Sains Malaysia, Health Campus, 16150 Kubang Kerian, Kelantan, Malaysia*
[2]*Department of Ophthalmology, Hospital Raja Permaisuri Bainun, 30990 Ipoh, Perak, Malaysia*
[3]*Department of Ophthalmology, Hospital Raja Perempuan Zainab 2, 15586 Kota Bharu, Kelantan, Malaysia*

Correspondence should be addressed to Evelyn Li Min Tai; daileid@yahoo.com

Academic Editor: Marcel Tanner

Background. Ocular bartonellosis can present in various ways, with variable visual outcome. There is limited data on ocular bartonellosis in Malaysia. *Objective.* We aim to describe the clinical presentation and visual outcome of ocular bartonellosis in Malaysia. *Materials and Methods.* This was a retrospective review of patients treated for ocular bartonellosis in two ophthalmology centers in Malaysia between January 2013 and December 2015. The diagnosis was based on clinical features, supported by a positive *Bartonella* spp. serology. *Results.* Of the 19 patients in our series, females were predominant (63.2%). The mean age was 29.3 years. The majority (63.2%) had unilateral involvement. Five patients (26.3%) had a history of contact with cats. Neuroretinitis was the most common presentation (62.5%). Azithromycin was the antibiotic of choice (42.1%). Concurrent systemic corticosteroids were used in approximately 60% of cases. The presenting visual acuity was worse than 6/18 in approximately 60% of eyes; on final review, 76.9% of eyes had a visual acuity better than 6/18. *Conclusion.* Ocular bartonellosis tends to present with neuroretinitis. Azithromycin is a viable option for treatment. Systemic corticosteroids may be considered in those with poor visual acuity on presentation.

1. Introduction

Cat-scratch disease is caused by the Gram-negative, intracellular bacteria *Bartonella henselae*. When ocular involvement is present, the disease is termed "ocular bartonellosis." The spectrum of ocular bartonellosis manifestation is wide, ranging from neuroretinitis to Parinaud's oculoglandular syndrome, which is an unusual syndrome characterized by granulomas in the eye, preauricular lymphadenopathy, and positive skin test to *Bartonella* spp. antigens [1–4]. In Malaysia, the data on cat-scratch disease, particularly ocular bartonellosis, is limited [5]. We aim to describe the clinical manifestations and visual outcome of ocular bartonellosis in Malaysia. We also outline the relevant investigations for this condition and discuss the management of this zoonotic disease.

2. Materials and Methods

We performed a retrospective review of medical records of patients with ocular bartonellosis treated in two ophthalmology centers in Malaysia, between 2013 and 2015. The conduct of the study followed the tenets outlined in the Declaration of Helsinki.

Selection criteria for this study were a diagnosis of ocular bartonellosis based on history of exposure to cats, ocular examination findings, and a single positive serology for *Bartonella* spp. Any two of these were sufficient to make the diagnosis. Patients suspected of ocular bartonellosis were also investigated for other possible infective causes (tuberculosis, syphilis). Serological tests were all performed via immunofluorescence assay (IFA) in the Bacteriology Unit, Institute for Medical Research, Ministry of Health

TABLE 1: Patient demographic profile.

Demographic data	n (%)
Age in year (mean, SD)	29.3, 13.2
Race	
Malay	19 (100.0)
Sex	
Male	7 (36.8)
Female	12 (63.2)
Cat exposure	
No	14 (73.7)
Yes (contact or scratch)	5 (26.3)
Systemic symptoms	
No	8 (42.1)
Yes	11 (57.9)
Headache	7 (43.8)
Upper respiratory tract infection	2 (12.5)
Fever	6 (37.5)
Lymphadenopathy	1 (6.2)

Malaysia. The cut off value was 1:12 for Ig M and 1:64 for Ig G using a commercial kit to detect *Bartonella henselae* and *Bartonella quintana* (Vircell IFA Bartonella, Paraque Tecnologico, Granada, Spain).

Data collected included onset and duration of visual disturbance, associated systemic symptoms, visual acuity, optic nerve function, anterior and posterior segment examination, treatment regime, and visual outcome. The latter was evaluated based on visual acuity at the last follow-up visit. Visual acuity was assessed monocularly, with the patient seated 6 meters from a Snellen chart. A 6/6 Snellen visual acuity means the patient can read at 6 meters a letter that a normal person would be able to read at 6 meters. The denominator in Snellen visual acuity notation describes the distance at which a normal individual is able to identify a certain symbol, while the numerator refers to the distance required by the patient to identify the same symbol. In this study, a visual acuity of 6/18 or better was considered good, while visual acuity worse than 6/18 was considered poor. Follow-up was until completion of the course of antibiotics, given for a minimum of six weeks.

The data were analyzed using the Statistical Package for Social Science, version 22.0 (SPSS Inc., Chicago, IL, USA). The results are presented as frequencies and percentages.

3. Results

A total of 19 patients (26 eyes) with ocular bartonellosis were diagnosed within the study period. The period of follow-up ranged from 3 to 68 weeks, with the mean duration of follow-up being 23.4 weeks. Two patients were lost to follow-up. The duration of symptoms ranged from 5 days to 1 month prior to their first consultation at eye clinic.

The demographic and clinical profile of our subjects is summarized in Table 1. The mean age was 29.3 years. All were Malay, and most of them were female (63.2%, $n = 12$). Only 5 (26.3%) patients gave a history of being scratched or bitten by a cat. The majority (63.2%, $n = 12$) had unilateral involvement.

The most common ocular complaint was blurring of vision, with 61.6% (16 eyes) presenting with a visual acuity worse than 6/18. About one-quarter (7 eyes) had a visual acuity of worse than 6/60. Approximately 62.5% of eyes presented with neuroretinitis. Optic disc edema was seen in 42.1% of patients. One patient presented with features of vasculitis complicated with central retinal vein occlusion, evidenced by macular edema, dilated and tortuous vessels, and flame-shaped hemorrhages. Six patients (31.6%) had signs of uveitis. Ocular findings on presentation and treatment regimes are shown for each patient in Table 2. Table 3 shows a summary of the ocular presentation and results of serological testing.

Approximately 57.9% of patients had prodromal symptoms, of which headache was the most common. Less common symptoms were fever and upper respiratory tract symptoms. *Bartonella* spp. Ig G serology was positive in all patients, while 68.4% ($n = 13$) had positive Ig M serology. Only a single serology test was performed, due to financial constraints. Hence, disease progression was assessed based on clinical response. The duration of ocular symptoms did not vary between patients with positive Ig G and negative Ig M and those who were positive for both of these.

All patients except two received treatment, which was initiated within the first week of diagnosis. In the case of the latter, this was due to spontaneous recovery before treatment could be initiated. Azithromycin was the most common antimicrobial agent used for treatment (42.1%). Doxycycline, ciprofloxacin, ceftazidime, and cotrimoxazole were other agents used. Approximately 57.9% ($n = 11$) received systemic corticosteroid therapy. Six of these patients were treated with pulsed intravenous corticosteroid therapy, followed by oral corticosteroids. The overall final visual acuity was good, with approximately 76.9% of eyes achieving a good visual outcome (visual acuity of 6/18 or better).

4. Discussion

Cat-scratch disease, that is, bartonellosis, is a self-limiting condition in immunocompetent individuals. The spectrum of systemic involvement in bartonellosis ranges from endocarditis to thyroiditis, arthritis, haemolytic anemia, and glomerulonephritis [6–10]. The ocular manifestations of *Bartonella* spp. infection are likewise myriad and have included scotomas [11], papillitis, [12] retinal artery occlusions [13], and even a macular hole [14]. Although systemic cat-scratch disease primarily affects young patients, ocular bartonellosis has a broader age distribution [15]. Our mean age of 29.3 years, with a range of 9 to 58 years, is similar to that of Curi et al. in Brazil [2].

Cats are the main reservoir for *Bartonella* spp., and the main vector of cat-scratch disease is the flea *Ctenocephalides felis* [16]. Cats are common in Malaysia, both as household pets and strays. The prevalence of *Bartonella henselae* in fleas from healthy cats and dogs has been shown to be approximately 33%, while among strays, almost a quarter of

TABLE 2: Ocular Presentation of Bartonellosis and Treatment Regime.

Case number	Lat	Initial VA	Final VA	Positive serology (titre)	Anterior uveitis	Neuroretinitis	Optic disc edema	Others	Rx	Corticosteroid therapy
(1)	B	RE 6/18 LE 6/24	RE 6/7.5 LE 6/7.5	Ig M (1:96) /Ig G (1:56)		Yes			Azi	Oral
(2)	R	6/120	6/21	Ig M (1:24) /Ig G (1:128)	Yes	Yes			Azi	IV then oral
(3)	R	6/24	6/6	Ig M (n/a) /Ig G (n/a)			Yes	Focal choroiditis	Azi	None
(4)	L	6/120	6/45	Ig M (1:24) /Ig G (1:128)			Yes	Retinal infiltrates	Azi	Oral
(5)	L	6/7.5	6/6	Ig M (1:48) /Ig G (1:256)			Yes		Azi	None
(6)	L	2/60	6/6	Ig M/(1:24) /Ig G (1:128)	Yes	Yes		CWS	Azi	Topical
(7)	B	RE 6/30 LE 6/21	RE 6/9 LE 6/6	Ig M/(1:48) /Ig G (1:128)		Yes			Cip	IV only
(8)	B	RE 6/7.5 LE 6/12	RE 6/7.5 LE 6/7.5	Ig G (1:128)		Yes			Dox	None
(9)	L	6/24	LE 6/6	Ig M (1:24) /Ig G (1:128)			Yes		Dox	Topical
(10)	B	RE 6/6 LE 6/6	RE 6/6 LE 6/6	Ig M (1:24) /Ig G (1:128)	Yes		Yes		None	None
(11)	B	RE 6/6 LE 2/60	RE 6/6 LE 6/9	Ig M (1:96) /Ig G (1:512)		Yes		Retinal infiltrates	Azi	Oral
(12)	B	RE CF LE 6/36	RE 6/9 LE 6/6	Ig G (1:128)		Yes		CWS/retinal hemorrhage	Ceft	None
(13)	B	RE 6/9 LE 6/60	RE 6/9 LE 6/24	Ig G (1:128)			Yes		Ceft/Azi	IV then oral
(14)	L	1/60	6/24	Ig M (1:24) /Ig G (1:128)		Yes			Cefu	Oral
(15)	R	HM	HM	Ig M (1:24) /Ig G (1:128)			Yes	Macular edema/ vasculitis/dilated vessels/retinal hemorrhage	Ceft/Dox	IV then oral
(16)	L	6/60	6/36	Ig M (1:24) /Ig G (1:128)		Yes			Dox	IV then oral
(17)	L	6/18	6/9	Ig G (1:128)			Yes	Vasculitis/ dilated vessels/ perivascular sheathing	Co-t	Oral
(18)	R	6/9	6/6	Ig G (1:128)	Yes				Ceft/Cefu	Topical
(19)	L	6/24	6/6	Ig G (1:128)	Yes	Yes		Retinal hemorrhage	None	IV then oral

Lat, laterality; R, right; L, left; B, bilateral; VA: visual acuity; CF, counting finger; HM, hand movement; Ig, immunoglobulin; Rx, antibiotic; Azi, azithromycin; Cip, ciprofloxacin; Dox, doxycycline; Ceft, ceftazidime; Cefu, cefuroxime; Co-t, cotrimoxazole; IV, intravenous.

TABLE 3: Presenting features of ocular bartonellosis.

Parameters	*n* (%)
Laterality	
Left	8 (42.1)
Right	4 (21.1)
Bilateral	7 (36.8)
Ocular presentation	
Anterior uveitis	6 (31.6)
Neuroretinitis	10 (62.5)
Optic disc edema	8 (42.1)
Focal choroiditis	1 (5.3)
Retinal infiltrates	2 (10.5)
Cotton wool spots	1 (5.3)
Retinal hemorrhages	3 (15.8)
Macular edema	1 (5.3)
Vasculitis	2 (10.5)
IFA serology positivity	
Ig M	13 (68.4)
Ig G	19 (100.0)

IFA, immunofluorescent assay; Ig, immunoglobulin.

them have been found to be seropositive for the bacterium [12, 17]. Exposure to cats or a history of cat-scratch or cat bite is usually present in more than 50% of reported cases of bartonellosis [2, 18–20]. A recent study among healthy blood donors in Brazil revealed that cat contact or a history of tick bite conferred an adjusted odds ratio of *Bartonella* spp. bloodstream infection of 3.4 (95% CI 1.1–9.6) and 3.7 (95% CI 1.3–13.4), respectively [21]. Our study results contradict those, as only approximately one-quarter of our patients had this history. We thus counsel the reader that although a history of cat exposure is common, it is not a prerequisite to make the diagnosis, especially in regions where cats abound [22].

Neuroretinitis in ocular bartonellosis is usually unilateral, but bilateral presentation has been reported [2, 23–25]. In our study, 63.2% of patients presented with unilateral involvement. This is similar to the percentage noted by Kerkhoff et al., who noted that 61.5% of ocular bartonellosis was unilateral [18]. Nearly all (8 out of 9) patients with neuroretinitis had unilateral involvement. Meanwhile, all those with panuveitis (4 patients) had bilateral involvement [18]. Our results differ from those of Curi et al., who reported that 13 out of 24 patients (54.2%) presented with bilateral disease [2].

Neuroretinitis and focal retinochoroiditis are the most common ocular manifestations of cat-scratch disease [2, 19, 20, 23, 24]. In our series, neuroretinitis remained the most common presentation, followed by optic disc swelling. This varies from the findings of Solley et al., who reported that, in his study of 24 patients, the most common finding was discrete retinal infiltrates or choroidal lesions, seen in 83% of patients, followed by optic disc swelling, in 63% of patients [1]. Curi et al. had similar findings to Solley et al., in which the most common ocular manifestation was a small area of retinal infiltrate, which occurred in 11 eyes [1, 2]. In that series, neuroretinitis occurred in only 6 out of 37 eyes (16.2%) [2].

The seroprevalence of antibodies to *Bartonella henselae* varies worldwide, ranging from 3.8% to 50% in various studies [26–28]. To the best of our knowledge, there is no available data on the seroprevalence of *Bartonella henselae* antibodies in our general population. Elevated immunoglobulin M (Ig M) or G (Ig G) for *Bartonella henselae* is suggestive of current or past infection [29]. However, the sensitivity of an Ig M assay using IFA has been found to be lower than that of enzyme immunoassay (EIA) Ig M (50% IFA versus 71.4% EIA) in patients who fulfilled two or more criteria for cat-scratch disease [30]. Despite this, IFA remains the only test of bartonella infection available in our setting. Unfortunately, the IFA used in our bacteriology unit measures antibodies to both *Bartonella henselae* and *Bartonella quintana*; therefore, we were unable to differentiate between these *Bartonella* spp. infections. Polymerase chain reaction (PCR) is emerging as an alternative, highly sensitive method of identifying *Bartonella* spp. in ocular specimens [18, 21]. PCR hybridization assay has shown 86.4% sensitivity in patients who fulfill two or more criteria for cat-scratch disease and 100% sensitivity in patients who fulfill three or more criteria [27]. However, routine PCR is not readily done in our setting due to high cost. We foresee the need for better serological diagnostic tests to guide the diagnosis and treatment of bartonella infection in our practice.

Generally, cat-scratch disease is a self-limiting disease, with good visual prognosis, but treatment may hasten recovery [20, 31]. Early antibiotic treatment may not only speed recovery, but also improve the final visual outcome [20]. According to Bass et al., the mean duration of illness was 2.8 weeks in those with treatment, compared to 14.5 weeks in those without treatment [32]. Rifampicin, gentamicin, cotrimoxazole, ciprofloxacin, and doxycycline have shown efficacy in the treatment of cat-scratch disease [20]. However, doxycycline is contraindicated in children and pregnant women. In mild to moderate disease, the use of oral azithromycin for five-day duration achieves more rapid resolution of lymphadenopathy than conservative management [33]. Azithromycin has become the preferred antimicrobial of choice in treating ocular bartonellosis in our setting due to issues with compliance (daily dosing) and its improved safety profile compared to doxycycline (which is given twice a day and tends to cause gastrointestinal upset). There is no prospective study on the efficacy of azithromycin in treating ocular bartonellosis. However, susceptibility evaluation of *Bartonella henselae* against macrolide antibiotics found that these antibiotics are useful in the treatment of cat-scratch disease [34].

The role of systemic corticosteroids in the treatment of cat-scratch disease is still controversial. Isolated case reports have demonstrated good response to corticosteroids, especially in cases where the presentation is atypical [35–38]. Only one study of ocular bartonellosis has discussed the role of corticosteroids, which gave a good outcome when used in combination with antibiotics, in a series of 14 patients in Japan [19]. Corticosteroids may help control the degree of intraocular inflammation and optic neuropathy due to cat-scratch disease. In our study, systemic corticosteroid therapy was used in patients who had significantly decreased visual acuity on presentation. However, we do not believe that topical corticosteroids play a significant role in the management of this condition, as their penetration to the posterior segment of the eye is limited.

Our study has several limitations. First, its retrospective nature limits the amount of information available. Secondly, although our data was collected from two institutions, the demographic and clinical features of this disease may show a wider global variation than currently reported, due to the different socioeconomic and bacteriology profile in different regions. Direct comparison with previous literature is also not possible due to the relatively small numbers of patients in most studies, as well as differences in study design, including inclusion criteria and type of serological assay used. Larger scale studies and standardized diagnostic criteria are required to consolidate our findings.

5. Conclusion

Ocular bartonellosis tends to present with blurring of vision, which is associated with prodromal symptoms in more than half of these cases. The most common ocular signs are neuroretinitis, papillitis, and uveitis. Azithromycin is a viable option for treatment. Systemic corticosteroids may be considered in those with poor visual acuity on presentation.

Competing Interests

The authors declare that there are no conflicts of interest in the publication of this paper.

References

[1] W. A. Solley, D. F. Martin, N. J. Newman et al., "Cat scratch disease: posterior segment manifestations," *Ophthalmology*, vol. 106, no. 8, pp. 1546–1553, 1999.

[2] A. L. L. Curi, D. MacHado, G. Heringer et al., "Cat-scratch disease: ocular manifestations and visual outcome," *International Ophthalmology*, vol. 30, no. 5, pp. 553–558, 2010.

[3] A. V. Gray, K. S. Michels, A. K. Lauer, and J. R. Samples, "Bartonella henselae infection associated with neuroretinitis, central retinal artery and vein occlusion, neovascular glaucoma, and severe vision loss," *American Journal of Ophthalmology*, vol. 137, no. 1, pp. 187–189, 2004.

[4] H. Martínez-Osorio, M. Calonge, J. Torres, and F. González, "Cat-scratch disease (ocular bartonellosis) presenting as bilateral recurrent iridocyclitis.," *Clinical Infectious Diseases*, vol. 40, no. 5, pp. e43–e45, 2005.

[5] A. Raihan, E. Zunaina, W. Wan-Hazabbah, H. Adil, and T. Lakana-Kumar, "Neuroretinitis in ocular bartonellosis: a case series," *Clinical Ophthalmology*, vol. 8, pp. 1459–1466, 2014.

[6] S. Rattanavong, P. E. Fournier, V. Chu et al., "Bartonella henselae endocarditis in Laos—'the unsought will go undetected'," *PLoS Neglected Tropical Diseases*, vol. 8, no. 12, article e3385, 2014.

[7] N. Sanchez Clemente, C. A. Ugarte-Gil, N. Solórzano et al., "Bartonella bacilliformis: a systematic review of the literature to guide the Research Agenda for Elimination," *PLoS Neglected Tropical Diseases*, vol. 6, no. 10, article e1819, 2012.

[8] A. R. Chaudhry, M. R. Chaudhry, J. C. Papadimitriou, and C. B. Drachenberg, "Bartonella henselae infection-associated vasculitis and crescentic glomerulonephritis leading to renal allograft loss," *Transplant Infectious Disease*, vol. 17, no. 3, pp. 411–417, 2015.

[9] G. Mirouse, A. Journe, L. Casabianca, P. E. Moreau, S. Pannier, and C. Glorion, "Bartonella henselae osteoarthritis of the upper cervical spine in a 14-year-old boy," *Orthopaedics & Traumatology: Surgery & Research*, vol. 101, no. 4, pp. 519–522, 2015.

[10] R. M. Chiuri, M. F. Matronola, C. Di Giulio, L. Comegna, F. Chiarelli, and A. Blasetti, "Bartonella henselae infection associated with autoimmune thyroiditis in a child," *Hormone Research in Paediatrics*, vol. 79, no. 3, pp. 185–188, 2013.

[11] J. A. Best and B. Price, "Central scotoma without prodromal illness caused by Bartonella henselae neuroretinitis," *The American Journal of Emergency Medicine*, vol. 31, no. 5, pp. 887.e1–887.e2, 2013.

[12] E. Brunetti, M. Fabbi, G. Ferraioli et al., "Cat-scratch disease in Northern Italy: atypical clinical manifestations in humans and prevalence of Bartonella infection in cats," *European Journal of Clinical Microbiology and Infectious Diseases*, vol. 32, no. 4, pp. 531–534, 2013.

[13] M. Eiger-Moscovich, R. Amer, M. Oray, K. F. Tabbara, I. Tugal-Tutkun, and M. Kramer, "Retinal artery occlusion due to Bartonella henselae infection: a case series," *Acta Ophthalmologica*, vol. 94, no. 5, pp. e367–e370, 2016.

[14] A. Seth, U. Raina, S. Thirumalai, S. Batta, and B. Ghosh, "Full-thickness macular hole in Bartonella henselae neuroretinitis in an 11-year-old girl," *Oman Journal of Ophthalmology*, vol. 8, no. 1, pp. 44–46, 2015.

[15] D. H. Hamilton, K. M. Zangwill, J. L. Hadler, and M. L. Cartter, "Cat-scratch disease—connecticut, 1992-1993," *Journal of Infectious Diseases*, vol. 172, no. 2, pp. 570–573, 1995.

[16] M. G. Pennisi, F. Marsilio, K. Hartmann et al., "Bartonella Species Infection in Cats: ABCD guidelines on prevention and management," *Journal of Feline Medicine and Surgery*, vol. 15, no. 7, pp. 563–569, 2013.

[17] C. Ishida, H. Tsuneoka, H. Iino et al., "Bartonella henselae infection in domestic cat and dog fleas," *Kansenshogaku Zasshi*, vol. 75, no. 2, pp. 133–136, 2001.

[18] F. T. Kerkhoff, A. M. C. Bergmans, A. Van Der Zee, and A. Rothova, "Demonstration of Bartonella grahamii DNA in ocular fluids of a patient with neuroretinitis," *Journal of Clinical Microbiology*, vol. 37, no. 12, pp. 4034–4038, 1999.

[19] T. Kodama, H. Masuda, and A. Ohira, "Neuroretinitis associated with cat-scratch disease in Japanese patients," *Acta Ophthalmologica Scandinavica*, vol. 81, no. 6, pp. 653–657, 2003.

[20] J. B. Reed, D. K. Scales, M. T. Wong, C. P. Lattuada Jr., M. J. Dolan, and I. R. Schwab, "Bartonella henselae neuroretinitis in cat scratch disease: diagnosis, management, and sequelae," *Ophthalmology*, vol. 105, no. 3, pp. 459–466, 1998.

[21] P. P. Diniz, P. E. Velho, L. H. Pitassi et al., "Risk factors for Bartonella species infection in blood donors from Southeast Brazil," *PLoS Neglected Tropical Diseases*, vol. 10, no. 3, Article ID e0004509, 2016.

[22] E. T. Cunningham Jr. and J. E. Koehler, "Ocular bartonellosis," *American Journal of Ophthalmology*, vol. 130, no. 3, pp. 340–349, 2000.

[23] S. L. Chi, S. Stinnett, E. Eggenberger et al., "Clinical characteristics in 53 patients with cat scratch optic neuropathy," *Ophthalmology*, vol. 119, no. 1, pp. 183–187, 2012.

[24] R. Ben-Ami, M. Ephros, B. Avidor et al., "Cat-scratch disease in elderly patients," *Clinical Infectious Diseases*, vol. 41, no. 7, pp. 969–974, 2005.

[25] T. A. Florin, T. E. Zaoutis, and L. B. Zaoutis, "Beyond cat scratch disease: widening spectrum of Bartonella henselae infection," *Pediatrics*, vol. 121, no. 5, pp. e1413–e1425, 2008.

[26] S. Bhengsri, H. C. Baggett, L. F. Peruski et al., "Bartonella seroprevalence in rural Thailand," *Southeast Asian Journal of Tropical Medicine and Public Health*, vol. 42, no. 3, pp. 687–692, 2011.

[27] H. Yoshida, N. Kusaba, K. Omachi et al., "Serological study of Bartonella henselae in cat scratch disease in Japan," *Microbiology and Immunology*, vol. 40, no. 9, pp. 671–673, 1996.

[28] A. Sander, M. Posselt, K. Oberle, and W. Bredt, "Seroprevalence of antibodies to Bartonella henselae in patients with cat scratch disease and in healthy controls: evaluation and comparison of two commercial serological tests," *Clinical and Diagnostic Laboratory Immunology*, vol. 5, no. 4, pp. 486–490, 1998.

[29] E. B. Suhler, A. K. Lauer, and J. T. Rosenbaum, "Prevalence of serologic evidence of cat scratch disease in patients with neuroretinitis," *Ophthalmology*, vol. 107, no. 5, pp. 871–876, 2000.

[30] A. M. C. Bergmans, M. F. Peeters, J. F. P. Schellekens et al., "Pitfalls and fallacies of cat scratch disease serology: evaluation of Bartonella henselae-based indirect fluorescence assay and enzyme-linked immunoassay," *Journal of Clinical Microbiology*, vol. 35, no. 8, pp. 1931–1937, 1997.

[31] J. Karolak and A. Gotz-Więckowska, "Neuroretinitis in cat scratch disease," *Klinika Oczna*, vol. 112, no. 4-6, pp. 131–134, 2010.

[32] A. M. Margileth, "Antibiotic therapy for cat-scratch disease: clinical study of therapeutic outcome in 268 patients and a review of the literature," *Pediatric Infectious Disease Journal*, vol. 11, no. 6, pp. 474–478, 1992.

[33] J. W. Bass, B. C. Freitas, A. D. Freitas et al., "Prospective randomized double blind placebo-controlled evaluation of azithromycin for treatment of cat-scratch disease," *Pediatric Infectious Disease Journal*, vol. 17, no. 6, pp. 447–452, 1998.

[34] T. J. Ives, P. Manzewitsch, R. L. Regnery, J. D. Butts, and M. Kebede, "In vitro susceptibilities of Bartonella henselae, B. quintana, B. elizabethae, Rickettsia rickettsii, R. conorii, R. akari, and R. prowazekii to Macrolide antibiotics as determined by immunofluorescent-antibody analysis of infected vero cell monolayers," *Antimicrobial Agents and Chemotherapy*, vol. 41, no. 3, pp. 578–582, 1997.

[35] K. Bryant and G. S. Marshall, "Hepatosplenic cat scratch disease treated with corticosteroids," *Archives of Disease in Childhood*, vol. 88, no. 4, pp. 345–346, 2003.

[36] E. M. Laswell, K. D. Chambers, D. R. Whitsel, and K. Poudel, "New-onset refractory status epilepticus in an adult with an atypical presentation of cat-scratch disease: successful treatment with high-dose corticosteroids," *Pharmacotherapy*, vol. 35, no. 6, pp. e106–e110, 2015.

[37] P. Lerdluedeeporn, P. Krogstad, R. L. Roberts, and E. R. Stiehm, "Oral se," *Clinical Pediatrics*, vol. 42, no. 1, pp. 71–73, 2003.

[38] K. D. Weston, T. Tran, K. N. Kimmel, and B. L. Maria, "Possible role of high-dose corticosteroids in the treatment of cat-scratch disease encephalopathy," *Journal of Child Neurology*, vol. 16, no. 10, pp. 762–763, 2001.

19

Molecular Characterization of *Cryptosporidium* spp. in Wild Rodents of Southwestern Iran Using 18s rRNA Gene Nested-PCR-RFLP and Sequencing Techniques

Jasem Saki,[1,2] Masoud Foroutan-Rad,[3] and Reza Asadpouri[2]

[1] *Health Research Institute, Infectious and Tropical Diseases Research Center, Ahvaz Jundishapur University of Medical Science, Ahvaz, Iran*
[2] *Department of Medical Parasitology, Faculty of Medicine, Ahvaz Jundishapur University of Medical Sciences, Ahvaz, Iran*
[3] *Department of Parasitology, Faculty of Medical Sciences, Tarbiat Modares University, Tehran, Iran*

Correspondence should be addressed to Masoud Foroutan-Rad; masoud_foroutan_rad@yahoo.com

Academic Editor: Jean-Paul J. Gonzalez

Background. Rodents could act as reservoir for *Cryptosporidium* spp. specially *C. parvum*, a zoonotic agent responsible for human infections. Since there is no information about *Cryptosporidium* infection in rodents of Ahvaz city, southwest of Iran, hence, this survey was performed to determine the prevalence and molecular characterization of *Cryptosporidium* spp. in this region. *Materials and Methods.* One hundred rodents were trapped from different regions of Ahvaz city. Intestine contents and fecal specimens of rodents were studied using both microscopy examination to identify oocyst and nested-polymerase chain reaction (PCR) technique for 18s rRNA gene detection. Eventually restriction fragment length polymorphism (RFLP) method using *SspI* and *VspI* restriction enzymes was carried out to genotype the species and then obtained results were sequenced. *Results.* Three out of 100 samples were diagnosed as positive and overall prevalence of *Cryptosporidium* spp. was 3% using both modified Ziehl-Neelsen staining under light microscope and nested-PCR (830 bp) methods. Afterwards, PCR-RFLP was performed on positive samples and *C. parvum* pattern was identified. Finally PCR-RFLP findings were sequenced and presence of *C. parvum* was confirmed again. *Conclusions.* Our study showed rodents could be potential reservoir for *C. parvum*. So an integrated program for control and combat with them should be adopted and continued.

1. Introduction

Cryptosporidium spp. are ubiquitous intracellular protozoan parasites that affect wide range of vertebrates like human and livestock [1]. Oocysts are infective stage of life cycle released via feces from infected hosts to environment in large amount. They are resistant to various environmental alterations and remain infective for long period in appropriate condition like surface of water and moist soils; thus, they are liable for transmission of disease to animals and humans [2, 3]. *Cryptosporidium* as an opportunistic agent infects the alimentary tract of hosts and have wide spectrum of clinical symptoms in human ranging from self-limiting and asymptomatic in immunocompetent individuals to severe and life-threatening in immunocompromised persons [2, 4, 5]. For first time, human cryptosporidiosis was diagnosed in individuals who had severe watery diarrhea during 1970s [6].

During past decades, numerous evidences have confirmed that small mammals such as rodents are considered as carrier or reservoir for several infectious agents. They can transmit the pathogens directly or indirectly. Also role of rodents in transferring the helminth and protozoan infections are clear [7–10]. Surveys in different zones of Iran indicate the existence of various rodent species such as the house mice (*Mus musculus*), the black rat (*Rattus rattus*), the brown rat (*Rattus norvegicus*), and the Himalayan rat (*Rattus pectoris*) in country [8, 10, 11]. Based on our previous survey in Ahvaz district, southwest of Iran, rodents could be considered as potential source of *Toxoplasma gondii* infection for definitive hosts [9].

Recently, several molecular studies have been conducted to determine the *Cryptosporidium* genotypes. Small subunit-rRNA (SSU 18s rRNA) gene is being utilized for identification of *Cryptosporidium* spp. worldwide extensively. According to SSU-rRNA gene sequencing, at least 20 *Cryptosporidium* species have been identified and more than sixty *Cryptosporidium* genotypes have undeterminate status till now. Approximately eight *Cryptosporidium* species/genotypes including *C. parvum*, *C. hominis*, *C. felis*, *C. meleagridis*, *C. ubiquitum*, *C. viatorum*, *C. canis*, and *C. cuniculus* are the main species responsible for human infections, although *C. hominis* and *C. parvum* account for over 90% of human cryptosporidiosis worldwide [1, 2].

Numerous epidemiological surveys have been performed throughout the globe and prevalence of *Cryptosporidium* infection in rodents was highly varied from 63% in UK [12], 32.8% in United States of America (USA) [13], 24.3% in Italy [14], 7.6% in Maryland [15], 11.5% in China [16], 25.8% in Philippines [17], 8.2% in northern Australia [18], 0% in northeast of Iran (Mashhad city) [19], and 27.3% in north of Iran (Tehran city) [20]. Due to lack of reports about *Cryptosporidium* infection in rodents of southwest of Iran till now, current study was aimed to determine the prevalence and molecular characterization of *Cryptosporidium* spp. in this region.

2. Materials and Methods

2.1. Study Area. Ahvaz city, capital of Khuzestan province which is located in the southwest of Iran (31°50′ N and 49° 11′ E), is ranked as the 7th largest city throughout the country and based on the latest census, its population was calculated at 1,395,184 in 352,128 families. Weather temperature is highly variable throughout the year so that in summer temperature exceeds 50°C whereas in winter it falls to 5°C. Also, annual average rainfall is approximately 230 mm. There is high density of rodents species and rat-man-domestic animals adjacency is remarkable in Ahvaz city [9, 11]. Rodents are additional reservoir for *Cryptosporidium* spp., mostly preyed on by cats and dogs, and, hence, could spread parasitic infections via other animals [8].

2.2. Rodents Collection. Ahvaz city initially divided into five geographical locations (north, west, south, east, and center). In each location Sherman live traps were placed outdoor at the entrance of rodent colonies and baited with favorite piece of foods (including cucumber pieces, tomato, and roasted almonds). The Sherman live traps were installed at sunset and gathered before sunrise. Overall, 100 rodents were collected from three different species (6 *M. musculus*, 73 *R. norvegicus*, and 21 *R. rattus*). Eventually trapped rodents were gathered and transferred to Department of Medical Parasitology of Ahvaz JundishapurUniversity of Medical Sciences. The trapped rodents were anaesthetized by putting the live traps in a thick transparent polythene bag and then a cotton swab was soaked in ether and placed near their nose. Afterwards, the anaesthetized rodents were dissected and fecal samples gathered from rectum or large intestinal section. Skull and tooth structures were used for species identification. The Iranian rodent key of Etemad was performed to identify the rodents [21].

2.3. Detection of Cryptosporidium spp. Oocysts. Samples were collected from intestine contents and fecal specimens of rodents. After sugar flotation (SG 1.266; 128 g sucrose and 100 distilled water) [22] and modified Ziehl-Neelsen staining, the samples were examined to find the *Cryptosporidium* spp. oocysts using optical microscope under ×1000 magnification. Diagnosis of oocysts was based on morphological features like red spherical shapes. Finally the samples were maintained at 2.5% potassium dichromate ($K_2Cr_2O_7$) [23] and kept in refrigerator (1-2 weeks) until DNA was extracted.

2.4. DNA Extraction and Nested-PCR. DNA extraction procedure was performed using QIAamp® DNA stool mini kit (QIAamp DNA Stool Mini Kit, USA) based on the manufacturer's guideline. The extracted DNA was kept in −20°C for next tests. For nested-PCR method, we used two specific primers to detect 18s rRNA gene whose length of produced fragments was 1325 bp and 830 bp. This dual stages technique was run using different primers that primary and secondary stages primers were as following: [4, 20, 23, 24].

First Stage Primers

Forward (F1): 5′-TTCTAGAGCTAATACATGCG-3′

Reverse (R1): 5′-CCCATTTCCTTCGAAACAGGA-3′

Second Stage Primers

Forward (F2): 5′-GGAAGGGTTGTATTTATT-AGATAAAG-3′

Reverse (R2): 5′-CTCATAAGGTGCTGAAGG-AGTA-3′

Finally PCR products after loading on 1.5% agarose gel and electrophoresis for 1.5 hours were stained with ethidium bromide and then visualized under UV light using Gel Doc device (Uvidoc, Gel Documentation System, Cambridge, UK) [25].

2.5. Genotyping Cryptosporidium spp. Using 18s rRNA PCR-RFLP and Sequencing. RFLP assay was done to determine the *Cryptosporidium* spp., using digestion of secondary PCR products. For this purpose, *SspI* and *VspI* endonuclease enzymes were employed for species recognition and genotyping, respectively, based on manufacturer's protocol as earlier described [20]. Then the mixture was incubated for approximately 8 hours at 37°C. Eventually visualization of the digested products was carried out under UV transilluminator after 1.5% agarose gel electrophoresis and ethidium bromide staining [20, 26]. The nested-PCR positive samples were purified using Bioneer kit corporation (Korea) and were sequenced by the same corporation. Sequence alignments were constructed by CLUSTAL W software (http://www.ddbj.nig.ac.jp/search/clustalwe.html).

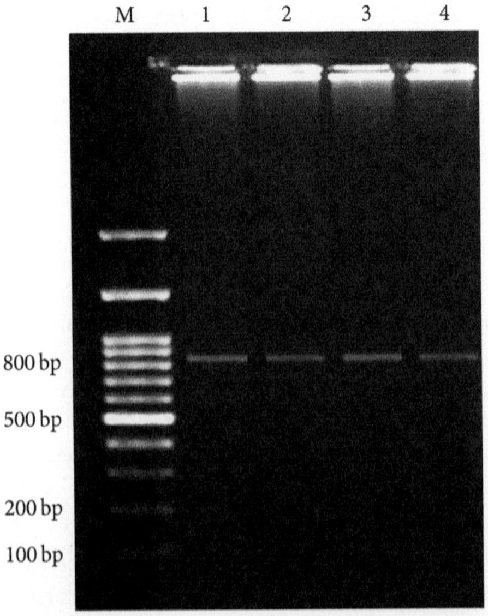

Figure 1: Secondary stage of nested-PCR findings on agarose gel. Lane M, DNA size marker. Lane 1, positive control for *Cryptosporidium*. Lanes 2–4, positive *Cryptosporidium* samples (830 bp).

Nucleotide sequence data reported in current article are available in the GenBank at accession numbers *AB986579*, *AB986580*, and *AB986581*.

3. Results

Three out of 100 samples were detected as positive for *Cryptosporidium* spp. using modified Ziehl-Neelsen staining under light microscope. In addition, nested-PCR was done and showed 830 bp band which confirmed only 3 samples as *Cryptosporidium* spp. (Figure 1). So, overall prevalence of *Cryptosporidium* infection in rodents of Ahvaz city was calculated at 3% using both methods. All positive samples belonged to *R. norvegicus* (3/73) and from *M. musculus* (0/6) and *R. rattus* (0/21) no positive cases were observed. In order to determine the genotype, PCR-RFLP technique using *SspI* and *VspI* restriction enzymes was utilized. With *SspI* restriction enzyme, three cuttings were seen in locations of 108, 258, and 421 bp visible on agarose gel after electrophoresis. Also after using from *VspI* enzyme, three cuttings happened in locations 104, 106, and 600 bp (Figure 2) and indicate *C. parvum* pattern. The amplified 18s rRNA genes from PCR-RFLP products of three *C. parvum* were sequenced. After submitting the results to the DDBJ/GenBank at accession numbers *AB986579*, AB986580, and *AB986581*, the nucleotide sequences were aligned with nucleotide sequences of *C. parvum* certified in GenBank with accession number AB986578 (Figure 3). Based on findings, *C. parvum* was recognized as infectious agent of Ahvaz rodents.

4. Discussion

Cryptosporidium spp. belong to Apicomplexa phylum with cosmopolitan distribution [1]. Rodents with maintaining the pathogens transmission cycle in surrounding regions play a key role in morbidity and mortality of human and livestock especially in areas with dense population [7].

The routine method for diagnosis of *Cryptosporidium* spp. is based on direct observation of oocysts in stool specimens using optical microscope. Since this method has low sensitivity and needs expertise, also it is unable to distinguish between different species of parasites; thus, molecular techniques like PCR have been used and developed recently. PCR-based techniques with high sensitivity, specificity, and rapidly features are capable of differentiating among species and genotypes in different specimens, that is, water, stool, and animal or human tissues, although they are expensive. Previously, genotyping of *Cryptosporidium* spp. has been done successfully by nested PCR-RFLP method according to SSU-rRNA (18S rRNA) gene [4, 18, 20, 24, 26, 27].

According to previous epidemiological reports, prevalence and rate of infection of *Cryptosporidium* spp. in rodents ranged from 0% to 63% and could be highly variable worldwide [12, 19]. Present investigation is the first report which focused on the prevalence and molecular detection of *Cryptosporidium* spp. in wild rodents of Ahvaz city, southwest of Iran. We found 3% (3/100) prevalence by both direct microscopic observations with Ziehl-Neelsen staining and nested-PCR (830 bp), while, in Bahrami et al. [20] survey in Tehran city (capital of Iran) using these methods, the prevalence was reported at 13% and 27.3%, respectively. Also all positive samples identified *C. parvum* by PCR-RFLP using *SspI* and *VspI* restriction enzymes and were confirmed by sequencing that is in agreement with our study. Differences between Tehran and Ahvaz findings could be justified with sample size, location of sampling, cities population, hygienic conditions, sewage systems, and so forth. It is worth mentioning that Tehran as capital of Iran is the most crowded city with highest density population over the country which is multifold than Ahvaz. In Mashhad city (northeast of Iran), prevalence of *Cryptosporidium* spp. with 0% [19] was lower than our study (3%), while higher prevalence was reported from USA 32.8% [13], China 11.5% [16], Australia 8.2% [18], Philippines 25.8% [17], and Tehran city (north of Iran) 27.3% [20].

Based on current study, 18s rRNA gene of *C. parvum* was detected only in *R. norvegicus* (3/73) and from *R. rattus* and *M. musculus* no positive samples were isolated. It should be mentioned that *R. norvegicus* is the most abundant rodent in southwest of Iran (73/100) and highest prevalence and rate of infection (4.1%, 3/73) allocate to this species which corresponds to previous investigations [9, 11]. The obtained results of amplifying 18s rRNA gene after sequencing were submitted to the DDBJ/GenBank under accession numbers *AB986579*, AB986580, and *AB986581* and then compared with AB986578 as control. Figure 3 illustrated several nucleotide replacements.

Lv and colleagues [16] studied the wild, laboratory, and pet rodents (totally 723 rodents from 18 species) in China and prevalence of *Cryptosporidium* spp. was reported at 11.5% and *C. parvum*, *C. muris*, *C. andersoni*, and *C. wrairi* were identified, as well. Prevalence in wild, laboratory, and pet rodents was 6.8%, 1.9%, and 21.8%, respectively.

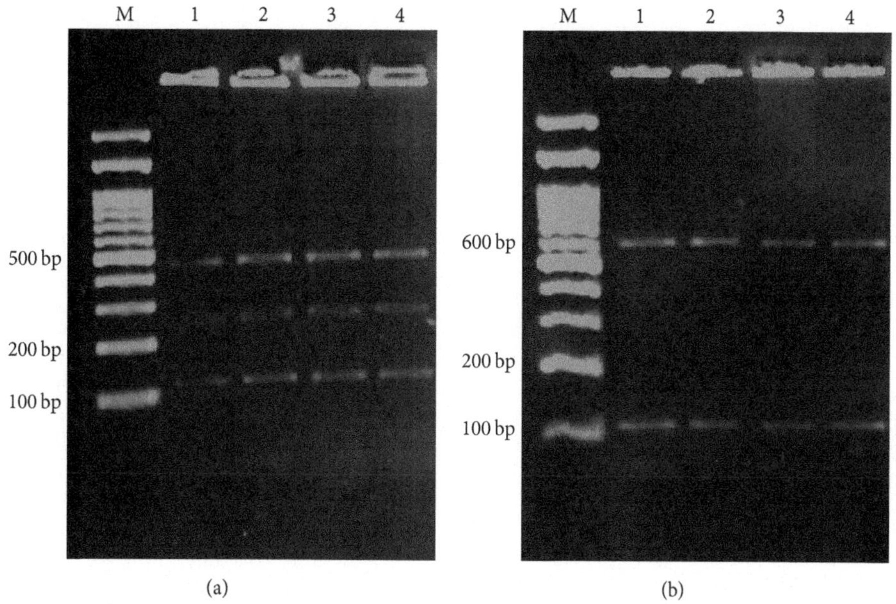

FIGURE 2: (a) PCR-RFLP products with *SspI* restriction enzyme. Three cuttings in locations 108, 258, and 421 bp are visible on gel electrophoresis. (b) PCR-RFLP products with *VspI* restriction enzyme. Three cuttings in locations 104, 106, and 600 bp are visible on agarose gel. Lane M, DNA size marker. Lane 1, positive control for *Cryptosporidium*. Lanes 2–4, positive *Cryptosporidium* samples.

```
AB986578.1GTAATTGGGGTGGCTCATAA   ATTGGAATGAGTTAAGTATAAACCCCTTTACAAGTATCAATTGGAGGGCA 242
AB986581.1CCTTTCGGGTAGGTGATGGT   ATTGGAATGAGTTAAGTATAAACCCCTTTACAAGTATCAATTGGAGGGCA 247
AB986579.1ACGGGTATAAATTGGGTTGA   ATTGGAATGAGTTAAGAATAAACCCCTTTACAAGTATCAATTGGAGGGCA 249
AB986580.1ACCCATTTTAAATTGGGTTG   ATTGGAATGAGTTAAGTATAAACCCCTTTACAAGTATCAATTGGAGGGCA 250
                                 ****************:*********************************

AB986578.1GTAATTGGGGTGGCTCATAA   AGTCTGGTGCCAGCAGCCGCGGTAATTCCAGCTCCAATAGCGTATATTAA 292
AB986581.1CCTTTCGGGTAGGTGATGGT   AGTCTGGTGCCAGCAGCCGCGGTAATTCCAGCTCCAATAGCGTATATTAA 297
AB986579.1ACGGGTATAAATTGGGTTGA   AGTCTGGTGCCAGCAGCCGCGGTAATTCCAGCTCCAATAGCGTATATTAA 299
AB986580.1ACCCATTTTAAATTGGGTTG   AGTCTGGTGCCTGCAGCCGCGGTAATTCCAGCTCCAATAGCGTATATTAA 300
                                 ***********:**************************************

AB986578.1GTAATTGGGGTGGCTCATAA   AGTTGTTGCAGTTAAAAAGCTCGTAGTTGGATTTCTGTTAATAATTTATA 342
AB986581.1CCTTTCGGGTAGGTGATGGT   AGTTGTTGCAGTTAAAAAGCTCGTAGTTGGATTTCTGTTAATAATTTATA 347
AB986579.1ACGGGTATAAATTGGGTTGA   AGTTGTTGCAGTTAAAAAGCTCGTAGTTGGATTTCTGTTAATAATTTATA 349
AB986580.1ACCCATTTTAAATTGGGTTG   AGTTGTTGCAGTTAAAAAGCTCGTAGTTGGATTTCTGTTAATAATTTATA 350
                                 **************************************************

AB986578.1GTAATTGGGGTGGCTCATAA   TAAAATATTTTGATGAATATTTATATAATATTAACATAATTCATATTACT 392
AB986581.1CCTTTCGGGTAGGTGATGGT   TAAAATATTTTGATGAATATTTATATAATATTAACATAATTCATATTACT 397
AB986579.1ACGGGTATAAATTGGGTTGA   TAAAATATTTTGATGAATATTTATATAATATTAACATAATTCATATTACT 399
AB986580.1ACCCATTTTAAATTGGGTTG   TAAAACATTTTGAGGAATATTTATATAATATTAACATAATTCATAGTGCT 400
                                 ***** ******* ******************************* *.**
```

FIGURE 3: Multiple alignments of 18s rRNA genes from three isolates which submitted to GenBank at accession numbers *AB986579*, *AB986580*, and *AB986581*. Asterisks (∗) show identical nucleotides.

In another survey by Ng-Hublin et al. [17] on 194 wild rats and mice from five species including the Asian house rat (*R. tanezumi*), the rice-field rat (*R. argentiventer*), the Pacific rat (*R. exulans*), *R. norvegicus*, and *M. musculus* in Philippines, overall prevalence was reported at 25.8%. In addition, based on sequencing and phylogenetic analysis of 18s rRNA gene and actin locus, *C. muris*, *C. parvum*, *C. scrofarum*, *C. suis*-like genotype, and rat genotypes I–IV were recognized. In current research, only *C. parvum* was identified using 18s rRNA gene sequencing. Throughout the world *C. parvum* have been isolated from numerous animals such as calves or cattle [24], some ruminants (goats and sheep) [28], horses [29], pigs [30], alpacas [31], some carnivores (gray wolves and dogs) [32, 33], reptiles [27], and rodents (rat, hamster, mice, nutria, chipmunk, squirrel, and capybara) [13, 16, 17, 20, 34–37]. In addition predominant *Cryptosporidium* species in Iran is *C. parvum* that has been verified frequently, for example, 73.3% in humans and animals [38], 83.3% in Tehran (human samples) [39], 100% in rodents of Tehran [20], 100% in cattle of Ilam [24], and 68.8% in Ahvaz (in immunocompromised patients and children) [4]. In Rafiei et al. investigation in southwest of Iran on immunocompromised patients and children (kidney transplant recipients, persons with hematological malignancies, HIV+ patients, and children less than 5 years old), 390 stool specimens were collected and examined. Prevalence of *Cryptosporidium* spp. was 4.1% (16/390). Moreover, 3 different species were identified using PCR-RFLP based on 18s rRNA gene including 11 *C. parvum*, 4 *C. hominis*, and 1 *C. meleagridis* [4] which was in consistent with our results. According to Rafiei et al. [4] survey and our study, *C. parvum* was identified as the most common species in both rodents and individuals in Ahvaz city. In past studies *C. parvum* transmission from rodents to human was reported repeatedly [17, 40].

5. Limitations

The present investigation was based on sampling of limited rodents species in limited areas. In future, for better understanding of exact burden of *Cryptosporidium* spp. and genetic diversity, studies should be designed on wide spectrum of both wild and pet rodents (rats, hamsters, mice, rabbits, etc.) in vast regions like throughout the Khuzestan province.

6. Conclusion

Present paper was the first report which focused on the prevalence and molecular characterization of *Cryptosporidium* spp. in wild rodents of Ahvaz city, southwest of Iran; that showed rate of infection in *R. norvegicus* is remarkable. Also, rodents could be potential reservoir for *C. parvum*. The results can help public health care to pursue new strategies (environmental sanitation, increasing the hygienic condition, increasing the hygienic condition, etc.). In future, adopting a suitable strategy for control and combat with rodents in order to decrease human cases is necessary and should be continued.

Ethical Approval

All applicable international, national, and/or institutional guidelines for the care and use of animals were followed.

Competing Interests

The authors declare that they have no conflict of interests.

Authors' Contributions

Jasem Saki contributed toward concept, design, and definition of intellectual content; Reza Asadpouri collected the samples and performed the experiments; Masoud Foroutan-Rad contributed to the literature search and manuscript preparation; Jasem Saki and Masoud Foroutan-Rad edited and reviewed the manuscript.

Acknowledgments

This study was conducted and financially supported by Ahvaz Jundishapur University of Medical Sciences, Grant no. CMRC-91. The authors appreciate the support of the staff of the Protozoology Laboratory at the Jundishapur University of Medical Sciences. They would like to thank Mr. Nezam Salehi for his help in collecting the samples.

References

[1] J. Plutzer and P. Karanis, "Genetic polymorphism in *Cryptosporidium* species: an update," *Veterinary Parasitology*, vol. 165, no. 3-4, pp. 187–199, 2009.

[2] M. Bouzid, P. R. Hunter, R. M. Chalmers, and K. M. Tyler, "*Cryptosporidium* pathogenicity and virulence," *Clinical Microbiology Reviews*, vol. 26, no. 1, pp. 115–134, 2013.

[3] K. Shi, F. Jian, C. Lv et al., "Prevalence, genetic characteristics, and zoonotic potential of *Cryptosporidium* species causing infections in farm rabbits in China," *Journal of Clinical Microbiology*, vol. 48, no. 9, pp. 3263–3266, 2010.

[4] A. Rafiei, Z. Rashno, A. Samarbafzadeh, and S. Khademvatan, "Molecular characterization of *Cryptosporidium* spp. Isolated from immunocompromised patients and children," *Jundishapur Journal of Microbiology*, vol. 7, no. 4, Article ID e9183, 2014.

[5] S. Gholami, M. Khanmohammadi, E. Ahmadpour et al., "*Cryptosporidium* infection in patients with gastroenteritis in Sari, Iran," *Iranian Journal of Parasitology*, vol. 9, no. 2, pp. 226–232, 2014.

[6] F. A. Nime, J. D. Burek, D. L. Page, M. A. Holscher, and J. H. Yardley, "Acute enterocolitis in a human being infected with the protozoan *Cryptosporidium*," *Gastroenterology*, vol. 70, no. 4, pp. 592–598, 1976.

[7] B. G. Meerburg, G. R. Singleton, and A. Kijlstra, "Rodent-borne diseases and their risks for public health," *Critical Reviews in Microbiology*, vol. 35, no. 3, pp. 221–270, 2009.

[8] R. Dehghani, H. Seyedi, S. Dehqan, and H. Sharifi, "Geographical distribution of mouse and mouse-borne diseases in Iran: a review article," *Feyz*, vol. 17, pp. 203–219, 2013.

[9] J. Saki and S. Khademvatan, "Detection of *Toxoplasma gondii* by PCR and mouse bioassay in rodents of Ahvaz District, Southwestern Iran," *BioMed Research International*, vol. 2014, Article ID 383859, 5 pages, 2014.

[10] Z. Seifollahi, B. Sarkari, M. H. Motazedian, Q. Asgari, M. J. Ranjbar, and S. Abdolahi Khabisi, "Protozoan parasites of rodents and their zoonotic significance in Boyer-Ahmad District, Southwestern Iran," *Veterinary Medicine International*, vol. 2016, Article ID 3263868, 5 pages, 2016.

[11] E. Kia, M. Homayouni, A. Farahnak, M. Mohebail, and S. Shojai, "Study of endoparasites of rodents and their zoonotic importance in Ahvaz, South West Iran," *Iranian Journal of Public Health*, vol. 30, pp. 49–52, 2001.

[12] J. P. Webster and D. W. Macdonald, "Cryptosporidiosis reservoir in wild brown rats (*Rattus norvegicus*) in the UK," *Epidemiology and Infection*, vol. 115, no. 1, pp. 207–209, 1995.

[13] Y. Feng, K. A. Alderisio, W. Yang et al., "*Cryptosporidium* genotypes in wildlife from a New York watershed," *Applied and Environmental Microbiology*, vol. 73, no. 20, pp. 6475–6483, 2007.

[14] M. Kváč, L. Hofmannová, S. Bertolino, L. Wauters, G. Tosi, and D. Modrý, "Natural infection with two genotypes of *Cryptosporidium* in red squirrels (*Sciurus vulgaris*) in Italy," *Folia Parasitologica*, vol. 55, no. 2, pp. 95–99, 2008.

[15] L. Zhou, R. Fayer, J. M. Trout, U. M. Ryan, F. W. Schaefer III, and L. Xiao, "Genotypes of *Cryptosporidium* species infecting

fur-bearing mammals differ from those of species infecting humans," *Applied and Environmental Microbiology*, vol. 70, no. 12, pp. 7574–7577, 2004.

[16] C. Lv, L. Zhang, R. Wang et al., "*Cryptosporidium* spp. in wild, laboratory, and pet rodents in China: prevalence and molecular characterization," *Applied and Environmental Microbiology*, vol. 75, no. 24, pp. 7692–7699, 2009.

[17] J. S. Y. Ng-Hublin, G. R. Singleton, and U. Ryan, "Molecular characterization of *Cryptosporidium* spp. from wild rats and mice from rural communities in the Philippines," *Infection, Genetics and Evolution*, vol. 16, pp. 5–12, 2013.

[18] A. Paparini, B. Jackson, S. Ward, S. Young, and U. M. Ryan, "Multiple *Cryptosporidium* genotypes detected in wild black rats (*Rattus rattus*) from northern Australia," *Experimental Parasitology*, vol. 131, no. 4, pp. 404–412, 2012.

[19] H. Borji, J. Khoshnegah, G. Razmi, H. Amini, and M. Shariatzadeh, "A survey on intestinal parasites of golden hamster (*Mesocricetus auratus*) in the northeast of Iran," *Journal of Parasitic Diseases*, vol. 38, no. 3, pp. 265–268, 2014.

[20] F. Bahrami, J. Sadraei, and M. Frozandeh, "Molecular characterization of *Cryptosporidium* spp. in Wild Rats of Tehran, Iran using 18s rRNA gene and PCR_RFLP method," *Jundishapur Journal of Microbiology*, vol. 5, no. 3, pp. 486–490, 2012.

[21] E. Etemad, Mammals of Iran, Vol. 1 (Rodents and their identification keys), A publication of the National Society for Natural Resource and Environment Conservation, Iran, 1978.

[22] T. Fujino, T. Matsuo, M. Okada, and T. Matsui, "Detection of a small number of *Cryptosporidium parvum* oocysts by sugar floatation and sugar centrifugation methods," *Journal of Veterinary Medical Science*, vol. 68, no. 11, pp. 1191–1193, 2006.

[23] M. Pirestani, J. Sadraei, A. Dalimi Asl, M. Zavvar, and H. Vaeznia, "Molecular characterization of *Cryptosporidium* isolates from human and bovine using 18s rRNA gene in Shahriar county of Tehran, Iran," *Parasitology Research*, vol. 103, no. 2, pp. 467–472, 2008.

[24] M. Mahami Oskouei, E. Fallah, M. Ahmadi et al., "Molecular and parasitological study of *Cryptosporidium* isolates from cattle in Ilam, west of Iran," *Iranian Journal of Parasitology*, vol. 9, no. 3, pp. 435–440, 2014.

[25] M. Foroutan-Rad, S. Khademvatan, J. Saki, and M. Hashemitabar, "*Holothuria leucospilota* extract induces apoptosis in *Leishmania major* promastigotes," *Iranian Journal of Parasitology*, vol. 11, pp. 339–349, 2016.

[26] K. Manouchehri Naeini, M. Asadi, and M. Hashemzade Chaleshtori, "Detection and molecular characterization of *Cryptosporidium* species in recreational waters of Chaharmahal va Bakhtiyari province of Iran using nested-PCR-RFLP," *Iranian Journal of Parasitology*, vol. 6, pp. 20–27, 2011.

[27] L. Xiao, U. M. Ryan, T. K. Graczyk et al., "Genetic diversity of *Cryptosporidium* spp. in captive reptiles," *Applied and Environmental Microbiology*, vol. 70, no. 2, pp. 891–899, 2004.

[28] J. Quílez, E. Torres, R. M. Chalmers, S. J. Hadfield, E. Del Cacho, and C. Sánchez-Acedo, "*Cryptosporidium* genotypes and subtypes in lambs and goat kids in Spain," *Applied and Environmental Microbiology*, vol. 74, no. 19, pp. 6026–6031, 2008.

[29] R. M. Chalmers, A. L. Thomas, B. A. Butler, and M. C. G. Morel, "Identification of *Cryptosporidium parvum* genotype 2 in domestic horses," *Veterinary Record*, vol. 156, no. 2, pp. 49–50, 2005.

[30] M. Kváč, B. Sak, D. Hanzlíková, J. Kotilová, and D. Květoňová, "Molecular characterization of *Cryptosporidium* isolates from pigs at slaughterhouses in South Bohemia, Czech Republic," *Parasitology Research*, vol. 104, no. 2, pp. 425–428, 2009.

[31] D. F. Twomey, A. M. Barlow, S. Bell et al., "Cryptosporidiosis in two alpaca (*Lama pacos*) holdings in the South-West of England," *Veterinary Journal*, vol. 175, no. 3, pp. 419–422, 2008.

[32] A. Giangaspero, R. Iorio, B. Paoletti, D. Traversa, and G. Capelli, "Molecular evidence for *Cryptosporidium* infection in dogs in Central Italy," *Parasitology Research*, vol. 99, no. 3, pp. 297–299, 2006.

[33] A. Paziewska, M. Bednarska, H. Niewęgłowski, G. Karbowiak, and A. Bajer, "Distribution of *Cryptosporidium* and *Giardia* spp. in selected species of protected and game mammals from north-eastern Poland," *Annals of Agricultural and Environmental Medicine*, vol. 14, no. 2, pp. 265–270, 2007.

[34] M. V. Meireles, R. M. Soares, F. Bonello, and S. M. Gennari, "Natural infection with zoonotic subtype of *Cryptosporidium parvum* in Capybara (*Hydrochoerus hydrochaeris*) from Brazil," *Veterinary Parasitology*, vol. 147, no. 1-2, pp. 166–170, 2007.

[35] A. Bajer, S. Cacciò, M. Bednarska, J. M. Behnke, N. J. Pieniazek, and E. Sinski, "Preliminary molecular characterization of *Cryptosporidium parvum* isolates of wildlife rodents from Poland," *Journal of Parasitology*, vol. 89, no. 5, pp. 1053–1055, 2003.

[36] U. Ryan, L. Xiao, C. Read, L. Zhou, A. A. Lal, and I. Pavlasek, "Identification of novel *Cryptosporidium* genotypes from the Czech Republic," *Applied and Environmental Microbiology*, vol. 69, no. 7, pp. 4302–4307, 2003.

[37] F. Berrilli, D. Di Cave, C. Orazi et al., "*Giardia* and *Cryptosporidium* in kennel dogs, pet rabbits and hamsters from Rome (Italy)," *Parassitologia*, vol. 48, no. 1-2, p. 261, 2006.

[38] A. R. Meamar, K. Guyot, G. Certad et al., "Molecular characterization of *Cryptosporidium* isolates from humans and animals in Iran," *Applied and Environmental Microbiology*, vol. 73, no. 3, pp. 1033–1035, 2007.

[39] A. Dalimi, F. Tahvildar-Biderouni, F. Ghaffarifar, and B. Kazemi, "The identification of human *Cryptosporidium* species in Tehran by PCR/RFLP," *Modares Journal of Medical Sciences: Pathobiology*, vol. 17, pp. 39–48, 2014.

[40] L. Xiao and R. Fayer, "Molecular characterisation of species and genotypes of *Cryptosporidium* and *Giardia* and assessment of zoonotic transmission," *International Journal for Parasitology*, vol. 38, no. 11, pp. 1239–1255, 2008.

20

Current Epidemiological Assessment of Bancroftian Filariasis in Tanga Region, Northeastern Tanzania

Happyness J. Mshana,[1,2] Vito Baraka,[1,3] Gerald Misinzo,[2] and Williams H. Makunde[1]

[1]National Institute for Medical Research, Tanga Research Centre, P.O. Box 5004, Tanga, Tanzania
[2]Sokoine University of Agriculture, Morogoro, Tanzania
[3]Global Health Institute, University of Antwerp, Antwerp, Belgium

Correspondence should be addressed to Happyness J. Mshana; jeremiahappiness@yahoo.com

Academic Editor: Jean-Paul J. Gonzalez

Background. Tanzania started a countrywide lymphatic filariasis elimination programme in 2000 adopting the mass drug administration (MDA) strategy. The drug used for the programme was the combination of ivermectin and albendazole. However, there is limited information on the current epidemiological trend of the infections, where MDA implementation is ongoing. The present study aimed at assessing the current status of Bancroftian filariasis infection rate and morbidity where MDA has been distributed and administered for over eight rounds. *Methodology.* The study was a cross-sectional descriptive study involving 272 individuals (>18 years) from endemic communities in Tanga region where MDA has been implemented. Clinical, sociodemographic, and circulating filarial antigen (CFA) test was undertaken using immune chromatographic card test according to the manufacturer's instructions. *Results.* A total of 472 individuals were screened: 307/472 (65.1%) were males while 165/472 (34.9%) were females. The overall prevalence of CFA was 5.51%, that of hydrocoele was 73.2%, and that of lymphoedema was 16.0%. The prevalence of hydrocoele combined with lymphoedema was 5.5%. *Conclusion.* Our findings demonstrate a considerable reduction in filarial infection. However, there is clear evidence of ongoing transmission despite the 8 rounds of MDA. It is unlikely that the annual MDA would interrupt filarial transmission; therefore, additional strategies are needed to accelerate lymphatic filariasis control and elimination.

1. Introduction

Lymphatic filariasis (LF) is the second leading cause of long-term disability globally due to lymphoedema, elephantiasis, and hydrocele [1]. The long-term disability is triggered through overt hydrocoele, lymphoedema, elephantiasis, repeated orchitis, and adenolymphangitis [2]. These acute and chronic pathologies impose a significant impediment to socioeconomic development and an extremely poor quality of life [3]. LF affects more than 120 million individuals globally [4]. It is estimated that around 20% of the world population in more than 83 countries are at risk of acquiring infection which is 1.1 billion people [5]. In the endemic communities, 7% of the adult population suffer from lymphoedema whereas 30–50% develop hydrocele [6]. In sub-Saharan Africa (SSA), the predominant parasite is filarial nematode *Wuchereria bancrofti (W. bancrofti)* which is estimated to affect 500 million people [7]. Epidemiological mapping in Tanzania has shown that the risk is particularly high in the coastal zone along the Indian Ocean although cases are also reported in other mainland regions [8].

In response to the World Health Organization (WHO) Global Programme to Eliminate Lymphatic Filariasis (GPELF) that aimed at filariasis elimination, Tanzania established the National Lymphatic Filariasis Elimination Programme (NLFEP) in 2000 where targeted communities were given a combination of ivermectin and albendazole (ALB+IV) annually [8]. The ivermectin dosage is administered according to body weight (150–200 μg/kg) while 400 mg of albendazole is given to individuals aged ≥5 years in all endemic districts. In some settings, it has shown a reduction of infections rate to low levels as 1%.

Conversely, the endemic areas along the coast of the Indian Ocean have shown a high prevalence of infection up to 63.3% despite the ongoing MDA for over eight years [8]. It was anticipated that using the MDA strategy as recommended in WHO guidelines on MDA coverage (>65%) through a variety of approaches will lead to interrupting transmission [3], whereby microfilariae (mf) levels will reach below 1%.

However, evidence in Tanga region has shown that, despite 8 rounds of MDA and supplementation with other interventions such as the provision of insecticide-treated nets (ITNs), still, both infection and clinical disease rates remain high especially along the coastline [8]. The prevalence in Tanga region before the MDA survey in 2004 of the community mf was 24.5%, that of CFA was 63.3%, and that of specific antibodies to recombinant filarial antigen was 78.9%. In comparison, after 8 rounds of MDA, the CFA and mf prevalence in combined study communities was reduced by 75.5% and 89.6%, respectively, compared to baseline levels, while the CFA prevalence in school children was reduced by 90.9% compared to baseline [8]. The present study was designed to ascertain the LF infections rates and morbidities after the MDA rounds in Tanga region.

2. Methods

2.1. Study Area and Population. The study was conducted in Tanga region in Northeastern Tanzania along the Indian Coast (05°04′S, 39°06′E). The region is characterised mainly by two rain seasons annually: the long rains from March to June and the less intensive short rains from November to December. The majority of the inhabitants practice subsistence farming, fishing, and livestock keeping. The climate in Tanga region is warm and wet. In most cases, there is no big variation of temperature at the coast due to the influence of the Indian Ocean. Also, the region is characterised by high humidity, which often goes up to 100% maximum and ranges from 65 to 70% minimum. There are health facilities in most villages in the regions, and the majority of the population have access to a health facility within a distance of 6 km. Most of the houses are made of mud walls with their roofs thatched with dried coconut leaves. This makes it easier for the vector to penetrate. Bancroftian filariasis control started in 2004 using MDA campaigns and advocacy with ivermectin and albendazole in all districts [8]. The estimated population size of the area was 2,045,205 inhabitants according to 2012 national census survey [9].

2.2. Study Design. The study was a cross-sectional, descriptive study conducted between April and May 2015. The study participants were selected using convenience sampling, a nonprobability sampling technique where individuals were selected based on their convenient accessibility and proximity.

2.3. Ethical Considerations. Ethical clearance for the study was granted by the Medical Research Coordinating Committee of the National Institute for Medical Research in Tanzania (NIMR-MRCC). The investigators explained the purpose of the study and all study participants consented orally and in writing.

TABLE 1: Sociodemographic characteristics of the study population.

Characteristics	Frequency (N)	Proportion (%)
Age group in years		
18–31	36	13.2
32–45	66	24.5
46–59	58	21.3
60–73	90	33.1
74–87	22	8.1
Sex ratio (female : male)	33 : 239	
Occupation		
Peasant farmers	102	37.5
Fishermen	170	62.5

N: number of individuals.

2.4. Clinical Examination. A clinician experienced in LF examined those patients and recorded the swelling of the lower limbs and scrotum in stages according to Meyrowitsch et al. [10]. Thereafter, a semistructured questionnaire was used to collect the demographic information and other clinical disease conditions. Individuals with lymphoedema and hydrocoele stages lower than III were treated with antibiotic (doxycycline or tetracycline) for 7 days and topical broad-spectrum antifungal cream as recommended by the study physician.

2.5. Parasitological Examination. Patients were then asked to donate 100 μL for circulating filarial antigen examination using immune chromatographic test cards. The BinaxNOW Filariasis immune chromatographic card test (Alere Inc., Scarborough, ME) was used to detect circulating filarial antigen as described in the WHO guidelines [11]. Briefly, 100 μL of finger-prick blood was collected from each individual and then transferred to an immune chromatographic card test using a calibrated capillary tube. The test was read 10 minutes after closing the card, as per the manufacturer's instructions. The antigen contains the epitope present in circulating *W. bancrofti* antigen that was detected by the BinaxNOW Filariasis test. The identification number and test result of each individual tested were recorded in the case report form.

3. Results

A total of 472 individuals were examined during the community survey, among whom 65.1% (307) were males while 34.9% (165) were females. Of those, 272 were recruited for the study, of whom 87.86% were males and 12.14% were females, $p \leq 0.0001$. The rest did not fulfil the inclusion criteria as presented in the flow diagram (Figure 1). The study population that was more frequently observed with high proportion was the 32–45-year age group with a rate of 24.2%, followed by the 60–73-year age group with a rate of 33.1%, and the majority of them were fishermen (62.5%) (Table 1).

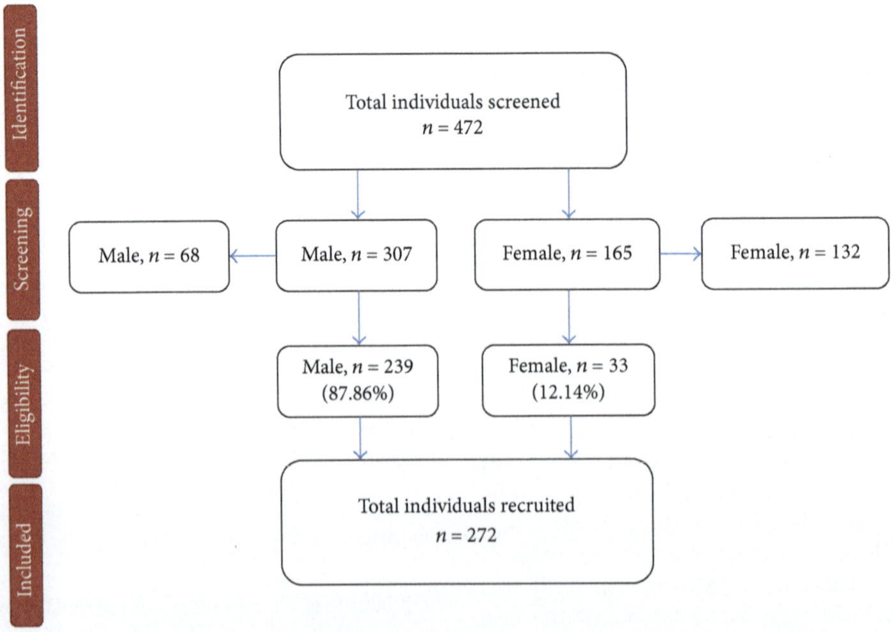

FIGURE 1: Study profile of the individuals recruited in the cross-sectional survey in Tanga region.

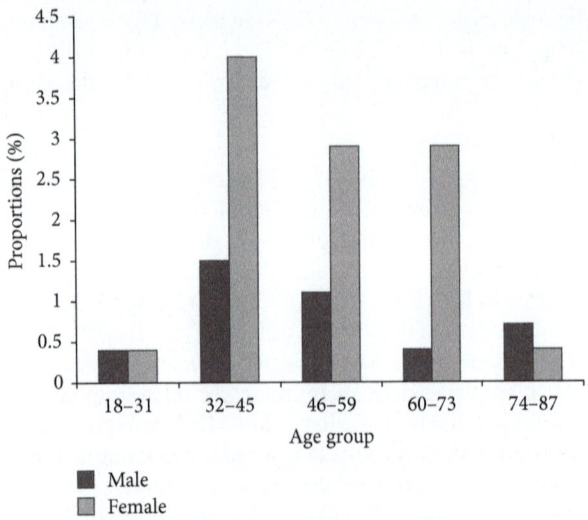

FIGURE 2: Age distribution of lymphoedema pathology according to stages in the examined individuals.

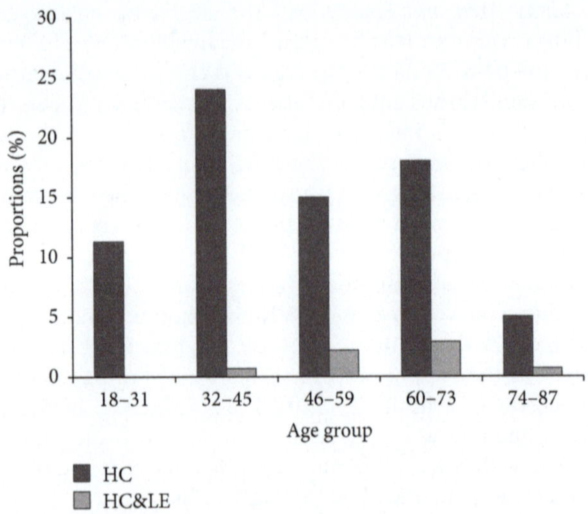

FIGURE 3: Age distribution of scrotal hydrocoele pathology according to stages in those examined individuals. HC: hydrocoele; HC&LE: hydrocoele and lymphoedema.

Females were observed to have a higher proportion of lymphoedema than males in the age group of 32–45 years (Figure 2). Figures 3 and 4 summarise the infection rates in the study group whereby 5.51% of the 272 individuals were CFA-positive and the majority of those were males (3.3%). Few of the confirmed CFA patients were females (2.21%). The proportions of scrotal hydrocele in males above 18 years old were high (73.2%) as compared to lymphoedema (15.8%). Conversely, the proportion of individuals with both lymphoedema and hydrocele was 5.51%.

4. Discussion

In our study, hydrocoele has been shown to be the main public health problem causing debilitation in males and similarly lymphoedema in females as observed elsewhere [12]. It has also been shown in our study that these conditions affect the 32–45-year age group. Recent studies focusing on the molecular mechanism regulating blood and lymphatic vessels growth have shown that vascular endothelial growth factors control angiogenesis and lymphangiogenesis in humans [13], which is a process of developing lymphangiectasia as a clinical

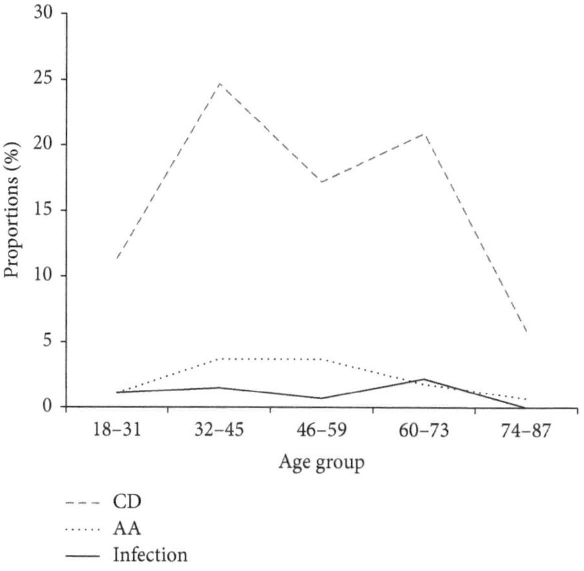

FIGURE 4: Acute and chronic clinical disease stratified into age groups. CD: chronic pathology (lymphedema, hydrocele, and lymphedema combined with hydrocele); AA: acute attacks (filarial fever); infection: circulating filarial antigen (CFA).

disease. Similarly, expression of VEGF-A and VEGF-C has been shown to be upregulated by proinflammatory cytokines affecting the lymphatic vessels in males [13]. However, currently, there is limited data on the heterogeneity of the disease. Since the pathogenesis and development of lymphoedema remain largely unknown, there is a need for future studies to explore the role of genetics in relation to clinical phenotypes to better understand the disease aetiology and optimise the control strategies. The results of this study suggest that, during the era of lymphatic filariasis control of infections, the disease has shown a clear reduction of acute infection and morbidity rates compared to the baseline study, especially in the older age group. This could have been triggered by the host human-immune and parasite interaction leading to the clearance of acute infection [12]. On the other hand, the presence of adult worms and their secretions and the death of such adult worms may lead to dilatation of scrotal lymphatic vessel causing dysfunction and accumulation of protein-rich fluid in the tissue causing lymphangiectasia [13]. However, there is still ongoing LF transmission in some of the studied communities in the region and it is unlikely that the annual single dose can interrupt the transmission and therefore other strategies such as biannual administration of MDA can be applied to interrupt the transmission as observed in other studies. In Figure 4, young age groups (18–31 years) have increasing acute and chronic infections. A similar observation has been shown in Fiji [14]. These are the productive segment in the communities indicating a shifting trend of the clinical disease into the lower age groups because low-level transmission continues in those communities. This could be possibly due to some existing hotspots in the communities whereby mosquito vectors pick infection from humans and maintain the local transmission [15]. It is also likely that the postponement of the MDA distribution within the timely scheduled period could have halted reaching the desired coverage of at least 65% according to the WHO, hence leading to LF resurgence [14]. It is vital to expand the frequency of drug administration to a maximum of three doses per year, expand the age range of the target population, and improve health education to the community with the aim of increasing coverage within the targeted areas. Similarly, we should conduct an anthropological study to find out why transmission continues although MDA is in place, tracking factors associated with that, such as the incentive to drug distributors, health system roles in the district, timely availability of drugs, financial resources, and advocacy and training of distributors. The need for adequate financial and logistics resources is paramount to successfully achieve the targeted coverage and reach the end goal of the programme. Adequate resources and infrastructural support should be available to ensure timely availability and supply of the MDA drugs to reach the implementation units in endemic communities. Moreover, more evidence is needed to assess whether parasite genetic variability has implications in the effectiveness of diagnostic test, epidemiology, and control of the disease [16], as well as cross-reactivity of the ICT card to non-*W. bancrofti* filariae that could reinforce doubts on the validity of the current map of LF as observed in other studies [17]. Formulation of guidelines for LF coendemic areas assessment is therefore very important. It is worth also addressing issues related to the vector for successful control of LF. MDA in combination with other interventions such as insecticide-treated nets will improve reduction of infection and interrupt transmission of the infection in the communities. However, insecticide resistance could lead to a substantial increase and persistence of filarial infection incidence [18].

5. Conclusion

Our findings have shown a considerable reduction in filarial infection. However, there is clear evidence of ongoing transmission despite the 8 rounds of MDA using ivermectin and albendazole. It is unlikely that annual mass drug administration would interrupt filarial transmission; therefore, optimised strategies are needed to accelerate control and elimination of targets.

Competing Interests

The authors declare that they have no competing interests.

Acknowledgments

The authors are grateful to the villagers in Tanga region for their dedicated cooperation and to the technical staff from NIMR-Tanga (Fidelis Mumburi, Xavaeli Ngowi, Charles Guzo, and Tembo) for their assistance in the field and the laboratory. This study received financial support from University Hospital Bonn, Institute for Medical Microbiology, Immunology and Parasitology (Grant Code PF 673/2-1).

References

[1] S. Wynd, W. D. Melrose, D. N. Durrheim, J. Carron, and M. Gyapong, "Understanding the community impact of lymphatic filariasis: a review of the sociocultural literature," *Bulletin of the World Health Organization*, vol. 85, no. 6, pp. 493–498, 2007.

[2] S. Babu and T. B. Nutman, "Immunopathogenesis of lymphatic filarial disease," *Seminars in Immunopathology*, vol. 34, no. 6, pp. 847–861, 2012.

[3] WHO, "Global programme to eliminate lymphatic filariasis," in *A Handbook of Practical Entomology for National Lymphatic Filariasis Elimination Programmes*, p. 1, WHO, 2013.

[4] K. Ichimori, "MDA—lymphatic filariasis," *Tropical Medicine and Health*, vol. 42, no. 2, supplement, pp. 21–24, 2014.

[5] E. A. Ottesen, "Editorial: the global programme to eliminate lymphatic filariasis," *Tropical Medicine and International Health*, vol. 5, no. 9, pp. 591–594, 2000.

[6] L. Batsa, *Anti-wolbachia treatment of lymphatic filariasis and genetic analysis of the pathology of lymphedema as a clinical manifestation of the disease [Ph.D. dissertations]*, 2012.

[7] P. J. Hotez and A. Kamath, "Neglected tropical diseases in sub-Saharan Africa: review of their prevalence, distribution, and disease burden," *PLoS Neglected Tropical Diseases*, vol. 3, no. 8, article e412, 2009.

[8] P. E. Simonsen, Y. A. Derua, S. M. Magesa et al., "Lymphatic filariasis control in Tanga Region, Tanzania: status after eight rounds of mass drug administration," *Parasites & Vectors*, vol. 7, no. 1, article 507, 2014.

[9] National Bureau of Statistics (NBS) and Office of Chief Government Statistician Zanzibar (OCGS), *2012 Population and Housing Census: Population Distribution by Administrative Units: Key Findings*, The United Republic of Tanzania, 2013.

[10] D. W. Meyrowitsch, P. E. Simonsen, and W. H. Makunde, "Bancroftian filariasis: analysis of infection and disease in five endemic communities of north-eastern Tanzania," *Annals of Tropical Medicine and Parasitology*, vol. 89, no. 6, pp. 653–663, 1995.

[11] L. Original, *Preparing and Implementing a National Plan to Eliminate Lymphatic Filariasis*, World Health, 2000.

[12] D. G. Addiss and M. A. Brady, "Morbidity management in the global programme to eliminate lymphatic filariasis: a review of the scientific literature," *Filaria Journal*, vol. 6, article 2, 2007.

[13] K. M. Pfarr, A. Y. Debrah, S. Specht, and A. Hoerauf, "Filariasis and lymphoedema," *Parasite Immunology*, vol. 31, no. 11, pp. 664–672, 2009.

[14] M. E. Mwakitalu, M. N. Malecela, E. M. Pedersen, F. W. Mosha, and P. E. Simonsen, "Urban lymphatic filariasis in the metropolis of Dar es Salaam, Tanzania," *Parasites and Vectors*, vol. 6, article 286, p. 13, 2013.

[15] R. T. Rwegoshora, E. M. Pedersen, D. A. Mukoko et al., "Bancroftian filariasis: patterns of vector abundance and transmission in two East African communities with different levels of endemicity," *Annals of Tropical Medicine and Parasitology*, vol. 99, no. 3, pp. 253–265, 2005.

[16] S. Nuchprayoon, A. Junpee, and Y. Poovorawan, "Random amplified polymorphic DNA (RAPD) for differentiation between Thai and Myanmar strains of *Wuchereria bancrofti*," *Filaria Journal*, vol. 6, no. 6, article 6, 2007.

[17] S. Wanji, N. Amvongo-Adjia, A. J. Njouendou et al., "Further evidence of the cross-reactivity of the Binax NOW® Filariasis ICT cards to non- *Wuchereria bancrofti* filariae: experimental studies with Loa loa and *Onchocerca ochengi*," *Parasites & Vectors*, vol. 9, article 267, pp. 1–10, 2016.

[18] N. Protopopoff, J. Matowo, R. Malima et al., "High level of resistance in the mosquito *Anopheles gambiae* to pyrethroid insecticides and reduced susceptibility to bendiocarb in north-western Tanzania," *Malaria Journal*, vol. 12, article 149, pp. 1–8, 2013.

21

Nitazoxanide in Acute Rotavirus Diarrhea: A Randomized Control Trial from a Developing Country

Samarendra Mahapatro,[1] Nijwm Mahilary,[2] Amit Kumar Satapathy,[1] and Rashmi Ranjan Das[1]

[1]*Department of Pediatrics, All India Institute of Medical Sciences, Bhubaneswar, India*
[2]*Department of Pediatrics, Hi-Tech Medical College and Hospital, Bhubaneswar, India*

Correspondence should be addressed to Rashmi Ranjan Das; dr_rashmipgi@yahoo.com

Academic Editor: Marcel Tanner

Background. Acute diarrhea is one of the leading causes of childhood mortality, with rotavirus being an important pathogen. Nitazoxanide, an antiparasitic agent, has been shown to inhibit rotavirus. *Objective.* This double-blind, randomized trial was designed to study the role of nitazoxanide in acute rotavirus diarrhea. *Methods.* Of 174 children (12 months to 5 years) with acute diarrhea, 50 rotavirus positive cases were randomized. The intervention group received syrup nitazoxanide twice daily (100 mg in 12–47 months, 200 mg in ≥4 yr) for 3 days along with standard treatment of diarrhea. Duration of diarrhea was the primary outcome measure. *Results.* The median duration (hrs) of diarrhea (54 versus 80; 95% CI: −26 [−13.2 to −38.8]) and hospitalization (68 versus 90; 95% CI: −22 [−12.98 to −31.02]) was significantly shorter in the nitazoxanide group. No significant difference was seen in the median duration (hrs) of fever or vomiting or the proportion of children requiring parenteral rehydration. There was no report of any adverse events. *Conclusions.* Oral nitazoxanide is effective and safe in the management of acute rotavirus diarrhea in Indian children (CTRI REF/2016/10/012507).

1. Introduction

Diarrheal illness is one of the six leading causes of childhood mortality. In developing countries among children under five, it causes 15% of the 10.5 million deaths annually [1]. In India, it constitutes 13% of the common illness in children under five [2]. The global burden of rotavirus diarrhea, predominantly in developing countries, is estimated to be more than 100 million episodes, over 20 million out-patient visits and more than 6,00,000 deaths (range 4,54,000 to 7,05,000) [3]. A multicentric study by the Indian Rotavirus Strain Surveillance Network reported the detection of rotavirus in stools of 39% children aged <5 years [4]. The disease is more severe in infants aged 3 to 24 months. Due to the high incidence of rotavirus infection in both developing and the developed countries, the development of vaccines took shape in the early 1980s. Data on rotavirus vaccine impact in developing countries including India are sparse due to limited use of rotavirus vaccines in this region [5]. Poor access to medical care, malnutrition, and illiteracy are the main factors leading to the higher disease burden in these regions.

The rotavirus diarrhea is treated like any other diarrhea in childhood with oral rehydration therapy (ORT) and zinc [6]. ORT aims to prevent or reverse dehydration and has no effect either on the duration or on the stool output. Zinc is also not universally effective and has been used mainly in developing country settings [7]. For this reason, various other modalities (e.g., probiotics, diosmectite) have been tried with some benefits [8, 9].

Nitazoxanide is an oral synthetic broad spectrum antiparasitic agent that acts by interfering with the pyruvate ferredoxin oxidoreductase (PFOR) enzyme-dependent electron transfer reaction, which is essential to anaerobic energy metabolism [10]. It was approved for pediatric use by the US Food and Drug Administration (FDA) in year 2002, and the first clinical trial on rotavirus diarrhea was conducted in year 2006 [11]. The trial was based on the fact that an active metabolite of nitazoxanide (tizoxanide) showed a cytoprotective effect in in vitro rotavirus infected cells. After that two more trials (each one in children and adult) have been published, all showing beneficial effect [12, 13]. This drug can be an effective low cost treatment to control rotavirus diarrhea till the vaccination is universal in developing countries. There is no published study from developing countries including India specifically assessing the therapeutic efficacy and safety of nitazoxanide in acute rotavirus diarrhea. Hence, the present study aimed at evaluating nitazoxanide as a possible therapeutic intervention in acute rotavirus diarrhea in Indian children.

2. Materials and Methods

This double-blind, randomized controlled trial was conducted in the Department of Pediatrics of Hi-Tech Medical College and Hospital, Bhubaneswar, India from April 2014 to August 2014. Children with acute onset diarrhea of <48 hrs duration, some to severe dehydration, and aged between 12 months to 5 years were eligible for inclusion. Diarrhea was defined as passage of ≥3 unformed or loose stools in the last 24 hours [6]. Children with dysentery, severe malnutrition (weight for height < 3 SD of WHO growth-chart), coexisting systemic illnesses, and chronic diseases were excluded from the study.

2.1. Methodology. Children with acute diarrhea and positive stool rotavirus antigen test (SD Bioline Rota kit test followed by RT-PCR) were included. They were randomized to receive either nitazoxanide (intervention group) or no nitazoxanide (control group) through a computer generated admission list. Sequence was generated by a person not directly involved in execution of the study. Allocation concealment was done using serially numbered opaque sealed envelopes. The study was approved by the institute ethics committee. Informed written consent was obtained from the parents/legal guardians prior to enrolment in the study.

Prior to admission into the study, history, physical examination, nutritional status, hydration status (as per WHO guidelines), fever, oral acceptance, and stool characteristics were recorded on a predesigned pro forma. Case management was done as per the WHO acute diarrhea guideline [6]. After clinical stabilization and hydration maintenance, children were randomized into two groups: intervention group received syrup nitazoxanide twice daily (100 mg in 12–47 months; 200 mg in ≥4 yrs) and control group received a similar product, both being administered twice daily for 3 days. Both intervention and control had similar color and taste. The children were discharged after improvement in their clinical condition and were followed till day 7. During hospitalization, they were monitored for frequency and consistency of stools and time since last loose stool (every six hours/24 hrs). They were also monitored for adverse events (fever, vomiting, pain abdomen, or any other symptom).

2.2. Sample Size. This was calculated as per the method adopted by Teran et al. [13]. In order to detect an average difference of 24 hrs between the intervention and the control group, we assumed a standard deviation for the duration of diarrhea in the control group of 30 hrs. To achieve the power of 80% and a significance level of 5%, a total of 50 cases were needed (25 in each group).

2.3. Outcome Measures

Primary

(1) Duration (in hrs) of acute diarrhea

Secondary

(1) Duration (in hrs) of hospitalization

(2) Duration (in hrs) of vomiting

(3) Duration (in hrs) of fever

(4) Proportion of children requiring parenteral rehydration

(5) Any adverse effects

Duration of acute diarrhea was defined as the time (in hrs) from the first to the last abnormal (loose or liquid) stools preceding a normal stool output. Consistency of stool was evaluated through a score system, as described by previously [15], and stool was graded as 1 (normal), 2 (loose), 3 (semiliquid), and 4 (liquid). Duration of hospitalization was defined as the time from admission till discharge. Children were discharged 24 hrs after resolution of diarrhea. Adverse effects of nitazoxanide were also studied.

2.4. Statistical Analysis. All the data were entered into the Microsoft excel sheet. The data were analysed using SPSS software (version 20.0 Chicago, IL, USA). Statistical tests used for comparison included Chi-Square and the Mann–Whitney *U* test. Because many of the continuous variables were not normally distributed, when a Mann–Whitney *U* test was used to compare the groups, the medians and interquartile ranges (IQR) were presented. Difference between the median and calculation of 95% CI (confidence interval) was done [14]. Intention-to-treat analysis was used for the primary outcome. A p value of < 0.05 was considered significant.

3. Results

Of 174 acute diarrhea cases, 109 were excluded for various reasons (details of the exclusion have been described in Figure 1). Of 65 eligible children, 50 finally enrolled in the study; 47 (94%) completed the day 7 follow-up (Figure 1). One child in the nitazoxanide group and 2 children in the control group did not come for day 7 follow-up. The clinical and demographic characteristics in the two groups were comparable. Demographic status and characteristics of acute diarrhea between the two groups were comparable (Table 1).

3.1. Primary Outcome Measures

Duration of Acute Diarrhea. In the nitazoxanide group, the median duration was significantly less by about 26 hrs [95% CI: −13.2 to −38.8] compared to the control group (Table 2).

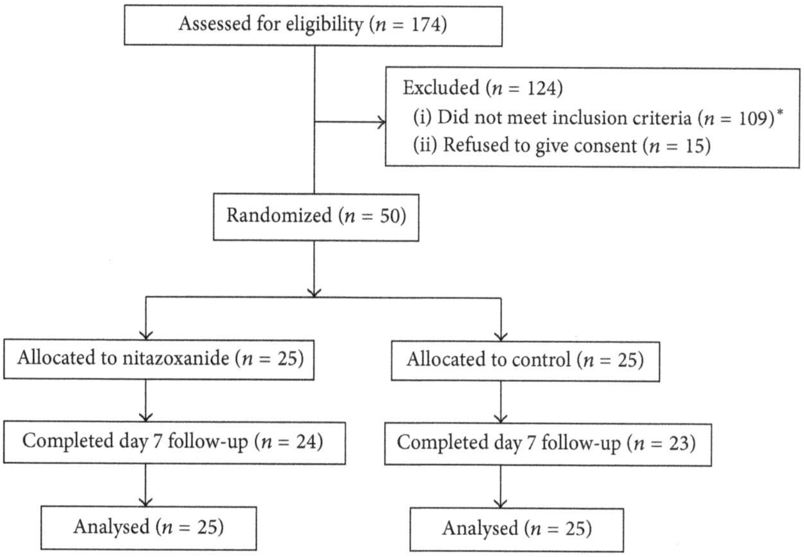

*Excluded: rotavirus not isolated (n = 74), acute dysentery (n = 19), severe malnutrition (n = 12), chronic illness (n = 3), and coexisting systemic illness (n = 1). Chronic illnesses were nephrotic syndrome in 2 cases and Pulmonary Tuberculosis (PTB) in 1 case. Coexisting systemic illness was pneumonia.

FIGURE 1: Flow of participants in the study.

TABLE 1: Baseline and demographic characteristics of the study population.

	Nitazoxanide group (n = 25)	Control group (n = 25)	p value
Age, months (IQR)	26 (8.7)	25 (8.3)	0.38
Males (%)	16 (64)	17 (68)	0.76
Weight (kg) (IQR)	11.3 (2.2)	11.1 (2.8)	0.28
Median duration (IQR) of diarrhea before treatment (hours)	42 (13)	45 (11)	0.35
Stool consistency at the time of enrolment (%)			
Liquid	11 (44)	10 (40)	
Semiliquid	05 (20)	07 (28)	0.24
Loose	09 (36)	08 (32)	
Number (%) of children vomiting	13 (52)	11 (44)	0.57
Median (IQR) duration of vomiting (hours)	28 (13)	30 (12)	0.4
Number (%) of children with fever	09 (36)	07 (28)	0.55
Median (IQR) duration of fever (hours)	30 (16)	33 (15)	0.47
Dehydration status (%)			
Mild	08 (32)	09 (36)	0.65
Moderate	13 (52)	11 (44)	

IQR: Interquartile range.

TABLE 2: Primary and secondary outcome measures.

	Nitazoxanide group (n = 25)	Control group (n = 25)	Difference [95% CI]
Median (IQR) hours of diarrhea[a]	54 (45–65)	80 (65–89)	−26 [−13.2 to −38.8]
Median (IQR) hours of hospitalization[a]	68 (57–75)	90 (77–93)	−22 [−12.98 to −31.02]
Median (IQR) duration of fever (hours)[a]	43 (35–48)	47 (42–52)	−4 [−10.89 to 2.89]
Median (IQR) duration of vomiting (hours)[a]	38 (33–41)	41 (35–46)	−3 [−8.84 to 2.84]
Proportion (%) of children requiring parenteral rehydration[b]	1 (4)	2 (8)	0.48 [0.04 to 5.65]

[a]The difference between the two medians and calculation of 95% CI (confidence interval) has been done by the method proposed by Bonett and Price [14].
[b]Data expressed in odds ratio (OR) and 95% CI.

3.2. Secondary Outcome Measures

Duration of Hospitalization. In the nitazoxanide group, the median duration was significantly less by about 22 hrs [95% CI: −12.98 to −31.02] compared to the control group (Table 2).

Duration of Fever. In the nitazoxanide group, the median duration was less by about 4 hrs [95% CI: −10.89 to 2.89] compared to the control group, but the result was nonsignificant (Table 2).

Effect on Vomiting. In the nitazoxanide group, the median duration was less by about 3 hrs [95% CI: −8.84 to 2.84] compared to the control group, but the result was nonsignificant (Table 2).

Proportion of Children Requiring Parenteral Rehydration. There was no significant difference between the two groups (odds ratio (OR) 0.48 [95% CI: 0.04 to 5.65]) (Table 2).

Adverse Events. There was no report of any adverse events in either of the groups.

4. Discussion

In this randomized controlled trial, nitazoxanide (100 mg in 12–47 months; 200 mg in ≥4 yrs) given orally twice daily for 3 days to children aged 12 months to 5 years during an acute episode of rotavirus diarrhea resulted in significant decrease in the duration of diarrhea and hospitalization without any adverse events. There was no effect on the duration of fever or vomiting or on the proportion of children requiring parenteral rehydration.

In the present study, the incidence of rotavirus diarrhea was 37.3%. Slightly lower or higher results (the range being 34% to 55%) have been obtained by others from India and outside [4, 16–19]. Now, there has been gradual introduction of rotavirus vaccine (monovalent, RV1, and pentavalent, RV5) in developing world, so the scenario might change in future. A Cochrane review found that in countries with high-mortality rates RV1 probably prevents 42% of severe rotavirus diarrhea cases, and RV5 prevents 41% of severe rotavirus diarrhea cases [20]. There has been a low but less variable efficacy of the vaccine in Indian setting. The efficacy is around 58% for Rotarix and 83% for Rotateq, by different ways of assessment [21, 22]. In 2014, another rotavirus vaccine (116E) showed 55% efficacy in a clinical trial in India [23]. Besides this, experience in other countries (Australian children) suggests that the vaccines are not targeting the proper strains of rotavirus, and some of the circulating serotypes are not responding to the vaccines or may be mutating. So, the vaccine alone may not be the answer for management of rotavirus diarrhea even after introduction of the vaccine.

Only two previous trials have been published till date on the role of nitazoxanide in treatment of acute rotavirus diarrhea in hospital settings from developed countries. In the first trial, 38 children (5 months to 7 years) were included and the intervention group received 7.5 mg/kg nitazoxanide orally twice daily for 3 days [11]. The median time to resolution of illness was 31 hrs for the nitazoxanide group compared with 75 hrs for the control group ($p = 0.0137$), and no significant adverse effect was reported. In the second trial, 75 children (28 days to 24 months) were included and the intervention group ($n = 25$) received oral nitazoxanide (15 mg/kg/day) twice daily for 3 days [13]. The median duration of hospitalization (nitazoxanide, 81 hrs, control, 108 hrs; $p = 0.017$) and diarrhea (nitazoxanide, 54 hrs, control, 79 hrs; $p = 0.009$) was significantly reduced in the nitazoxanide group. The only adverse event noted was greenish discoloration of body fluid that spontaneously disappeared in follow-up. The present study result was in accordance with these trials without report of any adverse event and provides evidence that nitazoxanide is helpful in hospitalized children with <10% dehydration.

The strength of the present study is that it studied the effect of nitazoxanide in Indian setting with high mortality due to rotavirus diarrhea. As previous trials have been conducted in western countries, their findings cannot be extrapolated on Indian children due to a higher breast feeding rate, poor hygienic condition, and a distinct gut colonization status. The age range included 12 months to 5 years which is important, as diarrhea is an important cause of under-five mortality in developing countries in this age group. The effect on the requirement of rehydration was evaluated which is important from public health point of view. Potential limitations include the following: no genotyping of rotavirus strain was done due to cost constraints. Measurement of the volume of stool output (g/kg) was also not done, which has been cited in different diarrhea research studies as an additional important outcome. Cost-effective analysis was not done.

5. Conclusion

Rotavirus as a single agent is the major cause of acute diarrhea (37.3%) in infants and under-five children. Oral nitazoxanide was found to be effective and safe in the management of acute rotavirus diarrhea in Indian children.

Competing Interests

The authors declare that they have no competing interests.

References

[1] I. Rudan, K. L. O'Brien, H. Nair et al., "Epidemiology and etiology of childhood pneumonia in 2010: estimates of incidence, severe morbidity, mortality, underlying risk factors and causative pathogens for 192 countries," *Journal of Global Health*, vol. 3, no. 1, Article ID 010401, 2010.

[2] D. Shah, P. Choudhury, P. Gupta et al., "Promoting appropriate management of diarrhea: a systematic review of literature for advocacy and action: UNICEF-PHFI series on Newborn and child health, India," *Indian Pediatrics*, vol. 49, no. 8, pp. 627–649, 2012.

[3] K. L. Kotloff, J. P. Nataro, W. C. Blackwelder et al., "Burden and aetiology of diarrhoeal disease in infants and young children in developing countries (the Global Enteric Multicenter Study, GEMS): a prospective, case-control study," *The Lancet*, vol. 382, no. 9888, pp. 209–222, 2013.

[4] G. Kang, R. Arora, S. D. Chitambar et al., "Multicenter, hospital-based surveillance of rotavirus disease and strains among Indian children aged <5 years," *Journal of Infectious Diseases*, vol. 200, no. 1, pp. S147–S153, 2009.

[5] C. Yen, J. E. Tate, T. B. Hyde et al., "Rotavirus vaccines: current status and future considerations," *Human Vaccines and Immunotherapeutics*, vol. 10, no. 6, pp. 1436–1448, 2014.

[6] World Health Organization (WHO), *The Treatment of Diarrhoea: A Manual for Physicians and Other Senior Health Workers*, WHO/COD/SER/80.2, WHO, Geneva, Switzerland, 4th edition, 2005, http://whqlibdoc.who.int/publications/2005/9241593180.pdf.

[7] R. R. Das, "Zinc in acute childhood diarrhea: is it universally effective," *Indian Journal of Pharmacology*, vol. 44, no. 1, p. 140, 2012.

[8] R. R. Das, J. Sankar, and S. S. Naik, "Efficacy and safety of diosmectite in acute childhood diarrhoea: a meta-analysis," *Archives of Disease in Childhood*, vol. 100, no. 7, pp. 704–712, 2015.

[9] S. Das, P. K. Gupta, and R. R. Das, "Efficacy and safety of saccharomyces boulardii in acute rotavirus diarrhea: double blind randomized controlled trial from a developing country," *Journal of Tropical Pediatrics*, vol. 62, no. 6, pp. 464–470, 2016.

[10] Y. Miyamoto and L. Eckmann, "Drug development against the major diarrhea-causing parasites of the small intestine, *Cryptosporidium* and *Giardia*," *Frontiers in Microbiology*, vol. 6, article 1208, 2015.

[11] J.-F. Rossignol, M. Abu-Zekry, A. Hussein, and M. G. Santoro, "Effect of nitazoxanide for treatment of severe rotavirus diarrhoea: randomised double-blind placebo-controlled trial," *Lancet*, vol. 368, no. 9530, pp. 124–129, 2006.

[12] J.-F. Rossignol and Y. M. El-Gohary, "Nitazoxanide in the treatment of viral gastroenteritis: a randomized double-blind placebo-controlled clinical trial," *Alimentary Pharmacology and Therapeutics*, vol. 24, no. 10, pp. 1423–1430, 2006.

[13] C. G. Teran, C. N. Teran-Escalera, and P. Villarroel, "Nitazoxanide vs. probiotics for the treatment of acute rotavirus diarrhea in children: a randomized, single-blind, controlled trial in Bolivian children," *International Journal of Infectious Diseases*, vol. 13, no. 4, pp. 518–523, 2009.

[14] D. G. Bonett and R. M. Price, "Statistical inference for a linear function of medians: confidence intervals, hypothesis testing, and sample size requirements," *Psychological Methods*, vol. 7, no. 3, pp. 370–383, 2002.

[15] A. Guarino, R. Berni Canani, M. I. Spagnuolo, F. Albano, and L. Di Benedetto, "Oral bacterial therapy reduces the duration of symptoms and of viral excretion in children with mild diarrhea," *Journal of Pediatric Gastroenterology and Nutrition*, vol. 25, no. 5, pp. 516–519, 1997.

[16] M. A. Mathew, A. Paulose, S. Chitralekha, M. K. C. Nair, G. Kang, and P. Kilgore, "Prevalence of rotavirus diarrhea among hospitalized under-five children," *Indian Pediatrics*, vol. 51, no. 1, pp. 27–31, 2014.

[17] A. A. Nunes, L. M. de Mello, R. N. Parrode, J. P. Maneira Bittar, and A. L. da Silva Domingues, "Prevalence of rotavirus in acute diarrhea and its association with clinical signs and symptoms," *Journal of Tropical Pediatrics*, vol. 56, no. 3, pp. 212–213, 2009.

[18] D. Prasetyo, I. M. Sabaroedin, Y. S. Ermaya, and Y. Soenarto, "Association between severe dehydration in rotavirus diarrhea and exclusive breastfeeding among infants at Dr. Hasan Sadikin General Hospital, Bandung, Indonesia," *Journal of Tropical Medicine*, vol. 2015, Article ID 862578, 4 pages, 2015.

[19] A. M. Kazi, G. J. Warraich, S. Qureshi et al., "Sentinel hospital-based surveillance for assessment of burden of rotavirus gastroenteritis in children in Pakistan," *PLoS ONE*, vol. 9, no. 10, Article ID e108221, 2014.

[20] K. Soares-Weiser, H. Maclehose, H. Bergman et al., "Vaccines for preventing rotavirus diarrhoea: vaccines in use," *Cochrane Database of Systematic Reviews*, vol. 11, Article ID CD008521, 2012.

[21] A. Narang, A. Bose, A. N. Pandit et al., "Immunogenicity, reactogenicity and safety of human rotavirus vaccine (RIX4414) in Indian infants," *Human Vaccines*, vol. 5, no. 6, pp. 414–419, 2009.

[22] M. R. Lokeshwar, S. Bhave, A. Gupta, V. K. Goyal, and A. Walia, "Immunogenicity and safety of the pentavalent human-bovine (WC3) reassortant rotavirus vaccine (PRV) in Indian infants," *Human Vaccines and Immunotherapeutics*, vol. 9, no. 1, pp. 172–176, 2013.

[23] N. Bhandari, T. Rongsen-Chandola, A. Bavdekar et al., "Efficacy of a monovalent human-bovine (116E) rotavirus vaccine in Indian infants: a randomised, double-blind, placebo-controlled trial," *The Lancet*, vol. 383, no. 9935, pp. 2136–2143, 2014.

22

Child Survival Strategies: Assessment of Knowledge and Practice of Rural Women of Reproductive Age in Cross River State, Nigeria

Aniekan Jumbo Etokidem[1] and Ofonime Johnson[2]

[1]*Department of Community Medicine, University of Calabar, Calabar 540001, Cross River State, Nigeria*
[2]*Department of Community Medicine, University of Uyo, Uyo 520101, Akwa Ibom State, Nigeria*

Correspondence should be addressed to Aniekan Jumbo Etokidem; etokidem@etokidem.com

Academic Editor: Marcel Tanner

Introduction. Nigeria is one of the five countries that account for about 50% of under-five mortality in the world. The objective of this study was to assess the knowledge and practice of child survival strategies among rural community caregivers in Cross River State of Nigeria. *Materials and Methods.* This descriptive cross-sectional survey used a pretested questionnaire to obtain information from 150 women of reproductive age. Data analysis was done using SPSS version 20. *Results.* The child survival strategy known to most of the respondents was oral rehydration therapy as indicated by 98% followed by female education by 73.3% and immunization by 67.3%. Only 20% of the respondents had adequate knowledge of frequency of weighing a child while only 32.7% knew that breastfeeding should be continued even if the child had diarrhea. More respondents with nonformal education (83.3%) practiced exclusive breastfeeding of their last children compared to respondents with primary education (77.3%), secondary education (74.2%), and tertiary education (72.2%). *Conclusion.* Although respondents demonstrated adequate knowledge and practice of most of the strategies, there was evidence of gaps, including myths and misconceptions that could mar efforts towards reducing child morbidity and mortality in the state.

1. Introduction

Worldwide, nearly 6.6 million under-five children die yearly, translating to about 18,000 under-five deaths every day [1]. About 50% of under-five child deaths occur in only five countries of the world, namely, India, Nigeria, Democratic Republic of the Congo, Pakistan, and China. Two of these countries, India and Nigeria, account for more than one-third of global under-five mortality, contributing 22 percent and 13 percent, respectively [1]. Sub-Saharan Africa and Southern Asia countries are witnessing an increase in under-five mortality despite a drop from 32 percent in 1990 to 18 percent in 2012 in the rest of the world [1]. Sub-Saharan Africa records the highest rates of under-five child mortality in the world, 98 deaths per 1,000 live births. This figure is 15 times the average for developed countries [1].

The 2007 State of the World's Children Report documented that Nigeria is the country with the 14th highest under-five mortality rate in the world [2]. Seven years after, the 2014 edition of the same report ranked Nigeria as the country with the 9th highest under-five mortality rate in the world, with 124 under-five children dying per 1,000 live births. Incidentally, some African countries fare better; for instance, according to the 2014 report, Libya with an under-five mortality of 15/1000 ranks 116th and Seychelles with 13/1,000 live births ranks 125th. Some of the West African countries that have fared better than Nigeria include Senegal and Ghana with under-five mortality rates of 60/1,000 and 72/1,000 live births and ranking of 43 and 36, respectively [2, 3].

Earlier studies on childhood morbidity and mortality and child survival strategies in Nigeria presented some noteworthy findings. According to Policy Project/Nigeria office, the main causes of infant and child mortality in Nigeria include pneumonia, malaria, diarrhea, undernutrition, and vaccine-preventable diseases [4].

Malaria has been reported as the leading cause of childhood morbidity and mortality in Nigeria, accounting for 25% of infant and 30% of childhood mortality [5, 6]. A study among children in Ilorin, Nigeria, found that pneumonia accounted for 13.3% of all hospital admissions during the study period with a male : female ratio of 1.5 : 1 and 60.5% of the children were infants [7].

Inadequate knowledge and practice of child survival strategies by caregivers, as well as myths and misconceptions, contribute to child morbidity and mortality. A study by Tobin et al. found that 90.2% of respondents indicated that when a child is being weaned from breast milk, the child should continue with breastfeeding when diarrhea occurs with 9.8% indicating that breastfeeding should be discontinued with the onset of diarrhea [8]. In a study in Sokoto, Nigeria, Abiola et al. found that 32.4% of mothers studied believed that "evil eye" was the cause of diarrhea [9].

Worried about the alarming under-five mortality rates in developing countries, the WHO in collaboration with UNICEF and the World Bank, developed a set of evidence-based interventions which, when properly implemented, would reduce under-five mortality. This package of interventions was named child survival strategies. Originally, there were four child survival strategies, namely, growth monitoring, oral rehydration therapy, breastfeeding, and immunization, giving the acronym "GOBI" [10]. With time, some other interventions like family planning, female education, food supplementation, and vitamin A administration were added, giving the acronym GOBIFFFA [11].

Currently, child survival centers around newer strategies such as antenatal care attendance, skilled birth attendance at delivery, and commencement of breastfeeding within one hour of delivery. Others include use of insecticide treated bed nets, management of fever, and treatment of acute respiratory infections, amongst others. According to the NDHS 2013 and the National Bureau of Statistics 2014, the percentage of women who had four or more antenatal clinic visits in Cross River State, 58.7%, was lower than the regional figure of 62.7% but higher than the national figure of 51.1% [12, 13]. Similarly, the percentage of children with fever for whom advice or treatment was sought from a health facility or provider was 21.0% which was lower than the regional figure of 28.2% and the national figure of 31.8% for males and 31.1% for females. However, Cross River State fared better in childhood immunization as the percentage of children aged 12–23 months who received specific vaccines at any time before the survey was higher than the national figures for the three vaccines considered, namely, BCG, DPT3, and OPV3.

2. Aim of the Study

The aim of this study was to determine the knowledge and practice of child survival strategies among rural community women in Cross River State, Nigeria.

3. Materials and Methods

3.1. Study Area. The study was carried out in Cross River State of Nigeria. Cross River State is one of the six states in Nigeria's South-South geopolitical zone. With a population of over 3 million, Cross River State is made up of 18 Local Government Areas which are further grouped into three senatorial districts. The low socioeconomic status of rural community dwellers in Cross River State influences the health-seeking behavior of the women both for themselves and for children in their care.

3.2. Study Design. This was a descriptive cross-sectional study.

3.3. Sample Size Determination and Sample Selection. The sample size for the study was calculated using Leslie Kish formula:

$$n = \frac{z^2 pq}{d^2}. \quad (1)$$

In a study by Tobin et al., 90.2% of respondents were of the opinion that a child being weaned from breast milk should continue to receive the same when he/she has diarrhea [8]. Thus, the proportion with the desired positive attribute was taken as 0.902.

Thus

$$n = \frac{(1.96 \times 1.96 \times 0.902 \times 0.098)}{0.0025} = 135. \quad (2)$$

Making provision for 10% nonresponse, the sample size became

$$n = 135 + 13.5 = 148.5 \text{ or approximately, } 150. \quad (3)$$

Convenience sampling method was used to select 150 rural women. A questionnaire was used to collect data from them. The variables in the questionnaire included sociodemographic variables like age, marital status, occupation, religion, educational status, and ethnic grouping. Other variables included knowledge of the strategies that facilitate child survival and practice of the different child survival strategies. Data obtained from the respondents were analyzed using SPSS software version 20. Both univariate and bivariate analysis were performed. Association between categorical variables was explored using Chi square test.

3.3.1. Ethical Consideration. The data for this study were collected in accordance with the Declaration of Helsinki. Informed consent was obtained from the respondents.

4. Results

4.1. Sociodemographic Variables. Twenty-six percent of the respondents were aged 45 and above while over 90% were Christians. Nearly 19% of the respondents were civil servants while only 8% were full-time housewives. Sixty-percent of the respondents were married. Fifty-four (36%) respondents had tertiary education. The Efiks constituted majority of the respondents, 77 (51.3%) (Table 1).

4.2. Knowledge of Child Survival Strategies and Sources of Information. As shown in Tables 2, 3, and 4, the child survival

Table 1: Sociodemographic characteristics.

Variable	Frequency ($n = 150$)	Percent
Age group		
15–19	12	8.0
20–24	18	12.0
25–29	18	12.0
30–34	18	12.0
35–39	28	18.7
40–44	17	11.3
45 and above	39	26
Religion		
Christianity	142	94.7
Others	8	5.3
Educational status		
Nonformal	12	8.0
Primary	22	14.7
Secondary	62	41.3
Tertiary	54	36.0
Occupation		
Farming	24	16.0
Trading	27	18.0
Civil servant	29	19.3
Student	24	16
Full-time housewife	12	8.0
Other	34	22.7

Table 2: Knowledge of child survival strategies.

Components of child survival strategies correctly indicated	Frequency*	Percent
Growth monitoring	64	42.7
Oral rehydration therapy	147	98
Breastfeeding	94	62.7
Immunization	101	67.3
Family planning	65	43.3
Female education	110	73.3
Food supplementation	40	26.7
Essential drugs program	34	22.7
Treatment of common ailments	64	42.7

*Multiple responses allowed.

Table 3: Source of information.

Source	Frequency*	Percent
Health talks in hospital/health center	113	75.3
Personal advice by health worker	77	51.3
Health books	43	28.7
Radio/TV	60	40
Village health worker	41	27.3
Friends and relatives	32	21.3
Patent medicine vendor	7	4.7
Traditional birth attendant	21	14

*Multiple responses allowed.

Table 4: Adequacy of knowledge of child survival strategies.

Aspect of knowledge	Correct response	
	Frequency ($n = 150$)	Percent
Frequency of weighing of child	30	20
Vitamin that prevents blindness	110	73.3
Food that contains vitamin D	67	44.7
When to commence breastfeeding	114	76
Should a child be given first milk?	119	79.3
Name of the first milk from mother's breast after childbirth	126	84
When should first polio vaccine be given?	105	70
What is exclusive breastfeeding?	117	78
Give salt sugar solution if child has diarrhea	123	82
Continue breastfeeding if child has diarrhea	49	32.7

strategy known to almost all of the respondents was oral rehydration therapy, 147 (98%), followed by female education, 110 (73.3%), and immunization, 101 (67.3%). The commonest source of information regarding child survival strategies indicated by the respondents was health talk in health facility, 113 (75.3%). Only 30 (20%) respondents had adequate knowledge of frequency of weighing a child. One hundred and ten (73.3%) respondents knew that vitamin A prevents blindness among children. The majority of respondents, 114 (76%), knew that breastfeeding should be commenced within the first hour of birth just as the majority, 119 (79.3%), agreed that a child should be given the first milk that the mother expresses after childbirth. Similarly, the majority of respondents, 123 (82%), knew that children should be given salt sugar solution when they have diarrhea. Only 49 (32.7%) respondents knew that breastfeeding should be continued even if the child has diarrhea.

4.3. Practice of Child Survival Strategies. As shown in Table 5, sixty-two percent of respondents had attended antenatal clinic in the last pregnancy while 88% indicated that their last children had received all age-appropriate vaccinations. With regard to child spacing, 74% of respondents indicated that the interval between their last two deliveries was at least 2 years while 25% practiced exclusive breastfeeding of their last children.

4.4. Some Myths and Misconceptions regarding Certain Aspects of Child Survival. Figure 1 shows that thirty-one respondents indicated various reasons why colostrum should not be given to the baby; 15 (48.4%) of these indicated that "it is not good for the child's health," 6 (19.4%) indicated that "it is not

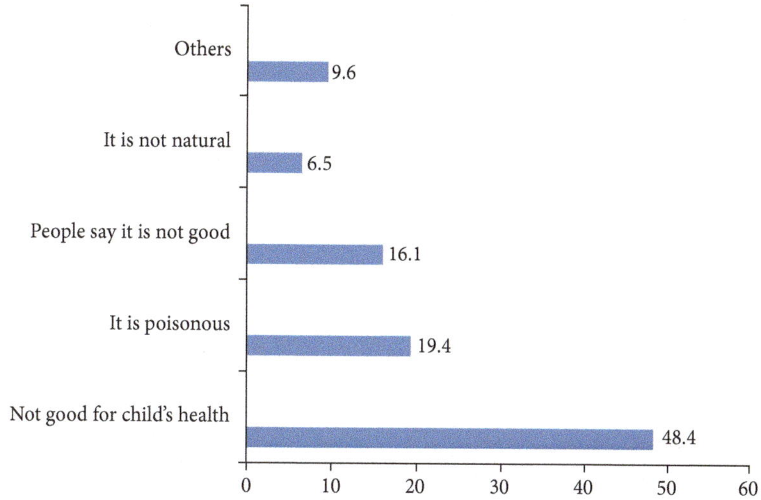

FIGURE 1: False beliefs about colostrum by respondents.

TABLE 5: Practice of child survival strategies in the last pregnancy and childbirth.

Child survival strategy practiced	Frequency	Percent
Antenatal clinic attendance	93	62
Last child received all immunizations	137	88
At least 2-year interval between last two deliveries	111	74
Exclusively breastfed last child	38	25
Given antimalarial in the last pregnancy	126	84

natural," 2 (6.5%) indicated that "it is poisonous," 5 (16.1%) indicated that "people say it is not good," and 3 (9.6%) gave various other reasons.

4.5. Association between Level of Education and Knowledge of Child Survival Strategies. Table 6 shows that more respondents with tertiary education (57.4%) knew that growth monitoring is a child survival strategy compared with those with secondary education (38.7%), primary education (31.8%), and nonformal education (16.7%). The difference in response between the four categories was statistically significant (Chi square = 9.568, df = 3, P = 0.022). Similarly, all respondents with tertiary education (100%) knew that oral rehydration therapy is a child survival strategy compared with 98.4% with secondary education, 95.5% with primary education, and 91.7% with nonformal education. There was no statistically significant difference in the response from the four groups (P = 0.1289).

4.6. Association between Level of Education and Practice of Child Survival Strategies. Table 7 shows that more respondents with tertiary education (66.7%) attended antenatal clinic in the last pregnancy than those with secondary education, (61.3%), primary education (59.1%), and nonformal education (50%). There was no statistically significant difference between respondents in the four levels of education (Chi square = 1.325; df = 3; P = 0.734). Similarly, all respondents with tertiary education (100%) indicated that their last children had received all vaccinations. When this was compared with respondents who had only secondary education (93.5%), primary education (77.3%), and nonformal education (66.7%), there was a statistically significant difference in the response between the four groups (Fisher's Exact Test, df = 3; P = 0.001). More respondents with nonformal education (83.3%) practiced exclusive breastfeeding of the last child compared to respondents with primary education (77.3%), secondary education (74.2%), and tertiary education (72.2%). However, there was no statistically significant difference in the response between the four groups (Chi square = 0.733; df = 3; P = 0.884). More respondents with tertiary education (87%) were likely to have interval between the last two deliveries equal to or greater than two years compared to those with secondary education (79%), primary education (54.5%), and nonformal education (25%). The difference between the responses from the four groups was statistically significant (Chi square = 24.889; df = 3; P = 0.000).

4.7. Association between Knowledge and Practice of Child Survival Strategies. As shown in Table 8, children of respondents who indicated that immunization is a child survival strategy were more likely to have been fully immunized than children of those who did not and the difference was statistically significant (χ^2 = 23.02; df = 1; P = 0.0000). There was no statistically significant association between knowledge of the correct definition of family planning and adequate spacing of the last two deliveries.

TABLE 6: Association between level of education and knowledge of child survival strategies.

Independent variable	Dependent variable Yes	No	Test statistic	df	*P*
Level of education	*Growth monitoring*				
Nonformal	2 (16.7%)	10 (83.3%)	Chi square = 9.568	3	0.022
Primary	7 (31.8%)	15 (68.2%)			
Secondary	24 (38.7%)	38 (61.3%)			
Tertiary	31 (57.4%)	23 (42.6%)			
Level of education	*Oral rehydration therapy*				
Nonformal	11 (91.7%)	1 (8.3%)	Fisher's Exact Test	3	0.1289
Primary	21 (95.5%)	1 (4.5%)			
Secondary	61 (98.4%)	1 (1.6%)			
Tertiary	54 (100%)	0 (0%)			
Level of education	*Breastfeeding*				
Nonformal	6 (50%)	6 (50%)	Chi square = 2.863	3	0.418
Primary	12 (54.5%)	10 (45.5%)			
Secondary	38 (61.3%)	24 (38.7%)			
Tertiary	38 (70.4%)	16 (29.6%)			
Level of education	*Immunization*				
Nonformal	6 (50%)	6 (50%)	Chi square = 7.210	3	0.066
Primary	12 (54.5%)	10 (45.5%)			
Secondary	40 (64.5%)	22 (35.5%)			
Tertiary	43 (79.6%)	11 (20.4%)			
Level of education	*Family planning*				
Nonformal	4 (33.3%)	8 (66.7%)	Chi square = 6.659	3	0.084
Primary	5 (22.7%)	17 (77.3%)			
Secondary	27 (43.5%)	35 (56.5%)			
Tertiary	29 (53.7%)	25 (46.3%)			

5. Discussion

Only 32.7% of respondents knew that breastfeeding should be continued even when the child has diarrhea. This is comparable to the finding by Tobin et al. that 35.3% of respondents in a related study in a rural community in South-South Nigeria indicated that a child that has diarrhea should be given more breast milk than usual [8]. The findings of these two studies reflect a deficiency in the knowledge and skill of home management of diarrhea among the respondents and are comparable to the finding of a study by Adimora et al. that only 39.4% of mothers of under-five children could correctly manage diarrhea at home while majority (60.6%) could not [14]. The finding of this study is also comparable to that of a related study where Okoh and Alex-Hart found that only 29.3% of respondents had good level of knowledge of home management of diarrhea while only 33.8% had good level of skill [15].

The majority of respondents, 79.3%, agreed that the baby should be given colostrum. This is contrary to the findings of Walia et al. where 66% of respondents withheld colostrums from neonates [16]. In a related study, Morse et al. found that, in 50 out of 120 cultural groups studied, initiation of breast-feeding was delayed by more than 2 days, thus withholding colostrum from the baby [17]. The idea that colostrum is not natural, as indicated by 19.4% of respondents, may be associated with the concept of witch's milk which is the local name given to the milk produced by the breasts of infants. This milk is believed to be abnormal and ancient folklore has blamed it as a source of nourishment for witches' familiar spirits [18]. The close resemblance of colostrum to the so-called witch's milk may explain why the respondents indicate that it is not natural [18]. Regarding reasons why colostrums should not be given to infants, in the study by Walia et al., 54.5% of respondents indicated that it causes obstructions in the intestine while 24.3% indicated that it would be difficult to digest [16].

The proportion of respondents who had antenatal care in the last pregnancy (62%) is comparable to the national average of 61% reported by NDHS 2013 [12]. The high ANC attendance in the state may be due to the free health care for pregnant women and under-five children instituted by the Cross River State Government [19]. Nearly all respondents (98%) knew that ORT is a child survival strategy. This is not surprising because, in Cross River State, the populace is so familiar with salt sugar solution that they even have an apt local name for it, "*mmong uwem*," which means "life giving

TABLE 7: Association between level of education and practice of child survival strategies.

Independent variable	Dependent variable		Test statistic	df	*P*
	Yes	No			
Level of education	*Attended antenatal care*				
Nonformal	6 (50%)	6 (50%)	Chi square = 1.325	3	0.734
Primary	13 (59.1%)	9 (40.9%)			
Secondary	38 (61.3%)	24 (38.7%)			
Tertiary	36 (66.7%)	18 (33.3%)			
Level of education	*Child received immunizations*				
Nonformal	8 (66.7%)	4 (33.3%)	Fisher's Exact Test	3	0.001
Primary	17 (77.3%)	5 (22.7%)			
Secondary	58 (93.5%)	4 (6.5%)			
Tertiary	54 (100%)	0 (0%)			
Level of education	*Interval between deliveries≥2 years*				
Nonformal	3 (25%)	9 (75%)	Chi square = 24.889	3	0.000
Primary	12 (54.5%)	10 (45.5%)			
Secondary	49 (79%)	13 (21%)			
Tertiary	47 (87%)	7 (13%)			
Level of education	*Exclusive breastfeeding*				
Nonformal	10 (83.3%)	2 (16.7%)	Chi square = 0.733	3	0.884
Primary	17 (77.3%)	5 (22.7%)			
Secondary	46 (74.2%)	16 (25.8%)			
Tertiary	39 (72.2%)	15 (27.8%)			
Level of education	*Being given antimalarial medicine during pregnancy*				
Nonformal	7 (58.3%)	5 (41.7%)	Fisher's Exact Test	3	0.023
Primary	16 (72.7%)	6 (27.3%)			
Secondary	55 (88.7%)	7 (11.3%)			
Tertiary	48 (88.9%)	6 (11.1%)			

TABLE 8: Association between knowledge and practice of child survival strategies.

Knowledge variable	Practice variable		df	Chi square	*P* value
Immunization as a child survival strategy	*Last child fully immunized*				
	Yes	*No*			
Yes	100	1	1	23.02	0.0000
No	37	12			
Correct definition of exclusive breastfeeding	*Last child was exclusively breastfed*				
	Yes	*No*			
Yes	20	97	1	19.087	0.0000
No	18	15			
Correct definition of family planning	*Spacing between last two deliveries is at least two years*				
	Yes	*No*			
Yes	31	6	1	2.44	0.1180
No	80	33			

water." This proportion is higher than that of a study by Sanusi and Gbadamosi which found that 78.3% of mothers in Oyo state, Nigeria, practiced ORT as a child survival strategy [20].

Education was found to be a determinant of knowledge and practice of some child survival strategies. It was a determinant of attendance of antenatal clinic although there was no statistically significant difference between the four levels of education ($P = 0.734$). A study by Joshi et al. showed that higher level of education was one of the predictors of both attendance at four or more antenatal visits and receipt of good quality care [21]. Education was a determinant of respondents' children having received all vaccinations, with children of respondents with tertiary education doing better than those of lower levels of education, with a statistically significant difference, $P = 0.001$. Educated women may want to have fewer children that they can cater for (in terms of health and social amenities) and help the children to also be as educated as them.

There was an association between level of education and having received antimalarial medicine in the last pregnancy with a statistically significant difference, $P = 0.023$. These findings compare favorably with those of the NDHS (2013) which documented that women with more than a secondary school education were more likely than other women to have received two or more tetanus toxoid injections during pregnancy. This positive effect of education on the quality of care obtained during antenatal care is further corroborated by another finding by NDHS 2013 that only 43 percent of women with no education used iron tablets or syrup, whereas 74 percent of women with a primary education, 86 percent of women with a secondary education, and 92 percent of women with more than a secondary education did so [12]. The observed inverse relationship between level of education and likelihood of exclusively breastfeeding the last child is likely because women with a higher level of education are more likely than those with lower levels to be employed in jobs that are so demanding that it is difficult for them to exclusively breastfeed their babies. One plausible reason why the breastfeeding prevalence recorded in this study (25%) is higher than the national prevalence (17%) is that 42% of respondents belong to the occupational category of farmers, traders, and full-time housewife. These occupations allow them more time to be within their communities and therefore have access to their babies for breastfeeding.

6. Conclusion

Respondents demonstrated adequate knowledge and practice of most of the child survival strategies, especially with regard to oral rehydration therapy. However, there was evidence of some gaps like majority of respondents not knowing that breastfeeding should be continued even when the child has diarrhea. Such inadequate knowledge and practice, including evidence of myths and misconceptions demonstrated by the respondents, could mar efforts to reduce child morbidity and mortality in the state. Education was associated with knowledge and practice of most child survival strategies. This may be an indication that the advocacy for girl child education, which has been intensified within the past 15 years, is gradually making the desired impact and should be encouraged. It is recommended that health care providers should do more to educate caregivers about the basic facts regarding child survival strategies.

Competing Interests

The authors declare that there is no conflict of interests regarding the publication of this paper.

References

[1] UNICEF, *Levels and Trends in Child Mortality. Report 2013 Estimates Developed by the UN Inter Agency Group for Child Mortality Estimation*, United Nations Children's Fund, New York, NY, USA, 2013.

[2] UNICEF, The State of the World's Children, 2007.

[3] UNICEF, *The State of the World's Children*, UNICEF, 2014.

[4] Policy Project/Nigeria, "Child Survival in Nigeria: Situation, Response, and Prospects Key Issues POLICY Project/Nigeria," October 2002, http://www.policyproject.com/pubs/countryreports/nig_csrevised.pdf.

[5] UNICEF Annual Report, "The inter-agency group for child mortality estimation (IGME). Estimates of under five mortality rates by country, the 2011 release," http://www.childmortality org/.

[6] FMOH, *Training Manual for Management of Malaria in Nigeria*, FMOH/National Malaria and Vector Control Division, Abuja, Nigeria, 2005.

[7] A. A. Abdulkarim, R. M. Ibraheem, A. O. Adegboye, W. B. R. Johnson, and M. A. N. Adeboye, "Childhood pneumonia at the University of Ilorin Teaching Hospital, Ilorin Nigeria," *Nigerian Journal of Paediatrics*, vol. 40, no. 3, pp. 284–289, 2013.

[8] E. A. Tobin, E. C. Isah, and D. A. Asogun, "Care giver's knowledge about childhood diarrheal management in a rural community in South-South Nigeria," *International Journal of Community Research*, vol. 3, no. 4, pp. 93–99, 2014.

[9] A. O. A. Abiola, A. L. Ndaman, S. H. Idris, N. M. Jiya, and M. T. O. Ibrahim, "Home management of childhood diarrhoea among mothers in Sokoto, Nigeria," *Tropical Journal of Health Sciences*, vol. 17, no. 1, 2015.

[10] The 1980s: Campaign for child survival, http://www.unicef.org/sowc96/1980s.htm.

[11] Choosing interventions to reduce specific risks, 2015, http://www.who.int/whr/2002/chapter5/en/index5.html.

[12] National Population Commission (NPC) (Nigeria) and ICF International, *Nigeria Demographic and Health Survey (NDHS) 2013*, NPC and ICF International, Abuja, Nigeria, 2014.

[13] NBS/UNICEF/USAID, *National Nutrition and Health Survey (NNHS)*, National Bureau of Statistics, Abuja, Nigeria, 2014.

[14] G. N. Adimora, A. N. Ikefuna, and G. Ilechukwu, "Home management of childhood diarrhoea: need to intensify campaign," *Nigerian Journal of Clinical Practice*, vol. 14, no. 2, pp. 237–241, 2011.

[15] B. A. N. Okoh and B. A. Alex-Hart, "Home management of diarrhoea by caregivers presenting at the diarrhoea training unit of a tertiary hospital in Southern Nigeria," *British Journal of Medicine & Medical Research*, vol. 4, no. 35, pp. 5524–5540, 2014.

[16] I. Walia, R. Kalia, and S. Chopra, "Initiation of breast feeding—the cultural factors," *Nursing and Midwifery Research Journal*, vol. 5, no. 1, pp. 10–18, 2009.

[17] J. M. Morse, C. Jehle, and D. Gamble, "Initiating breastfeeding: a world survey of the timing of postpartum breastfeeding," *International Journal of Nursing Studies*, vol. 27, no. 3, pp. 303–313, 1990.

[18] Galactorrhea of the newborn (witch's milk), 2015, http://www.pediatricsconsultantlive.com/photoclinic/galactorrhea-newborn-witch%E2%80%99s-milk.

[19] CRSG, "Maternal health services," http://www.crossriverstate.gov.ng/index.php?option=com_content&view=article&id=152:maternal-health-services&catid=88:healthcare&Itemid=754.

[20] R. A. Sanusi and A. O. Gbadamosi, "Do Mothers' knowledge and practice of 'Child Survival Strategies' affect the nutritional status of their children?" *Pakistan Journal of Nutrition*, vol. 8, no. 9, pp. 1506–1511, 2009.

[21] C. Joshi, S. Torvaldsen, R. Hodgson, and A. Hayen, "Factors associated with the use and quality of antenatal care in Nepal: a population-based study using the demographic and health survey data," *BMC Pregnancy and Childbirth*, vol. 14, article 94, 2014.

23

Antimalarial Properties of Aqueous Crude Extracts of *Gynostemma pentaphyllum* and *Moringa oleifera* Leaves in Combination with Artesunate in *Plasmodium berghei*-Infected Mice

Voravuth Somsak, Preeyanuch Borkaew, Chokdee Klubsri, Kittiyaporn Dondee, Panatda Bootprom, and Butsarat Saiphet

Department of Clinical Chemistry, Faculty of Medical Technology, Western University, Kanchanaburi 71170, Thailand

Correspondence should be addressed to Voravuth Somsak; voravuthsomsak@gmail.com

Academic Editor: Sukla Biswas

Due to the emergence and spread of malaria parasite with resistance to antimalarial drugs, discovery and development of new, safe, and affordable antimalarial are urgently needed. In this respect, medicinal plant extracts are targets to optimize antimalarial actions and restore efficacy of standard antimalarial drugs. The present study was aimed at determining the antimalarial activities of *Gynostemma pentaphyllum* and *Moringa oleifera* leaf extracts in combination with artesunate against *Plasmodium berghei*-infected mice. *P. berghei* ANKA maintained by serial passage in ICR mice were used based on intraperitoneal injection of 1×10^7 parasitized erythrocytes and subsequent development of parasitemia. These infected mice were used to investigate the antimalarial activity of artesunate (6 mg/kg) in combination with 500, 1,000, and 2,000 mg/kg of *G. pentaphyllum* and *M. oleifera* leaf extracts using 4-day suppressive test. It was found that these extracts showed significant ($P < 0.05$) antimalarial activity in dose-dependent manner with percentage of suppression of 45, 50, and 55% for *G. pentaphyllum* leaf extract and 35, 40, and 50% for *M. oleifera* leaf extract. Additionally, artesunate combined with these extracts presented higher antimalarial activity, compared to extract treated alone with percentage of suppression of 78, 91, and 96% for *G. pentaphyllum* leaf extract and 73, 82, and 91% for *M. oleifera* leaf extract. The results indicated that combination treatment of *G. pentaphyllum* or *M. oleifera* leaf extracts with artesunate was able to increase the antimalarial activity by using low dose of artesunate. Hence, these results justified the combination of these extracts and artesunate in antimalarial herbal remedies.

1. Introduction

Malaria is a major parasitic disease with high mortality and morbidity, especially in the sub-Saharan Africa, Latin America, and Asia. About 3 billion people worldwide are exposed annually, with 1.2 billion at high risk, and some 200 million developed symptomatic malaria. Moreover, it was estimated that 1 million deaths have occurred in the world [1]. This disease is caused by malarial protozoa parasite from genus *Plasmodium* and transmitted by female *Anopheles* mosquito. Due to the lack of effective vaccine to prevent malaria, the global strategy for malaria mainly focuses on case management through provision of antimalarial drugs which are capable of reducing or eliminating malaria parasites. Unfortunately, malaria parasite has developed resistance to drugs used in malarial therapy except the artemisinin [2]. However, artemisinin produces fast recrudescence when used alone due to its short half-life. Hence, artemisinin used in combination with other antimalarials, a combination known as artemisinin-combination therapy (ACT), has been recommended [3]. In addition, resistance of mosquitoes to insecticides has led to an increase in severe malaria, complicating the eradication of the disease, and the resurgence of malaria [4]. Moreover, many antimalarials in use today have high toxicity that exposes patients' health expenditure [5]. In this respect, medicinal plant extracts are potential targets [6]. Although up to 80% of Thailand population uses traditional medicinal plants for management of diseases, these plants are not yet fully explored [7]. Various researches have been conducted to investigate the antimalarial efficacy of traditionally used plants in Asia and Africa. For example, Ramazani et al. worked on ten Iranian plant species but only *Boerhavia elegans*, *Solanum surattense*, and *Prosopis juliflora* showed a promising antimalarial activity *in vitro* and *in vivo* with no toxicity [8]. Verma et al. reported that *Holarrhena antidysenterica* and *Viola canescens* exhibited *in vitro* antimalarial activity [9].

Gynostemma pentaphyllum and *Moringa oleifera* have been used traditionally for treatment of several diseases involving oxidative stress and infection [10, 11]. Many reports have described the activities of these plant extracts, including antioxidant, anti-inflammation, anticancer, antiparasitic, antidiabetes, antibacterial activities, and homeostasis of biomolecules in blood [12–16]. Recently, these plant extracts were reported to exert antimalarial activity in mouse model [17]. However, combination therapy with standard antimalarial drug, artesunate, has not yet been studied using these plant extracts. Therefore, the aim of the present study is to investigate antimalarial activities of *G. pentaphyllum* and *M. oleifera* extracts in combination with artesunate in *P. berghei*-infected mice.

2. Materials and Methods

2.1. Artesunate. The pure artesunate powder used in this study was a gift from Dr. Chairat Uthaipibull, National Center for Genetic Engineering and Biotechnology (BIOTEC). It was dissolved in 7% Tween 80 and 3% ethanol in distilled water to provide dose of 6 mg/kg. This dose was based on the ED50 of artesunate on *P. berghei*-infected mice [18].

2.2. Plant Materials. Dried leaves of *G. pentaphyllum* and *M. oleifera* were purchased from the Royal Project Foundation shop at Suphan Buri province. The plant materials were identified by Dr. Sakaewan Ounjaijean at Faculty of Pharmacology, Payap University, and voucher specimens were deposited in Department of Clinical Chemistry, Faculty of Medical Technology, Western University, with voucher numbers CC-MT-WTU01 (*G. pentaphyllum*) and CC-MT-WTU02 (*M. oleifera*).

2.3. Preparation of Aqueous Crude Extracts. For preparation of crude extract, microwave-associated hot water extract was carried out as previously described [19]. Briefly, dried leaves of plant materials were ground using electric blender to obtain the powdered dried plant materials and subsequently dissolved in distilled water at the proportion of 1 : 10. The mixtures were heated in microwave at 360 W for 5 min and incubated at room temperature for overnight to obtain complete extraction. Filter through Whatman no. 1 filter paper was done, and filtrate was then freeze-dried to obtain aqueous crude extracts of *G. pentaphyllum* (GPE) and *M. oleifera* (MOE). The extracts were stored at −20°C until used. Before use, the extracts were dissolved in a mixture of 7% Tween 80 and 3% ethanol in distilled water to provide appropriate doses.

2.4. Experimental Mice. Pathogen-free female ICR mice, 4 weeks old, weighting 20–25 g, obtained from the National Laboratory Animal Center, Mahidol University, Thailand, were used. They were kept at the animal room with temperature within 25–28°C and 12 h light/12 h dark cycle. They were fed with standard diet pellet CP082 and drinking water *ad libitum*. All experiments involving animals were approved and ratified by the Animal Ethical Committee, Western University.

2.5. Acute Toxicity Test. GPE and MOE were evaluated for their acute toxicity in experimental mice as previously described with some modification [20]. Briefly, the mice were starved for 3-4 h before the experiment with only drinking water allowed and 1-2 h after the administration of the extracts. In the evaluation for each extract, 25 mice were randomly divided into 5 groups of 5 mice/group and were given orally 500, 1,000, 2,000, and 4,000 mg/kg body weight in single dose volume of 0.2 mL of the extracts. The control group received 0.2 mL of respective vehicle of each extract (7% Tween 80 and 3% ethanol in distilled water). Then, these mice were observed continuously for 1 h, intermittently for 4 h, and for a period of 24 h for any gross behavioral changes including rigidity, sleep, mortality, and other signs of toxicity, and follow-up continued for 30 days.

2.6. Rodent Malaria Parasite. Drug sensitive-*Plasmodium berghei* strain ANKA (PbANKA) obtained from MR4 (Malaria Research and Reference Reagent Resource Center, EBI Resources, University Boulevard, Manassas, VA, USA) was used in this study. The cryopreservation stock was injected intraperitoneally to naïve ICR mice. Parasitemia was determined by microscopy of Giemsa stained thin blood smear. The parasite was maintained by serial passage of 1×10^7 parasitized erythrocytes on a weekly basis. Percent parasitemia was calculated using the following formula:

$$\% \text{ parasitemia} = \frac{\text{Number of parasitized erythrocytes}}{\text{Number of erythrocytes}} \times 100. \quad (1)$$

2.7. In Vivo Antimalarial Activity. The efficacy test of GPE, MOE, and combination with artesunate was carried out using standard protocol following Peter's 4-day suppressive test [21]. Groups of naïve ICR mice (5 mice/group) were inoculated intraperitoneally with 1×10^7 parasitized erythrocytes of PbANKA. Then, GPE (500, 1,000, and 2,000 mg/kg), MOE (500, 1,000, and 2,000 mg/kg), combination of GPE (500, 1,000, and 2,000 mg/kg) and artesunate (6 mg/kg), and combination of MOE (500, 1,000, and 2,000 mg/kg) and artesunate (6 mg/kg) were administered orally to the individual groups. The control groups were also used including artesunate (6 mg/kg) treated and untreated mice as positive and negative controls, respectively. Treatment was started 3 h after infection on day 0 and then continued daily (every

24 h) as a single dose for 4 days (days 0–3). On day 4, parasitemia was estimated by microscopy of Giemsa thin blood smear, and suppression percentage was subsequently calculated using the formula given below:

$$\% \text{ suppression} = \frac{(\text{parasitemia of untreated group} - \text{parasitemia of treated group})}{\text{parasitemia of untreated group}} \times 100. \quad (2)$$

2.8. Statistical Analysis. GraphPad Prism software was used to analyze this study. All results were expressed as mean ± standard error of mean (SEM). One-way ANOVA with Tukey *post hoc* test was used to compare several treated groups, and significant differences were considered at 95% confidence, $P < 0.05$.

3. Results

3.1. Acute Toxicity Test. The GPE and MOE administered orally in a single dose of up to 4,000 mg/kg showed no lethal effect within 24 h of observation. Gross physical and behavioral observation of these experimental mice revealed no visible signs of toxicity such as paw licking, salivation, stretching, urination, lacrimation, hair erection, and reduction in feeding activity. Generally, the mice were physically active. Additionally, no mortality occurred within the observation period of 30 days.

3.2. Antimalarial Activity of G. pentaphyllum. The effect of GPE on PbANKA infected mice, parasitemia measurement obtained from 4-day suppressive test, and percentage of suppression of parasitemia by GPE were summarized in Figure 1. Accordingly, 500, 1,000, and 2,000 mg/kg doses of GPE significantly ($P < 0.01$) inhibited parasitemia by 45, 50, and 55%, respectively, in a dose-dependent manner. The reference drug, artesunate (6 mg/kg), caused 60% suppression, which was higher than that of the extract treated groups. For combination treatment, the results indicated that GPE performed better antimalarial activity when combined with artesunate. The combination caused more significant ($P < 0.001$) suppression in parasitemia burden with 78, 91, and 96%, at 6 mg/kg of artesunate combined with 500, 1,000, and 2,000 mg/kg of GPE, respectively.

3.3. Antimalarial Activity of M. oleifera. As shown in Figure 2, the percentage of suppression at the doses of 500, 1,000, and 2,000 mg/kg of MOE was 35, 40, and 50%, respectively, while that of artesunate treated group was 60%. The extract caused significant ($P < 0.05$) suppression in a dose-dependent manner, compared to untreated control. In addition, combination of MOE with artesunate showed enhancement in antimalarial activity in a dose-dependent manner with significant ($P < 0.01$). The percentage of suppression at the doses of 6 mg/kg of artesunate combined with 500, 1,000, and 2,000 mg/kg of MOE was 73, 82, and 91%, respectively. Hence, antimalarial activity of MOE combined with artesunate was greater than the effect of artesunate or selected doses of the MOE when used singly in PbANKA infected mice.

4. Discussion

P. berghei-infected mice as rodent malaria model has been employed in this study. Several standard antimalarial drugs have been identified using this rodent model; therefore, it was the appropriate malarial model for the study [22–27]. Additionally, *in vivo* models are usually employed in antimalarial studies because they take into account the possible effect of prodrug and probable involvement of immune system in eradication of the parasite [28]. Moreover, the choice of 4-week-old mice for this study was used to avoid the effect of anemia in old mice and the effect of possible physiological changes associated with aging-related effects on the treatment result [29].

The present study assessed the antimalarial properties of two plant extracts, *G. pentaphyllum* and *M. oleifera*, individually and in combination with artesunate. The choice of these plants was based on the remarkable activity of quinine and the success of artemisinin [30]. However, reported cases of antimalarial resistance to these drugs made the search and development of new antimalarial drugs. The aqueous crude extracts of *G. pentaphyllum* and *M. oleifera* leaves showed high antimalarial properties with dose-dependent manner against *P. berghei* infection in mice as evidenced by the percent inhibition of parasitemia development. These extracts exhibited a dose-dependent manner. As the dose increased, likewise the antimalarial activity increased significantly. It has been described that plant extracts contain active compounds that have great potential for medicinal use, and both traditional healers and pharmaceutical drug companies make use of these plant extracts. The extracts of *G. pentaphyllum* and *M. oleifera* leaves were reported to contain different classes of active compounds such as tannins, alkaloids, quinines, saponins, flavonoids, polyphenols, terpenoids, quercetin, kaempferol, and gypenoside [31, 32]. Terpenoids, flavonoids, alkaloids, quinines, quercetin, and kaempferol were known to have antimalarial activity [33–36]. Moreover, polyphenol and flavonoids in these extracts which have antioxidant activity may also contribute to the antimalarial activity [37]. It has been described that antioxidant activity can inhibit hemozoin formation, and free heme is very toxic for the malaria parasite [38]. These active compounds which are found in the extracts may be acting singly or in synergy with other compounds to exert the antimalarial activity. In addition, quercetin, kaempferol, and gypenoside were found evidently on the ring stage of the parasite [39]. The mode of action corresponds with the nucleic acid and protein synthesis. Furthermore, anti-inflammation of quercetin, kaempferol, and gypenoside includes the nuclear transcription factor-kappa B (NF-κB) inhibition, making therapeutic target for cancer treatment. The role of NF-κB is also important in malaria growth and

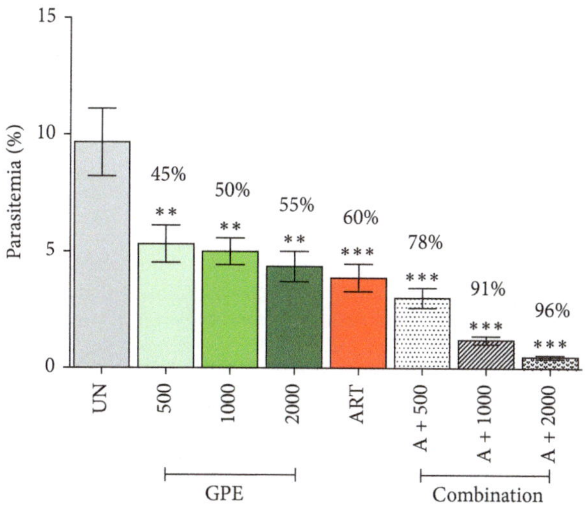

FIGURE 1: Antimalarial activity of *Gynostemma pentaphyllum*. Groups of naïve ICR mice (5 mice each) were infected intraperitoneally with 1×10^7 parasitized erythrocytes of PbANKA. They were then given orally the extract (500, 1,000, and 2,000 mg/kg) either alone or in combination with artesunate (6 mg/kg) for 4 consecutive days. Untreated and artesunate treated mice were used as negative and positive controls, respectively. Parasitemia and suppression percentage were subsequently measured. $^{**}P < 0.01$, and $^{***}P < 0.001$, compared to untreated control. UN: untreated control; GPE: *G. pentaphyllum* extract; ART: 6 mg/kg of artesunate; A + 500: combination of 6 mg/kg of artesunate and 500 mg/kg of GPE; A + 1000: combination of 6 mg/kg of artesunate and 1000 mg/kg of GPE; A + 2000: combination of 6 mg/kg of artesunate and 2000 mg/kg of GPE. The results came from 3 independent experiments.

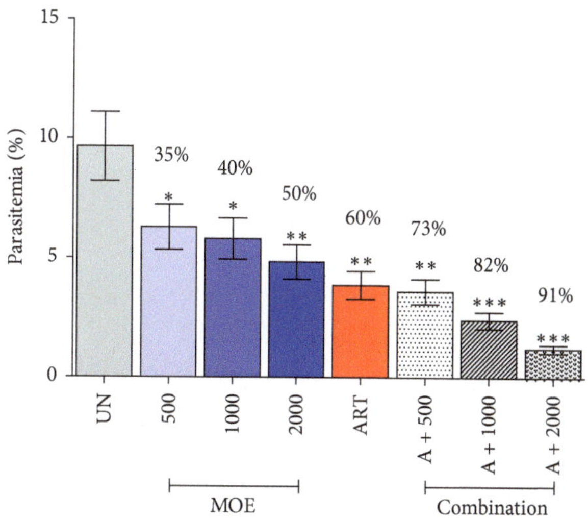

FIGURE 2: Antimalarial activity of *Moringa oleifera*. Groups of naïve ICR mice (5 mice each) were infected intraperitoneally with 1×10^7 parasitized erythrocytes of PbANKA. They were then given orally the extract (500, 1,000, and 2,000 mg/kg) either alone or in combination with artesunate (6 mg/kg) for 4 consecutive days. Untreated and artesunate treated mice were used as negative and positive controls, respectively. Parasitemia and suppression percentage were subsequently measured. $^{*}P < 0.05$, $^{**}P < 0.01$, and $^{***}P < 0.001$, compared to untreated control. UN: untreated control; MOE: *M. oleifera* extract; ART: 6 mg/kg of artesunate; A + 500: combination of 6 mg/kg of artesunate and 500 mg/kg of MOE; A + 1000: combination of 6 mg/kg of artesunate and 1000 mg/kg of MOE; A + 2000: combination of 6 mg/kg of artesunate and 2000 mg/kg of MOE. The results came from 3 independent experiments.

development [40]. The deciphering of antimalarial property in these extracts lays the foundation for the need to reevaluate their possible role in this transcription factor regulation for malarial control.

There are several reports on antimalarial drug combination showing their *in vitro* and *in vivo* on malaria parasites [41–45]. The aqueous crude extracts of *G. pentaphyllum* and *M. oleifera* leaves exhibited high level of antimalarial activity in *P. berghei*-infected mice when administered with artesunate. The significant decrease in parasitemia levels in response to combination treatment compared to the control, observed with the mice, was the main finding in this study. Hence, the addictive effect of these extracts with artesunate is important in the context that offers opportunities to further standardize new artemisinin-based combination therapy as possible antimalarial combination [46].

The aqueous crude extracts of *G. pentaphyllum* and *M. oleifera* leaves were well tolerated by the mice up to the dose level of 4,000 mg/kg within 24 h and up to 30 days. In acute toxicity, doses higher than 5,000 mg/kg are generally not considered as dose related, which is in accordance with the Organization for Economic Corporation and Development (OECD) Guidance Document for Acute Oral Toxicity Testing [47]. The oral median dose of these extracts were estimated to be greater than 4,000 mg/kg which was 8 times greater than the minimum effective dose of 500 mg/kg. Previous reports have shown that the median lethal dose of a test compound is 3 times more than the minimum effective dose. This compound is considered a good candidate for future studies [48]. Therefore, these aqueous crude extracts can be considered as nontoxic at acute oral administration, and the mice were safe with the different doses of these extracts administered to them.

5. Conclusions

This study has shown that aqueous crude extracts of *G. pentaphyllum* and *M. oleifera* leaves exhibited a significant antimalarial activity. Moreover, these extracts were safe at the highest tested dose of 4,000 mg/kg. Additionally, artesunate enhanced the antimalarial activity of these extracts. Hence, *G. pentaphyllum* and *M. oleifera* leaf extracts and their combination with artesunate show strong promise for development as antimalarial combination therapy.

Appendix

See Figures 1 and 2.

Competing Interests

The authors have declared that no competing interests exist.

Acknowledgments

The authors are grateful to Dr. Chairat Uthaipibull and Associate Professor Dr. Somdet Srichairatanakool for their excellent suggestion. They thankfully acknowledge the contribution of National Center for Genetic Engineering and Biotechnology (BIOTEC), particularly for the parasite strain. Moreover, They also thank the students who helped and offered support in animal experiments.

References

[1] N. J. White, S. Pukrittayakamee, T. T. Hien, M. A. Faiz, O. A. Mokuolu, and A. M. Dondorp, "Malaria," *The Lancet*, vol. 383, no. 9918, pp. 723–735, 2014.

[2] H. A. Antony and S. C. Parija, "Antimalarial drug resistance: an overview," *Tropical Parasitology*, vol. 6, no. 1, pp. 30–41, 2016.

[3] D. Sinclair, B. Zani, S. Donegan, P. Olliaro, and P. Garner, "Artemisinin-based combination therapy for treating uncomplicated malaria," *The Cochrane Database of Systematic Reviews*, no. 3, Article ID CD007483, 2009.

[4] J. R. D. A. Silva, A. D. S. Ramos, M. Machado et al., "A review of antimalarial plants used in traditional medicine in communities in Portuguese-Speaking countries: Brazil, Mozambique, Cape Verde, Guinea-Bissau, São Tomé and Príncipe and Angola," *Memorias do Instituto Oswaldo Cruz*, vol. 106, supplement 1, pp. 142–158, 2011.

[5] D. J. Sullivan Jr., N. Kaludov, and M. N. Martinov, "Discovery of potent, novel, non-toxic anti-malarial compounds via quantum modelling, virtual screening and *in vitro* experimental validation," *Malaria Journal*, vol. 10, article 274, 2011.

[6] T. J. Schmidt, S. A. Khalid, A. J. Romanha et al., "The potential of secondary metabolites from plants as drugs or leads against protozoan neglected diseases—part I," *Current Medicinal Chemistry*, vol. 19, no. 14, pp. 2128–2175, 2012.

[7] A. Thiengsusuk, W. Chaijaroenkul, and K. Na-Bangchang, "Antimalarial activities of medicinal plants and herbal formulations used in Thai traditional medicine," *Parasitology Research*, vol. 112, no. 4, pp. 1475–1481, 2013.

[8] A. Ramazani, S. Zakeri, S. Sardari, N. Khodakarim, and N. D. Djadid, "*In vitro* and *in vivo* anti-malarial activity of *Boerhavia elegans* and *Solanum surattense*," *Malaria Journal*, vol. 9, article 124, 2010.

[9] G. Verma, V. K. Dua, D. D. Agarwal, and P. K. Atul, "Anti-malarial activity of *Holarrhena antidysenterica* and *Viola canescens*, plants traditionally used against malaria in the Garhwal region of north-west Himalaya," *Malaria Journal*, vol. 10, article 20, 2011.

[10] Y. H. Liu, Y. F. Liu, and X. X. Guo, "Current studies on anti-endotoxic chemical components of traditional Chinese medicine in China," *Acta Pharmacologica Sinica*, vol. 22, no. 12, pp. 1071–1077, 2001.

[11] A. F. Abdull Razis, M. D. Ibrahim, and S. B. Kntayya, "Health benefits of *Moringa oleifera*," *Asian Pacific Journal of Cancer Prevention*, vol. 15, no. 20, pp. 8571–8576, 2014.

[12] S. J. Stohs and M. J. Hartman, "Review of the safety and efficacy of *Moringa oleifera*," *Phytotherapy Research*, vol. 29, no. 6, pp. 796–804, 2015.

[13] Y. Li, J. Huang, W. Lin et al., "*In vitro* anticancer activity of a nonpolar fraction from *Gynostemma pentaphyllum* (Thunb.) Makino," *Evidence-Based Complementary and Alternative Medicine*, vol. 2016, Article ID 6308649, 11 pages, 2016.

[14] D. Gao, M. Zhao, X. Qi et al., "Hypoglycemic effect of *Gynostemma pentaphyllum* saponins by enhancing the Nrf2 signaling pathway in STZ-inducing diabetic rats," *Archives of Pharmacal Research*, vol. 39, no. 2, pp. 221–230, 2016.

[15] S. H. Park, T. L. Huh, S. Y. Kim et al., "Antiobesity effect of *Gynostemma pentaphyllum* extract (actiponin): a randomized, double-blind, placebo-controlled trial," *Obesity*, vol. 22, no. 1, pp. 63–71, 2014.

[16] D. Srichana, R. Taengtip, and S. Kondo, "Antimicrobial activity of *Gynostemma pentaphyllum* extracts against fungi producing aflatoxin and fumonisin and bacteria causing diarrheal disease," *The Southeast Asian Journal of Tropical Medicine and Public Health*, vol. 42, no. 3, pp. 704–710, 2011.

[17] S. Ranasinghe, R. Ansumana, J. M. Lamin et al., "Herbs and herbal combinations used to treat suspected malaria in Bo, Sierra Leone," *Journal of Ethnopharmacology*, vol. 166, pp. 200–204, 2015.

[18] O. O. Abiodun, N. Gbimadee, and G. O. Gbotosho, "Lopinavir/ritonavir enhanced the antimalarial activity of amodiaquine and artesunate in a mouse model of *Plasmodium berghei*," *Journal of Chemotherapy*, pp. 1–5, 2016.

[19] C. Rodriguez-Perez, B. Gilbert-Lopez, J. A. Mendiola, R. Quirantes-Pine, A. Segura-Carretero, and E. Ibanez, "Optimization of microwave-assisted extraction and pressurized liquid extraction of phenolic compounds from *Moringa oleifera* leaves by multiresponse surface methodology," *Electrophoresis*, vol. 37, pp. 1938–1946, 2016.

[20] D. Lorke, "A new approach to practical acute toxicity testing," *Archives of Toxicology*, vol. 54, no. 4, pp. 275–287, 1983.

[21] W. Peters, "The chemotherapy of rodent malaria, XXII. The value of drug-resistant strains of *Plasmodium berghei* in screening for blood schizontocidal activity," *Annals of Tropical Medicine and Parasitology*, vol. 69, no. 2, pp. 155–171, 1975.

[22] V. Somsak, N. Polwiang, and S. Chachiyo, "*In vivo* antimalarial activity of *Annona muricata* leaf extract in mice infected with *Plasmodium berghei*," *Journal of Pathogens*, vol. 2016, Article ID 3264070, 5 pages, 2016.

[23] N. Nutham, S. Sakulmettatham, S. Klongthalay, P. Chutoam, and V. Somsak, "Protective effects of *Tinospora crispa* stem extract on renal damage and hemolysis during *Plasmodium berghei* infection in mice," *Journal of Pathogens*, vol. 2015, Article ID 738608, 5 pages, 2015.

[24] V. Somsak, S. Chachiyo, U. Jaihan, and S. Nakinchat, "Protective effect of aqueous crude extract of neem (*Azadirachta indica*) leaves on *Plasmodium berghei*-induced renal damage in mice," *Journal of Tropical Medicine*, vol. 2015, Article ID 961205, 5 pages, 2015.

[25] S. Audomkasok, W. Singpha, S. Chachiyo, and V. Somsak, "Antihemolytic activities of green tea, safflower, and mulberry extracts during *Plasmodium berghei* infection in mice," *Journal of Pathogens*, vol. 2014, Article ID 203154, 4 pages, 2014.

[26] W. Khobjai, U. Jaihan, W. Watcharasamphankul, and V. Somsak, "Protective effect of *Thunbergia laurifolia* extract on hemolysis during *Plasmodium berghei* infection," *Parasitology Research*, vol. 113, no. 5, pp. 1843–1846, 2014.

[27] V. Somsak, U. Jaihan, S. Srichairatanakool, and C. Uthaipibull, "Protection of renal function by green tea extract during *Plasmodium berghei* infection," *Parasitology International*, vol. 62, no. 6, pp. 548–551, 2013.

[28] P. J. Waako, B. Gumede, P. Smith, and P. I. Folb, "The *in vitro* and *in vivo* antimalarial activity of *Cardiospermum halicacabum*

L. and *Momordica foetida* Schumch. Et Thonn," *Journal of Ethnopharmacology*, vol. 99, no. 1, pp. 137–143, 2005.

[29] C. Pierrot, E. Adam, S. Lafitte et al., "Age-related susceptibility and resistance to *Plasmodium berghei* in mice and rats," *Experimental Parasitology*, vol. 104, no. 1-2, pp. 81–85, 2003.

[30] J. Karbwang and T. Harinasuta, "Overview: clinical pharmacology of antimalarials," *The Southeast Asian Journal of Tropical Medicine and Public Health*, vol. 23, supplement 4, pp. 95–109, 1992.

[31] P. T. Ky, P. T. Huong, T. K. My et al., "Dammarane-type saponins from *Gynostemma pentaphyllum*," *Phytochemistry*, vol. 71, no. 8-9, pp. 994–1001, 2010.

[32] G. Karthivashan, M. Tangestani Fard, P. Arulselvan, F. Abas, and S. Fakurazi, "Identification of bioactive candidate compounds responsible for oxidative challenge from hydro-ethanolic extract of *Moringa oleifera* leaves," *Journal of Food Science*, vol. 78, no. 9, pp. C1368–C1375, 2013.

[33] T. Murata, T. Miyase, F. W. Muregi et al., "Antiplasmodial triterpenoids from *Ekebergia capensis*," *Journal of Natural Products*, vol. 71, no. 2, pp. 167–174, 2008.

[34] A. Yenesew, H. M. Akala, H. Twinomuhwezi et al., "The antiplasmodial and radical scavenging activities of flavonoids of *Erythrina burttii*," *Acta Tropica*, vol. 123, no. 2, pp. 123–127, 2012.

[35] I. C. Ezenyi, O. A. Salawu, R. Kulkarni, and M. Emeje, "Antiplasmodial activity-aided isolation and identification of quercetin-4'-methyl ether in *Chromolaena odorata* leaf fraction with high activity against chloroquine-resistant *Plasmodium falciparum*," *Parasitology Research*, vol. 113, no. 12, pp. 4415–4422, 2014.

[36] M. Barliana, E. Suradji, R. Abdulah et al., "Antiplasmodial properties of kaempferol-3-O-rhamnoside isolated from the leaves of *Schima wallichii* against chloroquine-resistant *Plasmodium falciparum*," *Biomedical Reports*, vol. 2, no. 4, pp. 579–583, 2014.

[37] F. El Babili, J. Bouajila, I. Fouraste, A. Valentin, S. Mauret, and C. Moulis, "Chemical study, antimalarial and antioxidant activities, and cytotoxicity to human breast cancer cells (MCF7) of *Argania spinosa*," *Phytomedicine*, vol. 17, no. 2, pp. 157–160, 2010.

[38] M. Y. Lubbad, S. Al-Quraishy, and M. A. Dkhil, "Antimalarial and antioxidant activities of *Indigofera oblongifolia* on *Plasmodium chabaudi*-induced spleen tissue injury in mice," *Parasitology Research*, vol. 114, no. 9, pp. 3431–3438, 2015.

[39] K. Mishra, A. P. Dash, B. K. Swain, and N. Dey, "Anti-malarial activities of *Andrographis paniculata* and *Hedyotis corymbosa* extracts and their combination with curcumin," *Malaria Journal*, vol. 8, article 26, 2009.

[40] M. A. Hidalgo, A. Romero, J. Figueroa et al., "Andrographolide interferes with binding of nuclear factor-κB to DNA in HL-60-derived neutrophilic cells," *British Journal of Pharmacology*, vol. 144, no. 5, pp. 680–686, 2005.

[41] A. O. Adepiti and E. O. Iwalewa, "Evaluation of the combination of *Uvaria chamae* (P. Beauv.) and amodiaquine in murine malaria," *Journal of Ethnopharmacology*, vol. 193, pp. 30–35, 2016.

[42] A. O. Adepiti, A. A. Elujoba, and O. O. Bolaji, "Evaluation of herbal antimalarial MAMA decoction-amodiaquine combination in murine malaria model," *Pharmaceutical Biology*, vol. 54, no. 10, pp. 2298–2303, 2016.

[43] R. Sahu, L. A. Walker, and B. L. Tekwani, "*In vitro* and *in vivo* anti-malarial activity of tigecycline, a glycylcycline antibiotic, in combination with chloroquine," *Malaria Journal*, vol. 13, article 414, 2014.

[44] C. Desgrouas, J. Dormoi, C. Chapus, E. Ollivier, D. Parzy, and N. Taudon, "*In vitro* and *in vivo* combination of cepharanthine with anti-malarial drugs," *Malaria Journal*, vol. 13, no. 1, article 90, 2014.

[45] O. L. Anagu, A. A. Attama, V. C. Okore, H. T. Gugu, A. A. Ngene, and C. O. Esimone, "*Azadirachta indica* extract-artesunic acid combination produces an increased cure rate of *Plasmodium berghei*-infected mice," *Pharmaceutical Biology*, vol. 52, no. 7, pp. 883–889, 2014.

[46] J. Pousibet-Puerto, J. Salas-Coronas, A. Sánchez-Crespo et al., "Impact of using artemisinin-based combination therapy (ACT) in the treatment of uncomplicated malaria from *Plasmodium falciparum* in a non-endemic zone," *Malaria Journal*, vol. 15, article 339, 2016.

[47] A. Hayes, *Guidelines for Acute Oral Toxicity Testing*, Raven Press, New York, NY, USA, 2nd edition, 1987.

[48] E. Schleyer, S. Kuhn, H. Ruhrs et al., "Oral idarubicin pharmacokinetics-correlation of trough level with idarubicin area under curve," *Leukemia*, supplement 5, no. 11, pp. S15–S21, 1997.

24

Neonatal Tetanus Immunity in Nigeria: The Effect of HIV Infection on Serum Levels and Transplacental Transfer of Antibodies

Muhammad Faruk Bashir,[1] Hassan Abdullahi Elechi,[2] Mohammed Garba Ashir,[2] Adamu Ibrahim Rabasa,[2] David Nadeba Bukbuk,[3] Ahmadu Baba Usman,[4] Modu Gofama Mustapha,[2] and Mohammad Arab Alhaji[2]

[1] *Department of Paediatrics, Abubakar Tafawa Balewa University Teaching Hospital, Bauchi 740222, Nigeria*
[2] *Department of Paediatrics, University of Maiduguri, Maiduguri 600243, Nigeria*
[3] *Department of Microbiology, University of Maiduguri, Maiduguri 600243, Nigeria*
[4] *Department of Paediatrics, Federal Medical Centre Yola, Yola 640101, Nigeria*

Correspondence should be addressed to Hassan Abdullahi Elechi; h3elechi@unimaid.edu.ng

Academic Editor: Marcel Tanner

Background. Tetanus toxoid immunisation of pregnant mother has remained the most effective strategy in eliminating neonatal tetanus. Impaired production and/or transplacental transfer of antibodies may affect the effectiveness of this strategy. We studied the effect of maternal HIV infection on serum levels and transplacental transfer of anti-tetanus antibodies. *Methods.* A total of 162 mother-baby paired serum samples were taken and analysed for anti-tetanus antibody levels using ELISA. Maternal HIV status was also determined by double ELISA technique. Maternal TT vaccination status was also documented. *Results.* Thirty-eight (23.5%) mothers and 41 (25.3%) babies were seronegative, out of whom 8 mothers were HIV positive and 9 babies were HIV exposed. HIV infected mothers and HIV exposed infants were, respectively, 16.27 times (OR = 16.27, 95% CI = 3.28 to 80.61) and 33.75 times (OR = 33.75, 95% CI = 4.12 to 276.40) more likely to be seronegative for anti-tetanus antibody. Similarly, HIV positive mother-newborn pairs were 7.46 times more likely to have a poor transplacental transfer of tetanus antibodies (OR = 7.46, 95% CI = 1.96 to 28.41). *Conclusions.* Maternal HIV infection is associated with impaired maternofoetal transfer of anti-tetanus antibodies and seronegativity among mothers and their newborns. Hence, this may hinder efforts to eliminate neonatal tetanus.

1. Introduction

In developing countries, Human Immunodeficiency Virus (HIV) infection and neonatal tetanus (NT) are among the leading causes of childhood morbidity and mortality. Understanding the interaction between HIV and NT is important since it may have a major implication for NT elimination program. Newborns are protected from NT by maternal anti-tetanus antibody (MTA) of the IgG class which is actively transferred across the placental barrier from third trimester of gestation following tetanus toxoid (TT) vaccination in pregnant women. Strengthening of immunisation for pregnant women with TT vaccine is reported to be the single most effective strategy independent of other interventions in eliminating neonatal tetanus [1]. Its efficacy and effectiveness has been convincingly demonstrated in many field trials and in hospital-based studies [2–6].

However, there are conflicting reports of the influence of maternal HIV infection on anti-tetanus antibody production by the mothers as well as its transfer through the placenta to their unborn babies. Whereas lower anti-tetanus antibody levels in HIV infected women were reported from Senegal [7], Brazil [8], and The Gambia [9], no such relationship was found in Malawi [10]. Similarly, Cumberland et al. [11] in Kenya reported a decrease in cord-maternal ratio (CMR) with 50% reduction in cord blood tetanus antibody concentration in babies born by HIV infected mothers. Similar conclusions were arrived at by Bonetti et al. [8] in Brazil. To the best of our knowledge, no such study was carried out in Nigeria which happens to be one of the 46 remaining countries yet to eliminate neonatal tetanus as at 2008 and among the 24 countries responsible for 90% of the global burden of the disease [12]. Moreover, Chama et al. in 2010 reported a high prevalence of HIV infection of 12.7% among women attending antenatal clinic of the University of Maiduguri Teaching Hospital (UMTH), Maiduguri, northeastern Nigeria, where this study was carried out. We thus aim to assess the effect of maternal HIV infection on the serum levels of anti-tetanus antibodies in mother-infant pairs and hence transplacental transfer of antibody.

2. Materials and Method

2.1. Study Area. The study was carried out at the Labour Ward of the UMTH, Nigeria. The UMTH is a tertiary-based care centre located in northeastern Nigeria and a centre of excellence for infectious diseases and immunology. It also serves as a referral site for the six northeastern states of Nigeria and the neighboring countries of Chad, Cameroon, and Niger.

2.2. Design. The study was a hospital-based descriptive and cross-sectional study of mother-newborn pairs recruited from the Labour Ward of the UMTH.

2.3. Ethical Consideration. The study protocol was reviewed and approved by the Medical Research and Ethics Committee of UMTH. Informed consent of the delivering other was also obtained. Participants had unlimited liberty to deny consent without any consequences and confidentiality was maintained.

2.4. Sample Size. The minimum sample size was determined using Cochran's sample size formula for categorical data [13] at alpha level of 0.05 and power of 95%. Proportion of newborns with protective level of tetanus IgG antibody (seropositives), value of p, was taken from a previous study in Jos by Adabara et al. [14] to be 88%. Therefore, the sample size for the study was one hundred and sixty-two mother-newborn pairs.

2.5. Data Collection. Mother-newborn pairs were enrolled in this study using the systematic random sampling method, in which the first of every three mother-newborn pairs was picked at the Labour Ward from the first day of data collection after fulfilling the eligibility criteria. Exclusion criteria were failure to give consent (0.05%), stillbirth and history of antitetanus serum (ATS), or blood transfusion during pregnancy. Mothers with diabetes mellitus, hypertension, eclampsia, or preeclampsia were also excluded. Upon enrolment, a questionnaire detailing sociodemographic variables was completed for each mother-newborn pair. This included biodata, pregnancy history and antenatal history, and gestational age as well as indicators of socioeconomic status like occupation and educational levels of both parents. History of TT vaccination during current pregnancy, verifiable from the patients' antenatal clinic records, where possible, was obtained, including how many doses and their interval as well as TT received before the index pregnancy (both during and outside pregnancy). Gestational age (GA) at delivery was determined by date using the last menstrual period or by first-trimester ultrasound scan, where available. Dubowitz Score was used to access the GA of the newborn infants at birth [15], and their birth weight (BW) was measured using a digital weighing scale that has a sensitivity of 0.01 kg. Newborn infants with GA less than 37 completed weeks were classified as preterm, those from 37 completed to less than 42 completed weeks were term, and those with 42 completed weeks or more were postterm [15]. Newborns weighing >3.99 kilograms were classified as macrosomia, those weighing 2.5–3.99 kilograms were classified as normal, and those <2.5 kilograms were termed low BW [15]. Socioeconomic status was assigned using Oyedeji's model [16].

2.6. Sample Collection and Processing. Maternal venous blood (2 mL) was collected from a peripheral vein following aseptic procedure. Two millilitres of cord blood from the placental end of the cord, after early clamping of the cord, was also collected and stored in a properly labelled sterile plain bottle. Sera were separated after centrifuging these blood samples at 5000 rpm for five minutes. Aliquots of serum samples were stored at −20°C until analysis. All mother-newborn pairs sera were assayed for tetanus IgG antibodies by Enzyme Linked Immunosorbent Assay (ELISA) technique [17]. The optical density at 450 nm (OD_{450}) was measured in an ELISA microplate reader. Standard curves were drawn for each plate and optical densities of the test serum dilutions falling within the linear part of the curve were extrapolated. The results were expressed as IU per millilitre. World Health Organization (WHO) guidelines proposed a cut-off of 0.1–0.2 IU/mL for a protective antibody concentration [18]. For this study, antibody level of 0.1 IU/mL was used as the cut-off, below which individuals were classified as being seronegative.

Maternal HIV status was defined by presence of serum HIV antibodies determined by two different ELISA tests, as recommended by WHO [19]. Any two of Determine, Stat-pack, or Unigold were used.

2.7. Data Analysis. Data obtained were entered into a computer that generated a computerized data base. Analysis was done using SPSS version 16.0 (SPSS, Chicago, Illinois, USA). Tables were used for data presentation as appropriate. Geometric means ± standard deviations of tetanus antibody titres were determined. Frequencies of tetanus antibody serostatus (seropositives and seronegatives) were compared using Fisher exact test. A p value of <0.05 was considered significant.

3. Results

A total of 162 mother-newborn pairs were enrolled into this study. The mean ± standard deviation (SD) age of the mothers

Table 1: Sociodemographic and obstetric characteristics of the mothers studied.

Characteristic	Frequency (N = 162)	Percent
Age (years)		
14–19	14	8.6
20–24	38	23.5
25–29	54	33.3
≥30	56	34.6
Mean (SD)	27.2 (6.0)	
Parity		
Primipara	41	25.3
Multipara	121	74.7
Socioeconomic status		
High	14	8.6
Middle	16	9.9
Low	132	81.5
TT vaccination status		
None	12	7.4
1	12	7.4
≥2	138	85.2
HIV status		
Positive	10	6.2
Negative	152	93.8

SD = standard deviation; TT = tetanus toxoid.

was 27.2 ± 6.0 years. Most of them were multipara (121 [74.7%]) and belonged to the low socioeconomic class (132 [81.5%]). One hundred and thirty-eight (85.2%) mothers had at least 2 tetanus toxoid (TT) vaccinations during the current pregnancy. Ten (6.2%) mothers were HIV infected and were on antiretroviral treatment (Table 1). Nine (90%) of the HIV positive mothers had at least 2 doses of TT vaccination; the remaining woman had only a single dose. There was no significant variation in doses of TT vaccination between the HIV positive and HIV negative mothers (p = 1.000).

Among the 162 babies enrolled in the study, 84 (51.9%) were males and 78 (48.1%) were females with a male to female ratio (M : F) of1.08 : 1. Most of them, 149 (92%), were term and the remaining 13 (8%) were preterm. None of the babies was postterm. Low birth weight was observed in 9 (5.6%) babies while the remaining 153 (94.4%) were of normal birth weight.

One hundred and twenty-four mothers (76.5%) and 121 (74.4%) babies were seropositive for tetanus antibodies (titre of ≥0.1 IU/mL). The remaining were seronegative (titre <0.1 IU/mL), out of whom 8 of the mothers were HIV positive and 9 of the babies were delivered by HIV positive mothers. The mean (SD) tetanus antibody titres of the studied mothers and their babies were 0.160 (0.122) and 0.230 (0.170) IU/mL, respectively. There was a significant strong positive correlation between maternal and cord blood levels of tetanus antibodies (r = +0.668, r^2 = 0.445, $p < 0.001$) with a shared variance of 44.6% (Figure 1).

One hundred and six pairs (65.4%) had cord-maternal ratios (CMR) of ≥1 with a mean (SD) of 1.499 (0.729), while the remaining 56 (34.6%) had ratios of <1 with a mean (SD) of 0.553 (0.232). The overall mean (SD) of the cord-maternal ratios was 1.062 (0.767). There was a significant but weak negative correlation between maternal tetanus antibody levels and cord-maternal ratios (r = −0.158, p = 0.045) with a shared variance of only 2% (Figure 2).

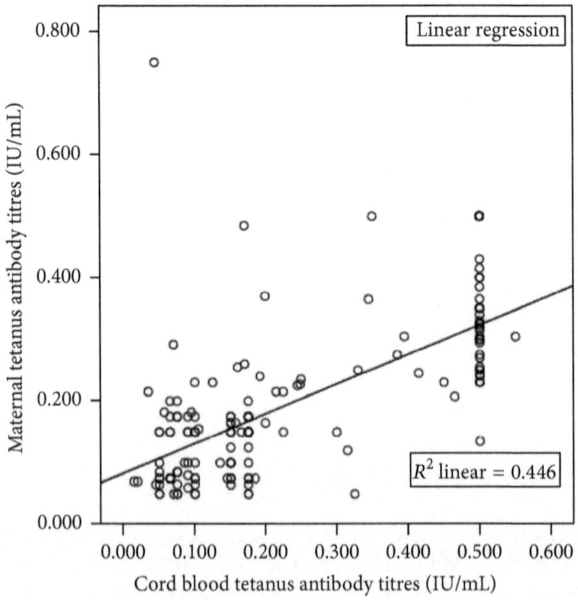

Figure 1: Pearson correlation between maternal and cord blood anti-tetanus antibody titres.

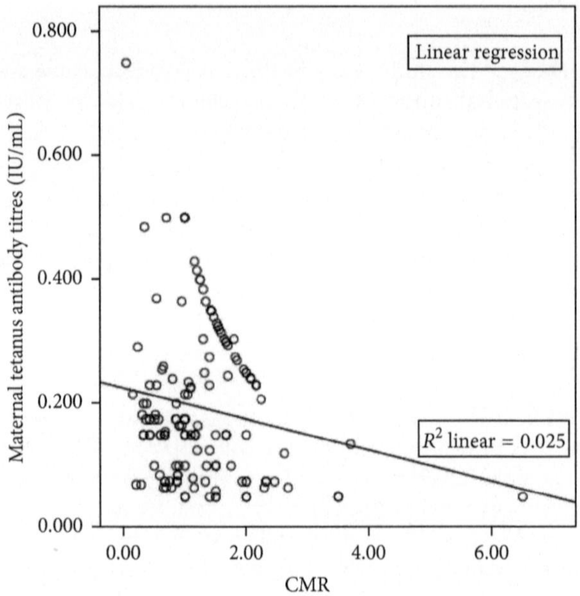

Figure 2: Pearson correlation between maternal anti-tetanus antibody titres and cord-maternal ratios (CMR).

On the effects of the various maternal and neonatal factors on the anti-tetanus antibody serostatus and CMR, only maternal TT vaccination and HIV status showed statistically significant association with maternal anti-tetanus antibody serostatus ($p \leq 0.001$) for both. Similarly, HIV exposure and gestational age at birth were the only factors

TABLE 2: Logistic regression analysis results exploring the predictive significance of maternal factors on maternal tetanus antibody serostatus.

Independent variables	Wald test	df	p value
Maternal age	0.876	3	0.831
SES	1.095	2	0.579
Parity	0.067	1	0.795
TT vaccination status	10.161	2	0.006[x]
HIV status	9.581	1	0.002[x]
Placental malaria	0.770	1	0.380
Constant	4.110	1	0.043

SES = socioeconomic status; df = degree of freedom; [x]significant relationship.

TABLE 3: Logistic regression analysis results exploring the predictive significance of some maternal and infant factors on cord-blood tetanus antibody serostatus.

Independent variables	Wald test	df	p value
Maternal age	2.050	3	0.562
SES	3.052	2	0.217
Parity	0.386	1	0.534
TT vaccination status	0.141	2	0.932
HIV status	10.950	1	0.001
Placental malaria	1.312	1	0.252
Birth weight	0.063	1	0.802
Gestational age	7.859	1	0.005
Gender	0.545	1	0.460
Constant	0.165	1	0.685

SES = socioeconomic status; df = degree of freedom; p significant at <0.05.

with statistically significant association with cord anti-tetanus antibody serostatus ($p \leq 0.001$ and 0.004), respectively. In both cases, these factors were still found to have a significant predictive value even after controlling for all the other variables using logistic regression analysis (Tables 2 and 3) for maternal serostatus and cord serostatus, respectively. Maternal HIV infection and neonatal gestational age at birth were the only factors with statistically significant association with CMR ($p = 0.001$ and 0.033) for maternal HIV and gestational age, respectively.

HIV infected mothers were 16.27 times more likely to have seronegative levels of tetanus antibody than HIV negative mothers. Similarly, HIV exposed babies were 33.75 times more likely to have seronegative cord blood than those delivered by HIV negative mothers. Again, HIV positive mother-newborn pairs were 4.91 times more likely to have a poorly efficient transplacental transfer of tetanus antibodies with CMR of <1.0 compared to HIV negative pairs (Table 4).

4. Discussion

The observed HIV prevalence of 6.2% among the mothers in this study is quite above the national average of 3.7% [20] This higher prevalence may be due to several factors. The UMTH antenatal clinic serves as a referral centre for HIV positive pregnant women from lower cadre health facilities for the purpose of enrolment into the PMTCT program. This will undoubtedly lead to concentration of HIV positive pregnant women in this hospital and hence the observed higher prevalence. Secondly, the child bearing age also corresponds to the age of maximal sexual activity and has been found to have the highest incidence of HIV infection [21]. This prevalence is, however, about half of 12.7% reported by Chama et al. [22] in 2010 among women attending antenatal clinic from the same hospital where this study was carried out. The lower prevalence observed in this study, compared to the one by Chama et al. [22] 4 years earlier, could be a reflection of the general decline in HIV prevalence being experienced in the country [23]. Secondly, while the study by Chama et al. considered all women attending ANC in UMTH over a 2-year period, this study enrolled 1 of every 3 women that delivered in UMTH over a period of 6 months until the required sample size was attained. Therefore, the difference in sampling technique might be a contributing factor.

The observed overall protective levels of tetanus antibodies (mean ≥0.1 IU/mL) for both mothers and infants are similar to the report of Cumberland et al. [11] in Kenya in 2007. They found that the geometric mean titres of both the mothers and their babies were within the protective range. Similarly, Hood et al. [24] found the geometric mean concentration of tetanus antibodies in Nigerian mothers and their infants to be within the protective range. The high proportion of tetanus antibody seropositivity among both the mothers and their babies in this study is similar to the findings in earlier studies from Kenya [11], Jos [14], and Ibadan [24]. Adabara et al. [14] at the Jos University Teaching Hospital, Nigeria, in 2010 also reported a highly significant positive correlation between the maternal tetanus antibody levels and those of the babies similar to our finding. These findings, however, are probably overestimates of the mean tetanus antibody titre and proportion of seropositivity in the general population, because women who deliver in hospital are more likely to have received TT vaccination than women who deliver at home [25], hence further underscoring the import of TT vaccination in attainment of anti-tetanus antibody seropositivity.

The mean cord-maternal ratio found in this study was higher than most previous studies reported from Kenya [11]; Ibadan, Nigeria [24]; Libreville, Gabon [26], as well as Thailand [27] and India [28]. While it was found to be >1.0 in this study signifying efficient placental transfer, the others reported <1.0, pointing to the earlier held view of poor placental transfer of tetanus antibodies in African mothers. However, besides the small sample size in the Ibadan study, most of the studies used *in vitro* technique to determine tetanus antibody levels which measures both IgG and IgM antibodies resulting in misleadingly high maternal titres and therefore low cord-maternal ratios, compared with standard ELISA (*in-vivo*) used in this study which measures only IgG.

The effect of maternal HIV infection on maternal serum and cord tetanus antibody levels as well as transplacental transfer of this antibody in this study is consistent with the findings of lower tetanus antibody levels in HIV infected women in Senegal [7], Brazil [8], and The Gambia [9]. It is also in agreement with data from Kenya, in the largest

TABLE 4: The effect of HIV infection on maternal and newborn anti-tetanus antibody status and cord-maternal ratio (CMR).

HIV status	Anti-tetanus antibody status		OR	CI	p value
	Seronegative (<0.1)	Seropositive (≥0.1)			
Mothers					
HIV positive	8	2	16.27	3.28–80.61	<0.001*
HIV negative	30	122			
Total	**38**	**124**			
Newborns					
HIV exposed	9	1	33.75	4.12–276.4	<0.001*
Not exposed	32	120			
Total	**41**	**121**			
	Cord-maternal ratio				
	Inefficient transfer (<1)	Efficient transfer (≥1)			
Mothers					
HIV positive	7	3	4.91	1.22–19.79	0.033*
HIV negative	49	103			
Total	**56**	**106**			

HIV, human immunodeficiency virus; OR, odds ratio; CI, confidence interval; *Fisher's exact test.

study of the association between maternal HIV infection and tetanus antibody levels by Cumberland et al. [11], where they found lower levels of tetanus antibody among HIV infected women, reduced transplacental transfer of tetanus antibody, and ~50% lower antibody levels in cord serum. In contrast, De Moraes-Pinto et al. from Malawi found that maternal HIV infection had no effect on maternal serum and cord anti-tetanus IgG levels as well as transplacental transfer of this antibody [10]. The reason for this contrasting finding is not clear but may be due to the fact that the authors did not adjust for TT vaccination status which has been demonstrated in this study and others [2–6] to be an important determinant of serum tetanus antibody status.

5. Conclusion

Maternal HIV infection was associated with significantly impaired maternofoetal transfer of tetanus antibody and seronegativity (unprotective) levels in both mother-newborn pairs at birth despite being on antiretroviral therapy for HIV. Hence, this may hinder efforts to eliminate neonatal tetanus. There is need to review and restrategize neonatal tetanus elimination program among this vulnerable population. Such strategies may include passive immunisation in addition to other elements of prevention among high risk groups.

Limitations

The study is hospital based and the studied population were skewed towards certain characteristics such as low socioeconomic class, multiparity, and term babies making generalization of the result difficult.

Conflict of Interests

The authors have no conflict of interests to disclose.

Acknowledgments

The authors would like to appreciate all the staff of Labour Ward, Special Care Baby Unit, and Immunology Laboratory of the University of Maiduguri Teaching Hospital for their immense contributions towards the success of this study.

References

[1] S. D. Gupta and P. M. Keyl, "Effectiveness of prenatal tetanus toxoid immunization against neonatal tetanus in a rural area in India," *Pediatric Infectious Disease Journal*, vol. 17, no. 4, pp. 316–321, 1998.

[2] K. W. Newell, L. A. Duenas, D. R. LeBlanc, and N. Garces Osorio, "The use of tetanus toxoid for the prevention of neonatal tetanus in developing countries for the prevention of tetanus neonatorum," *Bulletin of the World Health Organization*, vol. 35, pp. 863–871, 1966.

[3] R. E. Black, D. H. Huber, and G. T. Curlin, "Reduction of neonatal tetanus by mass immunization of non-pregnant women: duration of protection provided by one or two doses of aluminium-adsorbed tetanus toxoid," *Bulletin of the World Health Organization*, vol. 58, no. 6, pp. 927–930, 1980.

[4] G. G. Berggren, W. Berggren, and A. Verly, "Traditional midwives, tetanus immunization, and infant mortality in rural Haiti," *Tropical Doctor*, vol. 13, no. 2, pp. 79–87, 1983.

[5] J. Cliff, "Neonatal tetanus in Maputo, Mozambique Part II. Preventative measures," *Central African Journal of Medicine*, vol. 31, no. 2, pp. 27–31, 1985.

[6] J. Vandelaer, M. Birmingham, F. Gasse, M. Kurian, C. Shaw, and S. Garnier, "Tetanus in developing countries: an update on the maternal and neonatal tetanus elimination initiative," *Vaccine*, vol. 21, no. 24, pp. 3442–3445, 2003.

[7] T. N. Dieye, P. S. Sow, T. Simonart et al., "Immunologic and virologic response after tetanus toxoid booster among HIV-1 and HIV-2-infected Senegalese individuals," *Vaccine*, vol. 20, no. 5-6, pp. 905–913, 2002.

[8] T. C. S. Bonetti, R. C. M. Succi, L. Y. Weckx, L. Tavares-Lopes, and M. I. De Moraes-Pinto, "Tetanus and diphtheria antibodies and response to a booster dose in Brazilian HIV-1-infected women," *Vaccine*, vol. 22, no. 27-28, pp. 3707–3712, 2004.

[9] B. J. Okoko, L. H. Wesuperuma, M. O. Ota et al., "Influence of placental malaria infection and maternal hypergammaglobulinaemia on materno-fetal transfer of measles and tetanus antibodies in a rural west African population," *Journal of Health, Population, and Nutrition*, vol. 19, no. 2, pp. 59–65, 2001.

[10] M. I. De Moraes-Pinto, F. Verhoeff, L. Chimsuku et al., "Placental antibody transfer: influence of maternal HIV infection and placental malaria," *Archives of Disease in Childhood: Fetal and Neonatal Edition*, vol. 79, no. 3, pp. F202–F205, 1998.

[11] P. Cumberland, C. E. Shulman, P. A. C. Maple et al., "Maternal HIV infection and placental malaria reduce transplacental antibody transfer and tetanus antibody levels in newborns in Kenya," *Journal of Infectious Diseases*, vol. 196, no. 4, pp. 550–557, 2007.

[12] WHO, "Immunisation, surveillance, assessment, and monitoring," Maternal and Neonatal Tetanus (MNT) Elimination: 1–7, 2010.

[13] W. G. Cochran, *Sampling Techniques*, John Wiley & Sons, New York, NY, USA, 3rd edition, 1977.

[14] N. U. Adabara, Y. T. Kandakai-Olukemi, M. N. Enenebeaku, and P. H. Daru, "Assessment of materno-foetal transfer of antitetanus immunoglobulin G in Jos University Teaching Hospital, Jos," *Shiraz E Medical Journal*, vol. 11, no. 2, pp. 1–8, 2010.

[15] B. J. Stoll and I. Adams-Chapman, "The high-risk infant," in *Nelson Textbook of Pediatrics*, R. M. Kliegman, R. E. Behrman, H. B. Jenson, and B. F. Stanton, Eds., p. 97, Saunders, 18th edition, 2007.

[16] G. A. Oyedeji, "Socioeconomic and cultural background of hospitalized children in Ilesha," *Nigerian Journal of Paediatrics*, vol. 12, no. 4, pp. 111–117, 1985.

[17] *Product Information Instruction Manual. Enzyme Immunoassay for the Detection and the Quantitative Determination of Human IGG Antibodies against Tetanus Toxoid in Serum and Plasma*, Demeditec Diagnostics, Kiel, Germany, 2009.

[18] WHO, "Tetanus vaccine: WHO position paper," *The Weekly Epidemiological Record*, vol. 81, pp. 198–208, 2006.

[19] WHO, "Global program on AIDS—recommendations for the selection and use of HIV antibody tests," *Weekly Epidemiological Record*, vol. 20, pp. 145–149, 1992.

[20] Federal Republic of Nigeria, *Global AIDS Response Country Progress Report, Nigeria*, 2012, http://www.avert.org/hiv-aids-nigeria.htm#sthash.vQ1BO9Bk.dpuf.

[21] C. T. Omisakin, A. J. Esan, K. A. Fasakin et al., "Syphilis and Human Immunodeficiency virus co-infection among pregnant women in Nigeria: prevalence and trend," *International STD Research & Reviews*, vol. 2, no. 2, pp. 94–100, 2014.

[22] C. M. Chama, M. Bello, B. A. Ajayi, S. Zarma, and W. Gashau, "The use of highly active antiretroviral therapy for the prevention of mother-to-child transmission of the human immunodeficiency virus in Nigeria," *Journal of Obstetrics and Gynaecology*, vol. 30, no. 4, pp. 362–366, 2010.

[23] NACP, "National HIV prevalence sentinels survey among pregnant women in Nigeria," Tech. Rep., Department of Public Health, NACP, FMOH, 2010.

[24] N. Hood, M. C. K. Chan, S. M. Maxwell, J. B. Familusi, and C. A. Hart, "Placental transfer of tetanus toxoid antibodies in Nigerian mothers," *Annals of Tropical Paediatrics*, vol. 14, no. 3, pp. 179–182, 1994.

[25] F. T. Cutts, L. C. Rodriguez, S. Colombo, and S. Bennett, "Evaluation of factors influencing vaccine uptake in Mozambique," *International Journal of Epidemiology*, vol. 18, no. 2, pp. 427–433, 1989.

[26] J. L. Michaux, J. F. Heremans, and W. H. Hitzig, "Immunoglobulin levels in cord-blood serum of negroes and Caucasians," *Tropical and Geographical Medicine*, vol. 18, no. 1, pp. 10–14, 1966.

[27] V. Sangpetchsong, S. Vichaikummart, A. Vichitnant, and A. Podhipak, "Transfer rate of transplacental immunity to tetanus from non-immunized and immunized mothers," *Southeast Asian Journal of Tropical Medicine and Public Health*, vol. 15, no. 3, pp. 275–280, 1984.

[28] S. Y. Maselle, "Maternal and foetal tetanus toxoid antibody levels following immunization in pregnancy," *Journal of Obstetrics and Gynaecology of Eastern and Central Africa*, vol. 8, pp. 11–14, 1989.

25

Loop-Mediated Isothermal Amplification Test for *Trypanosoma gambiense* Group 1 with Stem Primers: A Molecular Xenomonitoring Test for Sleeping Sickness

Zablon K. Njiru,[1,2] Cecilia K. Mbae,[3] and Gitonga N. Mburugu[1]

[1]*School of Health Sciences, Meru University of Science and Technology, P.O. Box 972-60200, Meru, Kenya*
[2]*School of Health Professions, Murdoch University, Mandurah Campus, Education Drive, Mandurah, WA 6210, Australia*
[3]*Kenya Medical Research Institute, Centre for Microbiology Research, P.O. Box 19464-00202, Nairobi, Kenya*

Correspondence should be addressed to Zablon K. Njiru; z.njiru@murdoch.edu.au

Academic Editor: Sukla Biswas

The World Health Organization has targeted Human African Trypanosomiasis (HAT) for elimination by 2020 with zero incidence by 2030. To achieve and sustain this goal, accurate and easy-to-deploy diagnostic tests for Gambian trypanosomiasis which accounts for over 98% of reported cases will play a crucial role. Most needed will be tools for surveillance of pathogen in vectors (xenomonitoring) since population screening tests are readily available. The development of new tests is expensive and takes a long time while incremental improvement of existing technologies that have potential for xenomonitoring may offer a shorter pathway to tools for HAT surveillance. We have investigated the effect of including a second set of reaction accelerating primers (stem primers) to the standard *T. brucei gambiense* LAMP test format. The new test format was analyzed with and without outer primers. Amplification was carried out using Rotorgene 6000 and the portable ESE Quant amplification unit capable of real-time data output. The stem LAMP formats indicated shorter time to results (~8 min), were 10–100-fold more sensitive, and indicated higher diagnostic sensitivity and accuracy compared to the standard LAMP test. It was possible to confirm the predicted product using ESE melt curves demonstrating the potential of combining LAMP and real-time technologies as possible tool for HAT molecular xenomonitoring.

1. Introduction

The Human African Trypanosomiasis (HAT) is caused by two subspecies of trypanosomes, namely, *Trypanosoma brucei gambiense* which is prevalent in west and central Africa and causes chronic disease and *T. brucei rhodesiense* which occurs in East and southern Africa and causes acute form of disease. The parasites are transmitted through the bite of tsetse flies (*Glossina* spp.). The disease has been earmarked by the World Health Organization (WHO) for elimination by 2020 [1]. The goal being defined as having less than 1 case per 10 000 of the population in 90% of all foci [2] and with zero incidences by 2030 [3]. There is optimism that elimination will be achieved due to the current renewed control activities led by WHO and other partners. Indeed, the number of HAT cases reported had gone down to less than 5000 by 2014. In the 1960s the colonial health systems brought HAT under control but relaxation of the surveillance programmes led to resurgence of the disease [4], a mistake that should not be repeated today. Sustaining elimination and eventual eradication of HAT will require, among others, diagnostic tests that are accurate and easy to apply in endemic areas and that can be mass-produced at low cost to cover many samples since infection rates will go down. Of interest will be xenomonitoring tests that can be used in detection of pathogen in vectors and reservoir host as an alternative to screening populations. This is because compliance to screening may be reduced after HAT elimination. Therefore, monitoring of vectors for human infective trypanosomes will be an important assessment component in HAT elimination/eradication programs. The advantages of xenomonitoring are that the method is noninvasive and efficient in determining the presence of the pathogen in the target area. This approach has proven successful in the control of vector transmitted lymphatic filariasis [5].

The algorithms to diagnose Gambian HAT are often complex due to the unsatisfactory sensitivity and specificity of available tests. The methods include serological, parasitological, and those for staging the disease [6]. Recently, more serological tests with improved sensitivity and specificity have been developed, namely, *T. brucei gambiense*-specific SD Bioline HAT test [7, 8] and HAT sero-k-seT [9, 10], although further improvement is still required. Other recently launched tests include the *T. brucei* specific simple LED fluorescence microscope [11] and nucleic acid detecting RIME loop-mediated isothermal amplification (LAMP) test [12]. In addition, other experimental subgenus *Trypanozoon* LAMP tests have been reported [13–15] as well as more recently a *T. brucei gambiense* LAMP test [16]. It is postulated that the current serological tests will continue to play a dominant role in screening of HAT in population even after elimination while the LED microscopy and RIME LAMP test may have limited application in xenomonitoring for HAT due to their inability to exclude *T. b. brucei*. Therefore, there is need to develop tests that will specifically detect human pathogenic trypanosomes in vectors and in potential hosts.

Molecular characterisation of trypanosomes from Gambian HAT cases shows the vast majority of isolates belong to the genetically homogeneous group, Group 1 *T. brucei gambiense* [17, 18], with Group 2 *T. brucei gambiense* accounting for a smaller percentage [19]. Moreover, the *T. brucei gambiense*-specific glycoprotein (TgsGP) gene [20] was identified to be specific for Group 1 isolates and absent in Group 2 isolates [21]. Overall the percentage of Group 2 infection is so low and considered negligible and so far, only a few isolates exist in the laboratories. It is difficult to get a specific marker for Group 2 since the isolates are heterogeneous and genetically indistinguishable from *T. b. brucei*. PCR tests for *T. brucei gambiense* Group 1 based on TgsGP [22] and a *T. brucei rhodesiense* based on Serum Resistance Associated (SRA) gene [23] exist. These tests have low sensitivity limiting their application in HAT xenomonitoring.

It may be more advantageous in terms of cost and time to improve the existing HAT tests that show potential for xenomonitoring than developing new ones. One such test is the TgsGP *T. brucei gambiense* LAMP test [24]. Unfortunately, TgsGP is a low copy gene implying that even efficient amplification platform such as LAMP will only marginally improve sensitivity. Nevertheless, the specificity of TgsGP marker and the reported salient advantages of LAMP technology as a point of use platform make it desirable to investigate methods that may improve *T. brucei gambiense* LAMP test performance. One way is the inclusion of a second set of reaction accelerating primers called stem primers [25]. The stem primers anneal to the stem section of the sequence and sequentially amplify the target DNA with loop primers which anneal to the loop section of the target sequence [26]. This significantly increases the test product and hence increases the sensitivity. The use of stem primers was shown to improve sensitivity of HIV-LAMP test [25]; however no more follow-up studies have been done. In the present study, we have incorporated stem primers and significantly improved the detection of *T. brucei gambiense* DNA in tsetse fly samples. In addition, it was possible to confirm the predicted product through melt curves acquired in a portable real-time unit. Such integration of new technologies will contribute towards making LAMP technology a realistic surveillance tool for HAT.

2. Materials and Methods

2.1. Ethical Clearance. The samples from Uganda used in this study were collected from 1990 to 2005. The DNA were contributed as part a collaborative study for development of LAMP test for HAT at Murdoch University, Australia, as reported earlier [12]. The institutional Ethical Clearance for collection of human samples had been obtained from the Livestock Health Research Institute (LIRI), Tororo, Uganda, and the Uganda National Council of Science and Technology (UNCST), Kampala, Uganda, which records and regulates all research activities in the country. The use of samples from a HAT patient in Australia was approved by Royal Perth Hospital, Perth, Western Australia, through Dr. Christopher Heath as reported earlier [24]. All the samples were analyzed anonymously.

2.2. Sample Preparations. Two well characterised *T. brucei gambiense* DNA from isolates PT41 and B014 [12] initially isolated in Ivory Coast and Cameroon were used for analytical sensitivity and to spike tsetse fly samples, respectively. Tsetse midguts were prepared as described [27]. Briefly, tsetse fly midguts from nonexposed *G. pallidipes* were pooled in 5, 10, 15, and 20 and the whole dewinged fly into pools of 1, 5, and 10. Approximately ~10 pg (~100 trypanosomes/mL) of DNA from isolate B014 and double distilled water were added to each tube (Table 1). The samples were fully homogenized and divided into two portions. The first portion was processed with commercial DNA extraction kit (Qiagen, Victoria, Australia) and the resulting DNA was divided into aliquots and stored at −20°C. The second portion was mixed with an in-house prepared buffer composed of detergent and salts (0.1 M Tris-HCl, 0.05 M EDTA, and 1% SDS), boiled for 8 minutes, and centrifuged at 14,000 rpm for 4 min. The resulting supernatants were aspirated, divided into aliquots, and stored at −80°C.

2.3. LAMP Primers. The LAMP and stem primers were manually designed based on the TgsGP sequence (Genbank accession number AJ27795) and following the published primer conditions [25, 28]. The primers were designed from the same sequence section as the previously published TgsGP LAMP test [24] (Figure 1). We could not insert the stem primers between the published standard LAMP primers because the stem section could not accommodate them. The primers included the outer forward and backward (F3/B3), forward and backward inner primers (FIP/BIP), loop forward and backward primers (LF/LB), and stem forward and backward primers (SF/SB) (Figure 1). All the primers were checked for specificity using the nucleotide basic local alignment search tool (BLASTn) against human DNA and other human infectious pathogens. The *T. brucei gambiense*

TABLE 1: The analysis of tsetse fly samples using *T. brucei gambiense* standard and stem LAMP test formats.

Source	Number of pools[a]	Template type	LAMP tests					
			Standard LAMP[b]	C_T value[c]	Stem LAMP$_w$	C_T value	Stem LAMP$_{wn}$	C_T value
Midgut	5	DNA	+	26	+	19	+	19
		Supernatant	+	23	+	15	+	15
	10	DNA	−	—	+	21	+	21
		Supernatant	+	25	+	18	+	18
	15	DNA	−	—	−	—	−	—
		Supernatant	−	—	+	24	+	24
	20	DNA	−	—	−	—	−	—
		Supernatant	−	—	−	—	−	—
Whole fly	1	DNA	+	28	+	20	+	20
		Supernatant	+	26	+	19	+	20
	5	DNA	−	—	−	—	−	—
		Supernatant	−	—	+	—	+	23
	10	DNA	−	—	−	—	−	—
		Supernatant	−	—	−	—	+	28[†]

[a]Insectary *G. pallidipes* (midguts or whole fly).
[b]Published TgsGP LAMP test [24].
[c]Cycle threshold (minutes).
[†]2 out of 6 replicates showed the predicted product.

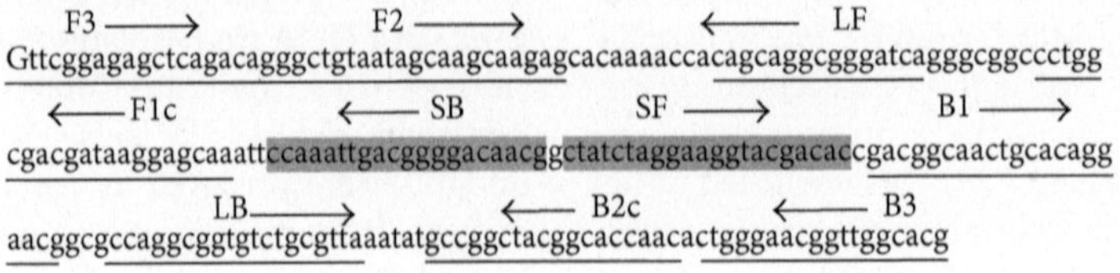

FIGURE 1: The position of LAMP and stem primers on *T. brucei gambiense*-specific glycoprotein (TgsGP) sequence section. The stem section lies between primers Flc and B1. The LAMP product is composed of the sequence between primers F2 and B2c. The outer forward and backward primers (F3/B3) displace the strand and therefore do not form part of the final LAMP product.

stem LAMP test was analyzed in the following combinations: (i) with outer primers, F3/B3, and (ii) without outer primers. The standard *T. brucei gambiense* LAMP consisted of F3/B3, FIP/BIP, and LF/LB primers [24].

2.4. The Real-Time LAMP Reactions. To improve the sensitivity of stem LAMP test, concentration of four reaction components was optimized using Taguchi method followed by regression analysis to select concentration optima for each reagent [29]. Briefly the concentration of FIP and BIP was varied from 30 to 60 pmoles, stem forward and backward (SF/SB) primers were varied from 10 to 30 pmoles, dNTPs were varied from 1 to 3 mM, and extra magnesium was varied from 0 to 3 mM. The 1x ThermoPol reaction buffer contained 20 mM Tris-HCl (pH 8.8), 10 mM KCl, 10 mM $(NH_4)_2SO_4$, 2 mM $MgSO_4$, and 0.1% Triton X-100. The *Bst* 3.0 DNA polymerase (New England Biolabs, MA, USA) was at 0.5 μL and SYTO-9 fluorescence dye was used at 3.0 μM (Molecular Probes, Oregon, USA). The template was ~100 pg of purified trypanosome DNA from *T. brucei gambiense* isolate PT41. The LAMP reactions were performed at 58, 63, and 65°C for 60 minutes using the Rotorgene 6000 (Qiagen, Victoria, Australia) and data acquired on HRM channel (460–510 nm) followed by reaction inactivation at 80°C for 5 minutes. Once the test conditions for stem LAMP test were selected, the test analytical sensitivity was determined and compared with standard LAMP test using tenfold serial dilution of PT41 DNA prepared from ~100 ng (1.0×10^6 trypanosomes/mL) to ~1 fg (0.01 trypanosomes/mL). All tests were done in duplicate and repeated once after two weeks. The LAMP test reaction conditions determined in the Rotorgene 6000 were duplicated using the portable and battery operated ESE Quant Tube Scanner amplification unit (Qiagen, Stockach, Germany) and used in analyses of tsetse samples. The results were obtained in real-time using the FAM channel in the scanner studio software. The template was set at 1 μL for the DNA and 2 μL for all other templates. The tests specificity was checked with tsetse DNA and the closely related *T. brucei rhodesiense* and *T. b. brucei* DNA.

2.5. Detection and Confirmation of LAMP Products. The formation of LAMP product was first monitored in real-time through fluorescence of SYTO-9 dye in Rotorgene 6000. To confirm that the stem LAMP test formats amplified the predicted target, melt curves were acquired after amplification using Rotorgene at 1°C steps, with a hold of 30 s, from 62°C to

TABLE 2: The diagnostic performance of TgsGP LAMP test formats and PCR using archived reference samples.

Indices (%)	LAMP tests			TgsGP-PCR
	Standard LAMP	Stem $LAMP_w$ [a]	Stem $LAMP_{wn}$ [b]	
Sensitivity	57.1	71.4	71.4	46.4
Specificity	79.4	74.6	88.9	95.2
Diagnostic accuracy	72.5	73.6	83.5	80.2
PPV	55.2	55.6	74.1	81.3
NPV	80.1	85.1	87.5	80

[a]Stem LAMP test with outer primers.
[b]Stem LAMP test without outer primers.

96°C [30]. The products were later analyzed in 2.0% agarose gels stained with SYBR® safe DNA gel stain. In the portable ESE Quant unit, the products were confirmed using the melt curves acquired using the ESE melt software as described by the manufacturer.

2.6. LAMP Diagnostic Performance. The tests diagnostic sensitivity, specificity, accuracy, and positive and negative predictive values were done using 28 archived DNA samples that had been prepared from microscopically positive patients and vectors (positive samples) [12, 27] and 63 microscopically negative samples from HAT foci (negative samples). In addition, a total of 19 DNA samples previously prepared from tsetse midguts of nonexposed tsetse flies were used as negative controls. The samples had been stored at −80°C for over 7 years. The performance indices were number of true positives (TP), true negatives (TN), false positives (FP), and false negatives (FN). The diagnostic sensitivity (ability of the test to detect a true positive) was expressed as TP/(TP + FN) and specificity (ability of the test to exclude a true negative) as TN/(TN + FP). The positive predictive value (PPV), negative predictive value (NPV), and diagnostic accuracy were also determined. The indices were calculated using the online statistical programme https://department.obg.cuhk.edu.hk/researchsupport/SenSpc.asp.

3. Results

The Taguchi method estimated the optimum concentration for the reaction components for *T. brucei gambiense* stem LAMP as follows: FIB/BIP at 35 pmol, SF/SB 15 pmol, 2 mM dNTPs, and 1.5 mM of extra magnesium sulphate. The optimum reaction temperature was determined at 63°C and 35 minutes was chosen as the test cut-off point since the lowest amplification level was recorded at 29 minutes. There was appearance of false positives (primer-dimers) when the reactions were ran beyond 48 min and 63 minutes for stem LAMP format with outer and without outer primers, respectively. The analytical sensitivity of both stem LAMP test formats was ~10 trypanosomes/mL (~1 pg) compared to ~100 trypanosomes/mL for standard LAMP test. Furthermore, we recorded sensitivity levels of ~1 trypanosome/mL (~100 fg) for stem LAMP test formats but results were inconsistent (i.e., 3 out of 6 replicates of 1.0×10^{-6} dilution were positive). The stem LAMP formats indicated faster time to results and with similar product with a melting temperature of ~89°C (Table 1 and Figures 2(a)–2(c)), though the amplicons for LAMP test without outer primers were less bright (Figure 2(d)). Overall the stem LAMP test formats recorded superior diagnostic sensitivity of 71.4% compared to standard LAMP test with 57.1% and PCR with 46.4%. Moreover the LAMP test format without outer primers showed higher diagnostic accuracy of 83.5%, positive predictive value of 74.1%, and negative predictive value of 87.5% (Table 2). These superior diagnostic indices translated into higher detection of pathogen DNA of 9/16 compared to standard LAMP test with 5/16 using tsetse fly samples spiked with trypanosome DNA (Table 1).

4. Discussion

The stem LAMP test formats described here indicated improved diagnostic performance compared to the standard LAMP test. This is attributed to the use of two sets of reaction accelerating primers (loop and stem primers) compared to one-set primers (loop primers) in the standard LAMP format. The loop primers accelerate the reaction by priming the stable loops between FIP/BIP primers [26] while the stem primers presumably work by priming off the newly generated amplicon as it is made transiently single-stranded during DNA replication [25]. This sequential amplification mimics nested PCR format and leads to increased formation of LAMP product and hence improvement in sensitivity. The use of both stem primers concurrently and in their reverse orientation indicated the best reaction performance (Figure 1). Any other combination and orientation increased reaction time and significantly reduced test sensitivity as much as 100-fold. The stem LAMP test formats amplified identical product with the standard LAMP test as indicated through melt curves. This is expected since the final LAMP product is between primers F2 and B2c and the stem primers are within this region. More promising is the ability of the new test to indicate a higher sensitivity with supernatant as compared to extracted DNA prepared from the same sample (Table 1). It appears that more DNA is lost through kit extraction than when the sample is processed through boiling. The ability to use supernatant shortens the experimental procedure; nevertheless before supernatant can be relied upon as template for LAMP reactions, protocols for template purification and buffers that stabilise DNA in the supernatant need to be developed.

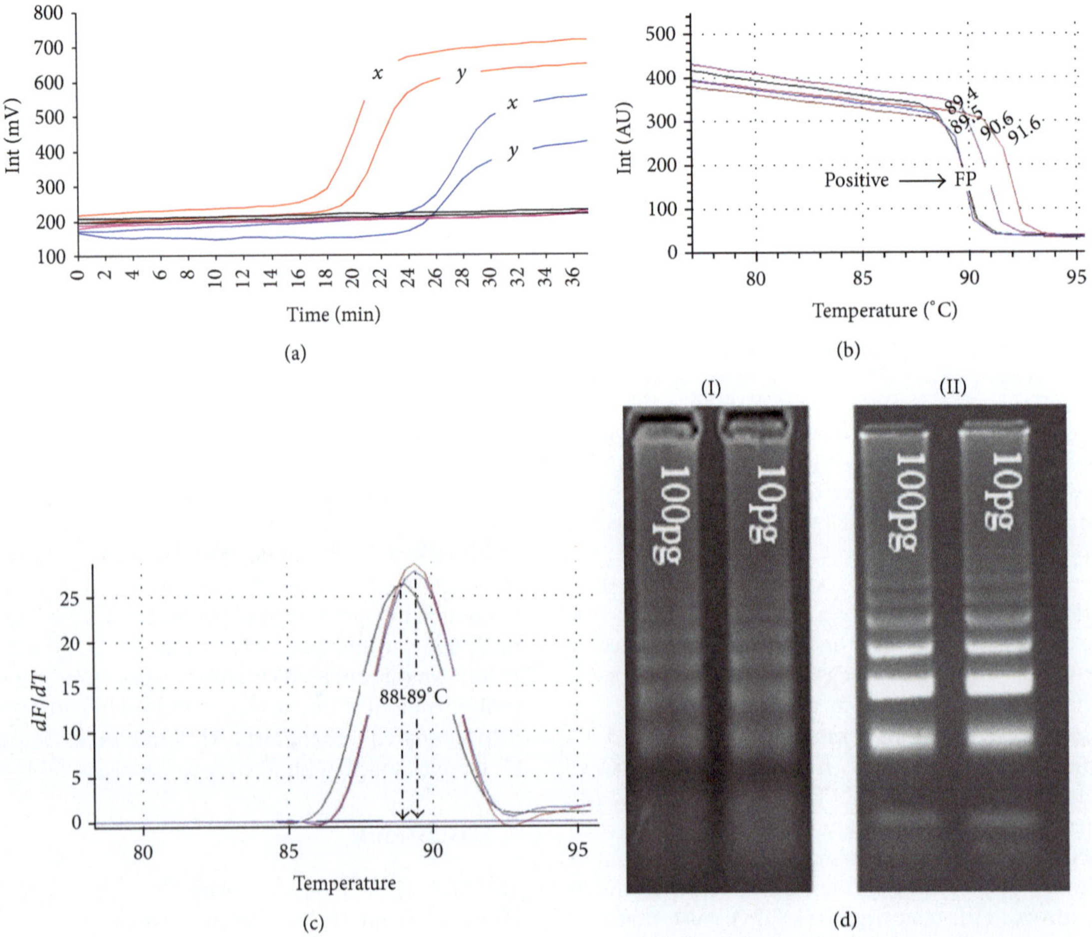

Figure 2: (a) The tube scanner fluorometric output of stem LAMP (red) and standard LAMP (blue) tests using ~10 pg of DNA from isolate PT41 (x) and DNA prepared from CSF (y) of a confirmed HAT patient. The unit reports the fluorescence in millivolts (mV) on y-axis and time in minutes on the x-axis. (b) The acquisition of melts curves for PT41, DNA prepared from CSF, and supernatant prepared from a tsetse fly sample spiked with B014 DNA. T_m was 89.5°C for PT41 and DNA from CSF patient and 89.4°C for B014 in tsetse fly sample. The nonspecific product (FP) is induced for illustration and showed T_m that ranged from 72 to 76°C and 90 to 92°C (c). The duplication of melts peaks for PT41, CSF, and B014 DNA samples using Rotorgene 6000. The melt peaks showed T_m of ~89°C for PT41 and CSF DNA and ~ 88°C for B014. (d) The amplicons for stem LAMP test (I) without outer primers and (II) with outer primers.

The omission of the outer primers in an optimized stem LAMP test format did not reduce the test sensitivity (Table 2) although the amplicons were less bright after electrophoresis (Figure 2(d)). Indeed the format without outer primers surprisingly showed superior diagnostic test performance compared to other LAMP test formats (Table 2). The use of four sets of primers (eight primers) in the stem LAMP format with outer primers increases the possibility of forming nonspecific products and hence the lower diagnostic accuracy of 73.6% and PPV value of 55.6%. The primary role of the outer primers is supposedly to displace the newly synthesised strands into a single strand making it available for extension by either inner primer [28]. It appears that other primers are able to displace and extend the strand in absence of outer primers albeit less efficiently. The possibility of omitting the outer primers is advantageous because it allows more flexibility of positioning both the loop and stem primers and especially in shorter sequences. We noted that the stem primers may not be appropriate for all LAMP tests. In separate studies, the inclusion of stem primers in the RIME LAMP test [12] did not alter the test sensitivity and lead to appearance of spurious products.

Since the inception of LAMP technology, the product detection formats have been developed towards visual inspection of result. Unfortunately most detection formats available are nonspecific and do not offer any step for confirming the predicted product. The real-time ESE Quant unit used in this study uses nonspecific fluorescence dye but provides a product confirmation step through acquisition of melt curves after amplification (Figure 2(b)). Melt curves can indicate different reaction products based on their shape and peaks (Figures 2(b) and 2(c)). In PCR the primer-dimers usually melt at lower temperatures since they are smaller than the desired product while the nonspecific product in LAMP can have either a lower or higher T_m than the desired product since more primers are used (Figure 1). Determination of nonspecific products is valuable since their presence reduces the amplification efficiency and ultimately the accuracy of the test. Ideally each LAMP test should give identical melt curves and/or peaks if the product is composed of identical sequence. Any base difference from the desired sequence will be detected as either a shift in the melt curve (Figure 2(b)) or peaks (Figure 2(c)) and hence the basis for determination of nonspecific product. The different melting temperatures observed in this study between B014 spiked samples and other positive samples may indicate a point mutation resulting in transversion of a single or more bases. Indeed transversion within TgsGP sequence has been reported in isolates from Cameroun [21] and B014 DNA was isolated from human in Fontem, Cameroon, in 1988. The reliability of the melt curves obtained here using ESE melt curve software was ascertained by duplication of similar results using Rotorgene 6000 (Figure 2(c)).

The detection of trypanosomes in the tsetse flies is routinely done through dissection followed by microscopic examination, methods that are time-consuming and more often inaccurate. This implies xenomonitoring through dissection is impractical. The stem TgsGP LAMP test reported here partly fills this gap since it is specific for *T. brucei gambiense* and shows improved diagnostic sensitivity and accuracy (Table 1) compared to the standard TgsGP LAMP test [24]. Similar LAMP test results were recorded albeit with higher sensitivity with RIME LAMP [27, 31]. Since RIME LAMP cannot differentiate human pathogenic trypanosomes from *T. b. brucei*, it is further proposed that the stem TgsGP LAMP test can be used in algorithm with RIME LAMP tests to identify *T. brucei gambiense* DNA among RIME LAMP positive samples.

5. Conclusions

This study provides a *T. brucei gambiense* stem LAMP test format that combines with real-time technology to detect and confirm pathogen DNA in tsetse samples. The stem LAMP test formats show improved diagnostic sensitivity and accuracy compared to the standard LAMP test. The LAMP format without outer primers indicated the best performance. The combination of LAMP test and real-time technology offers visual inspection and confirmation of results at the point of use, characteristics that are ideal for a surveillance test. Such combination can provide data on the distribution of trypanosomes and hence play a crucial role in guiding the vector control strategies since not all the vector population will carry infections.

Disclosure

The views expressed in this article do not reflect the views of the authors' respective institutions.

Competing Interests

The authors declare that there is no conflict of interests regarding the publication of this paper.

Acknowledgments

The authors acknowledge the provision of samples from Professor Wendy Gibson, University of Bristol, UK, and Professor John C. Enyaru, Uganda, through Professor Joseph M Ndung'u of Foundation for Innovative New Diagnostics, Geneva, as mentioned [12]. They thank Christopher Heath, Royal Perth Hospital, Western Australia, and Trypanosomiasis Research Centre, Kenya. They also thank David Berryman, State Agricultural Biological Centre, Murdoch University, for sample storage.

References

[1] World Health Organization, *2013 Report of a WHO Meeting on Elimination of African Trypanosomiasis (Trypanosoma brucei gambiense)*, World Health Organization, Geneva, Switzerland, 2013.

[2] J. Maurice, "New WHO plan targets the demise of sleeping sickness," *The Lancet*, vol. 381, no. 9860, pp. 13–14, 2013.

[3] P. Holmes, "First WHO meeting of stakeholders on elimination of *Gambiense* Human African Trypanosomiasis," *PLoS Neglected Tropical Diseases*, vol. 8, no. 10, Article ID e3244, 2014.

[4] World Health Organisation, "Trypanosomiasis, Human African Trypanosomiasis (sleeping sickness)," http://www.who.int/mediacentre/factsheets/fs259/en/.

[5] H. A. Farid, Z. S. Morsy, H. Helmy, R. M. R. Ramzy, M. El Setouhy, and G. J. Weil, "A critical appraisal of molecular xenomonitoring as a tool for assessing progress toward elimination of lymphatic filariasis," *American Journal of Tropical Medicine and Hygiene*, vol. 77, no. 4, pp. 593–600, 2007.

[6] F. Checchi, F. Chappuis, U. Karunakara, G. Priotto, and D. Chandramohan, "Accuracy of five algorithms to diagnose *Gambiense* human african trypanosomiasis," *PLoS Neglected Tropical Diseases*, vol. 5, no. 7, Article ID e1233, 2011.

[7] FIND Diagnostics, *The First Rapid Test to Screen for Sleeping Sickness Is Launched*, FIND Diagnostics, 2012.

[8] S. Bisser, C. Lumbala, E. Nguertoum et al., "Sensitivity and specificity of a prototype rapid diagnostic test for the detection of trypanosoma brucei gambiense infection: a multi-centric prospective study," *PLoS Neglected Tropical Diseases*, vol. 10, no. 4, Article ID e0004608, 2016.

[9] P. Büscher, Q. Gilleman, and V. Lejon, "Rapid diagnostic test for sleeping sickness," *New England Journal of Medicine*, vol. 368, no. 11, pp. 1069–1070, 2013.

[10] P. Büscher, P. Mertens, T. Leclipteux et al., "Sensitivity and specificity of HAT Sero-K-SeT, a rapid diagnostic test for serodiagnosis of sleeping sickness caused by *Trypanosoma brucei gambiense*: a case-control study," *The Lancet Global Health*, vol. 2, no. 6, pp. e359–e363, 2014.

[11] S. Biéler, E. Matovu, P. Mitashi et al., "Improved detection of *Trypanosoma brucei* by lysis of red blood cells, concentration and LED fluorescence microscopy," *Acta Tropica*, vol. 121, no. 2, pp. 135–140, 2012.

[12] Z. K. Njiru, A. S. J. Mikosza, E. Matovu et al., "African trypanosomiasis: sensitive and rapid detection of the subgenus *Trypanozoon* by loop-mediated isothermal amplification (LAMP) of parasite DNA," *International Journal for Parasitology*, vol. 38, no. 5, pp. 589–599, 2008.

[13] N. Kuboki, N. Inoue, T. Sakurai et al., "Loop-mediated isothermal amplification for detection of African trypanosomes,"

Journal of Clinical Microbiology, vol. 41, no. 12, pp. 5517–5524, 2003.

[14] O. M. M. Thekisoe, N. Kuboki, A. Nambota et al., "Species-specific loop-mediated isothermal amplification (LAMP) for diagnosis of trypanosomosis," *Acta Tropica*, vol. 102, no. 3, pp. 182–189, 2007.

[15] K. Hayashida, K. Kajino, L. Hachaambwa, B. Namangala, and C. Sugimoto, "Direct blood dry LAMP: a rapid, stable, and easy diagnostic tool for Human African Trypanosomiasis," *PLoS Neglected Tropical Diseases*, vol. 9, no. 3, Article ID e0003578, 2015.

[16] O. V. Nikolskaia, O. M. Thekisoe, J. S. Dumler, and D. J. Grab, "Loop-mediated isothermal amplification for detection of the 5.8S ribosomal ribonucleic acid internal transcribed spacer 2 gene found in *Trypanosoma brucei gambiense*," *The American Journal of Tropical Medicine and Hygiene*, vol. 96, no. 2, pp. 275–279, 2017.

[17] P. Paindavoine, F. Zampetti-Bosseler, H. Coquelet, E. Pays, and M. Steinert, "Different allele frequencies in *Trypanosoma brucei brucei* and *Trypanosoma brucei gambiense* populations," *Molecular and Biochemical Parasitology*, vol. 32, no. 1, pp. 61–71, 1989.

[18] G. D. Kanmogne, J. R. Stevens, T. Asonganyi, and W. C. Gibson, "Characterization of Trypanosoma brucei gambiense isolates using restriction fragment length polymorphisms in 5 variant surface glycoprotein genes," *Acta Tropica*, vol. 61, no. 3, pp. 239–254, 1996.

[19] D. Mehlitz, U. Zillmann, C. M. Scott, and D. G. Godfrey, "Epidemiological studies on the animal reservoir of gambiense sleeping sickness. Part III. Characterization of trypanozoon stocks by isoenzymes and sensitivity to human serum," *Tropenmedizin und Parasitologie*, vol. 33, no. 2, pp. 113–118, 1982.

[20] M. Berberof, D. Pérez-Morga, and E. Pays, "A receptor-like flagellar pocket glycoprotein specific to *Trypanosoma brucei gambiense*," *Molecular and Biochemical Parasitology*, vol. 113, no. 1, pp. 127–138, 2001.

[21] W. Gibson, L. Nemetschke, and J. Ndung'u, "Conserved sequence of the TgsGP gene in Group 1 *Trypanosoma brucei gambiense*," *Infection, Genetics and Evolution*, vol. 10, no. 4, pp. 453–458, 2010.

[22] M. Radwanska, F. Claes, S. Magez et al., "Novel primer sequences for polymerase chain reaction-based detection of *Trypanosoma brucei gambiense*," *The American Journal of Tropical Medicine and Hygiene*, vol. 67, no. 3, pp. 289–295, 2002.

[23] W. Gibson, T. Backhouse, and A. Griffiths, "The human serum resistance associated gene is ubiquitous and conserved in *Trypanosoma brucei rhodesiense* throughout East Africa," *Infection, Genetics and Evolution*, vol. 1, no. 3, pp. 207–214, 2002.

[24] Z. K. Njiru, R. Traub, J. O. Ouma, J. C. Enyaru, and E. Matovu, "Detection of group 1 *Trypanosoma brucei gambiense* by loop-mediated isothermal amplification," *Journal of Clinical Microbiology*, vol. 49, no. 4, pp. 1530–1536, 2011.

[25] O. Gandelman, R. Jackson, G. Kiddle, and L. Tisi, "Loop-mediated amplification accelerated by stem primers," *International Journal of Molecular Sciences*, vol. 12, no. 12, pp. 9108–9124, 2011.

[26] K. Nagamine, T. Hase, and T. Notomi, "Accelerated reaction by loop-mediated isothermal amplification using loop primers," *Molecular and Cellular Probes*, vol. 16, no. 3, pp. 223–229, 2002.

[27] I. I. Malele, J. O. Ouma, J. C. K. Enyaru et al., "Comparative diagnostic and analytical performance of PCR and LAMP-based trypanosome detection methods estimated using pooled whole tsetse flies and midguts," *Veterinary Parasitology*, vol. 197, no. 3-4, pp. 549–556, 2013.

[28] T. Notomi, H. Okayama, H. Masubuchi et al., "Loop-mediated isothermal amplification of DNA," *Nucleic Acids Research*, vol. 28, no. 12, p. E63, 2000.

[29] B. D. Cobb and J. M. Ciarkson, "A simple procedure for optimising the polymerase chain reaction (PCR) using modified taguchi methods," *Nucleic Acids Research*, vol. 22, no. 18, pp. 3801–3805, 1994.

[30] P. T. Monis, S. Giglio, and C. P. Saint, "Comparison of SYTO9 and SYBR Green I for real-time polymerase chain reaction and investigation of the effect of dye concentration on amplification and DNA melting curve analysis," *Analytical Biochemistry*, vol. 340, no. 1, pp. 24–34, 2005.

[31] L. J. Cunningham, J. K. Lingley, L. R. Haines, J. M. Ndung'u, S. J. Torr, and E. R. Adams, "Illuminating the prevalence of *Trypanosoma brucei* s.l. in *Glossina*using LAMP as a tool for xenomonitoring," *PLoS Neglected Tropical Diseases*, vol. 10, no. 2, Article ID e0004441, 2016.

26

Atherogenic Risk Assessment among Persons Living in Rural Uganda

Clara Wekesa,[1] Gershim Asiki,[1] Ivan Kasamba,[1] Laban Waswa,[1] Steven J. Reynolds,[2,3] Rebecca N. Nsubuga,[1] Rob Newton,[1] and Anatoli Kamali[1]

[1] *Medical Research Council/Uganda Virus Research Institute Uganda Research Unit on AIDS, Entebbe, Uganda*
[2] *Division of Intramural Research, National Institute of Allergy and Infectious Diseases, National Institutes of Health, Bethesda, MD 20892, USA*
[3] *Johns Hopkins School of Medicine, Baltimore, MD 21205, USA*

Correspondence should be addressed to Clara Wekesa; clara.wekesa@gmail.com

Academic Editor: Marcel Tanner

Background. Hypertension and dyslipidemia are independent risk factors for coronary heart disease and commonly coexist. Cardiovascular risk can be reliably predicted using lipid ratios such as the atherogenic index, a useful prognostic parameter for guiding timely interventions. *Objective.* We assessed the cardiovascular risk profile based on the atherogenic index of residents within a rural Ugandan cohort. *Methods.* In 2011, a population based survey was conducted among 7507 participants. Sociodemographic characteristics, physical measurements (blood pressure, weight, height, and waist and hip circumference), and blood sampling for nonfasting lipid profile were collected for each participant. Atherogenic risk profile, defined as logarithm base ten of (triglyceride divided by high density lipoprotein cholesterol), was categorised as low risk (<0.1), intermediate risk (0.1–0.24), and high risk (>0.24). *Results.* Fifty-five percent of participants were female and the mean age was 49.9 years (SD ± 20.2). Forty-two percent of participants had high and intermediate atherogenic risk. Persons with hypertension, untreated HIV infection, abnormal glycaemia, and obesity and living in less urbanised villages were more at risk. *Conclusion.* A significant proportion of persons in this rural population are at risk of atherosclerosis. Key identified populations at risk should be considered for future intervention against cardiovascular related morbidity and mortality. The study however used parameters from unfasted samples that may have a bearing on observed results.

1. Background

Globally, cardiovascular disease (CVD) is the leading cause of death with up to 80% occurring in low and middle income countries (LMICs) [1]. Premature death due to CVD is rapidly growing in Sub-Saharan Africa (SSA) [2]. Hypertension and dyslipidemia are thought to be the major risk factors for CVD [3]. A systematic review on hypertension in SSA yielded 17 studies conducted between 1998 and 2008 in 11 countries and found an overall prevalence of 16.2%, with small variation between urban and rural communities [4]. In Uganda, the prevalence of hypertension ranges from 14.6% in the rural areas [5] to 27.2% in the periurban area [6]. In Western populations, dyslipidemia among patients with hypertension is a common finding. The prevalence of dyslipidemia coexisting with hypertension has been estimated at 15–24% [3, 7]. Over 40% of all newly diagnosed hypertensive patients have at least one lipid abnormality [8]. There is dearth of data on the burden of dyslipidemia among patients with hypertension in SSA.

Hypertension and dyslipidemia are both independent modifiable risk factors for CVD. However, some studies suggest that dyslipidemia may play a role in the development of hypertension via endothelial damage [9]. The risk for CVD is higher in the presence of both hypertension and dyslipidemia than by the individual disease entities [10]. In high income countries, strategies targeting the reduction of serum cholesterol levels provide the single most important benefit against CVD resulting from coronary heart disease (CHD) when evaluated in a cohort setting [11]. A review on a number of cohort studies and randomised clinical trials found that a 10% decrease in cholesterol reduced the risk of CHD by 50% at the age of 40 and this benefit reduces to 20% by the age of 70 [12]. In contrast, blood pressure control provides only a 20% risk reduction of mortality due to CHD in high income settings.

Current medical practice encourages risk stratification for all persons at risk of CHD including those with hypertension. This is advantageous for timely intervention in preventing CHD and its sequelae. Cardiovascular risk assessment based solely on serum low density lipoprotein cholesterol (LDL-C) has been found to be inadequate [13, 14] and even in persons on statin therapy with normal or near normal LDL-C serum levels, there remains risk for future cardiovascular events. Hypertriglyceridemia has been identified as an independent cardiovascular risk factor [15, 16]. Hypertriglyceridemia is a proxy for atherogenic dyslipidemia (elevated TG (triglyceride) and low high density lipoprotein cholesterol) [16, 17], a component of the metabolic syndrome and a known risk factor for CHD. Despite interaction with other lipids that might increase atherogenic risk and in-subject variation, elevated TG has been shown to be a good predictor of CHD in consideration of the high density lipoprotein cholesterol (HDL-C) levels [17] and is used in clinical practice to predict atherosclerosis [17, 18]. The lipid ratio log [TG/HDL-C] (atherogenic index) provides an alternative simple option for risk stratification. The use of this ratio is to reflect the balance between risk and protective lipoprotein forces [15] as well as acting as a correlate with LDL-C particle size [19], LDL-phenotype B, and small HDL-C particles [16]. This ratio has also been evaluated as a prognostic tool in predicting CHD [16] and its predictive value far outweighs that of absolute lipid parameters [20, 21] as well as the TC (total cholesterol)/HDL ratio [21] given its strong correlation with lipoprotein particle size.

Uganda bears a significant burden of hypertension [22] and like other SSA countries is not presently equipped with the necessary resources, expertise, and technology to manage the CVD sequelae. A recent study done within a rural population reflected the dominant dyslipidemic pattern to be that of low serum HDL-C levels and a good proportion with hypertriglyceridemia [23]. Whereas there are well-recognised recommendations on the use of serum LDL-C and TC for cardiovascular risk assessment, there is limited progress in addressing concerns with low serum HDL-C which may lead to underestimation of CHD risk [24]. The atherogenic index provides a simple and reliable method for point of care risk assessment that can be done by nonspecialists even within hard-to-reach areas. The aim of this study was to assess the atherogenic risk profile using the atherogenic index among people living in rural Uganda.

2. Methods

2.1. Design and Setting. A population based survey was conducted in 2011 among 7507 individuals aged 13 years and above living in an established rural cohort in southwestern Uganda, the General Population Cohort (GPC) consisting of 25 villages. This cohort has been in existence for the last 25 years and was initially established for the purpose of investigating HIV trends in rural Uganda. Research activities have since been broadened to include noncommunicable diseases, assessing burden and risk factors [25].

2.2. Study Procedures

2.2.1. Questionnaire. Sociodemographic information was collected for each participant and entered into an electronic questionnaire. This information included age, sex, and occupation, level of education, marital status, smoking history, and use of alcohol. The level of urbanicity was determined and presented as described elsewhere [26].

2.2.2. Physical Measurements. Blood pressure measurement, height, weight, and hip and waist circumferences were measured as described by Riha et al. 2014 [26]. Participants found to have systolic blood pressure ≥140 mmHg and/or diastolic pressure ≥90 mmHg were referred to as having hypertension. Participant categorisation using body mass index (BMI) was as follows: BMI ≤ 18.5, "underweight," BMI 18.5–24.9, "normal weight," BMI 25–29.9, "overweight," and BMI ≥ 30, "obese". Categorisation by waist-hip ratio (WHR) was as follows: abnormal in male if >0.95 and abnormal in females if >0.8.

2.2.3. Laboratory Measurements. Participants underwent phlebotomy for purposes of a nonfasting lipid profile (TC, TG, HDL-C, and low density lipoprotein cholesterol (LDL-C)), HIV serology, and glycated haemoglobin (HbA1c). All blood samples were transported on the same day to a central laboratory for sample processing and testing. Lipid profile analysis was done using the enzymatic colorimetric assay by the Cobas Integra 400 Plus. Cut-off values for the different lipid parameters representative of dyslipidemia were as follows: TC > 5.2 mmol/L, TG > 2.3 mmol/L, LDL-C > 3.4 mmol/L, and HDL-C < 1.04 mmol/L, male, and <1.3 mmol/L, female. Participants with HbA1c ≥ 6.5% were termed as diabetic, HbA1c 6–6.49% were termed as high risk for diabetes, and HbA1c < 6% were termed as low risk for diabetes [27]. HIV testing was done in accordance with the Ministry of Health guidelines [28].

2.3. Data Analysis. To assess the atherogenic risk we used the atherogenic index defined as log(triglycerides/HDL-C). The risk was categorised into low (<0.1), intermediate (0.1–0.24), and high (>0.24) [21].

The sample was described using proportions by sex. Age and systolic and diastolic blood pressure were summarized with means and corresponding standard deviations (SD). Atherogenic risk was determined using proportions in each category and the chi-squared test was used to compare proportions. We used the ordered logistic regression model to evaluate the effect of demographic characteristics, blood pressure, lipid profiles, and HIV status on atherogenic risk and the results were presented by sex. To avoid residual confounding and loss of power, continuous lipid measures were modelled as continuous rather than categorised.

The continuous variables were included into the model as centered and assessed for nonlinearity by fitting a first-order fractional polynomial to the data. The proportional odds assumption in using the ordered logistic regression was tested. Analysis was done using STATA 13 (Stata Corp, College Station, TX).

2.4. Ethical Consideration. The study was conducted in accordance with the principles of the Declaration of Helsinki and was approved by the Uganda Virus Research Institute Research Ethics Committee (UVRI REC) in Entebbe, Uganda, and by the Uganda National Council of Science and Technology (UNSCT). Written informed consent was obtained from all study participants. For participants below the age of 18 years, parental consent and formal assent to participate in the study were obtained as per the Ugandan National Guidelines for Research Involving Humans as Research Participants [29]. Participants with hypertension and raised serum lipids were referred to a care clinic for further management and received standard of care (health education on risk factor prevention and/or control and drug therapy with statins).

3. Results

3.1. Baseline Characteristics. The study enrolled 7507 participants, the majority were females (55%), and the mean age was 49.9 years (SD ± 20.2). There were equal distributions of participants across the different levels of urbanicity, most of the participants were under the age of 30, and the use of alcohol and tobacco was more common among the male participants (Table 1).

From the physical and laboratory measurements we found more female participants to be overweight and obese and have an abnormal WHR. Approximately 18% of participants were identified as having hypertension and only 2% had controlled hypertension on treatment. The most common form of dyslipidemia was low serum HDL-C levels (Table 1).

3.2. Atherogenic Risk. The proportion of participants with intermediate and high atherogenic risk was 17% and 25%, respectively, with the greater proportion at high risk being male participants (Figure 1).

3.3. Risk Factors for High Atherogenic Risk. Participants with hypertension (particularly those with suboptimal control on treatment), residents from less urbanised villages, HIV-infected participants not on antiretroviral therapy (ART), overweight and obese participants, and participants with abnormal HbA1c had significantly higher odds of having high atherogenic risk (Table 2).

Being female, 30 years of age and above, having attained higher level of education, current consumption of alcohol, and being on ART were significantly associated with lower odds of having high atherogenic risk. Abnormal total cholesterol serum levels and history of smoking had no association with atherogenic risk.

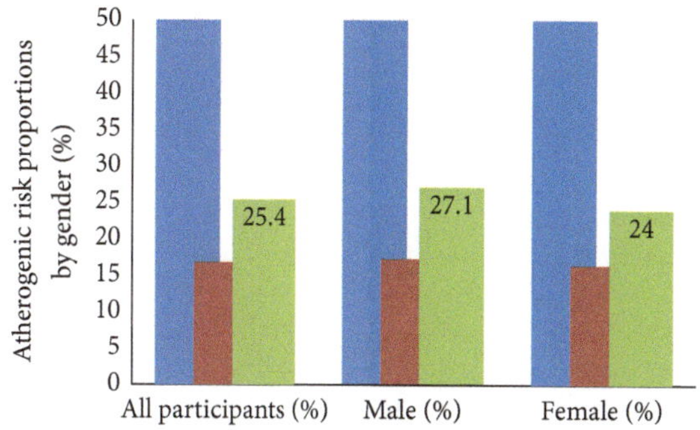

	All participants (%)	Male (%)	Female (%)
Low risk	57.8	55.6	59.7
Intermediate risk	16.8	17.3	16.4
High risk	25.4	27.1	24

FIGURE 1: Atherogenic risk profile among study participants stratified by gender.

4. Discussion

With increasing globalisation, varying degrees of urbanisation exist even within rural areas [26]. Urbanisation influences environmental and individual factors that may have impact on cardiovascular risk. In this study we assessed the risk for atherosclerosis using the atherogenic index in a rural Ugandan cohort. The atherogenic index in comparison to absolute lipid parameters and to TC/HDL-C ratio provides more accurate estimates of cardiovascular risk [30] and is more likely to be a better screening tool. Our study is one of the few studies in the region that provides insight into the use of the atherogenic index and having a cohort already in establishment provides the unique opportunity to conduct pilot studies that generate hypotheses to guide future research in this field. This study also assesses the use of the atherogenic index in a widely distributed rural population and is not only restricted to most at-risk populations. The atherogenic index requires minimal expertise and can be widely implemented as a screen method for cardiovascular disease even within remote locations.

A significant proportion of participants were at risk of atherosclerosis. A population based survey done in Iran and using the atherogenic index found a similar high estimate of atherogenic risk [31]. The INTERHEART study, an observational study involving 52 countries spread across all continents, found that persons with history of myocardial infarction had three times the odds of having a raised ApoB/ApoA1 ratio (surrogate for atherogenic dyslipidemia) compared to persons without history of myocardial infarction [32]. An observational study done in Brazil found that persons with coronary disease had two times the odds of having an abnormal TG/HDL-C ratio [33]. In our study participants with hypertension had higher odds of risk for atherosclerosis. We found that 27% of participants with hypertension had a high atherogenic risk, a higher estimate compared to a Nigerian study that found a lower proportion of patients with hypertension at risk for CHD using LDL-C/HDL-C ratios for risk stratification [30]. We attributed this difference in proportions to the atherogenic index being a correlate to

TABLE 1: Sociodemographic, clinical, physical, and biochemical characteristics of cohort by gender.

	All participants n (%)	Sex	
		Male, n (%)	Female, n (%)
All	7507	3378	4129
Demographic characteristics			
Age, in years			
13–29	3679 (49.0)	1804 (53.4)	1875 (45.4)
30–59	2978 (39.7)	1226 (36.3)	1752 (42.4)
60+	850 (11.3)	348 (10.3)	502 (12.2)
*Urbanicity score**			
Quartile 1 (least urban)	1978 (26.4)	884 (26.2)	1094 (26.5)
Quartile 2	1893 (25.2)	848 (25.1)	1045 (25.3)
Quartile 3	1946 (25.9)	888 (26.3)	1058 (25.6)
Quartile 4 (most urban)	1690 (22.5)	758 (22.4)	932 (22.6)
Highest education level			
None/up to P4	2112 (28.1)	876 (25.9)	1236 (29.9)
P5–P7	3365 (44.8)	1579 (46.7)	1786 (43.3)
Secondary+	2030 (27.0)	923 (27.3)	1107 (26.8)
Occupation			
Subsistence crop	2975 (39.6)	1102 (32.6)	1873 (45.4)
Cash crop cultivator	934 (12.4)	491 (14.5)	443 (10.7)
Noncrop	1043 (13.9)	625 (18.5)	418 (10.1)
Unemployed/full-time education	2555 (34.0)	1160 (34.3)	1395 (33.8)
*Marital status***			
Not married/divorced	3861 (51.5)	1842 (54.6)	2019 (48.9)
Married/living	3638 (48.5)	1532 (45.4)	2106 (51.1)
Lifestyle characteristics			
Smoking			
Never smoked	6747 (89.9)	2707 (80.1)	4040 (97.8)
Ever smoked daily	760 (10.1)	671 (19.9)	89 (2.2)
Alcohol consumption			
Never drinker	4844 (64.5)	2032 (60.2)	2812 (68.1)
Ex-drinker	583 (7.8)	235 (7.0)	348 (8.4)
Current drinker	2080 (27.7)	1111 (32.9)	969 (23.5)
Biophysical characteristics			
BMI group			
Underweight (<18.5)	1701 (22.7)	1022 (30.3)	679 (16.4)
Normal (18.5–24.9)	4878 (65.0)	2179 (64.5)	2699 (65.4)
Overweight (≥25)	730 (9.7)	156 (4.6)	574 (13.9)
Obese	198 (2.6)	21 (0.6)	177 (4.3)
Waist-hip ratio (WHR)			
Normal (≤0.95-m, ≤0.80-f)	4440 (59.1)	3257 (96.4)	1183 (28.7)
Abnormal (>0.95-m, >0.80-f)	3067 (40.9)	121 (3.6)	2946 (71.3)
Biochemical characteristics			
Total cholesterol			
Desirable (≤5.2 mmol/L)	7084 (94.4)	3270 (96.8)	3814 (92.4)
High (>5.2 mmol/L)	423 (5.6)	108 (3.2)	315 (7.6)
Triglycerides			
Desirable (≤2.3 mmol/L)	7190 (95.8)	3261 (96.5)	3929 (95.2)
High (>2.3 mmol/L)	317 (4.2)	117 (3.5)	200 (4.8)
LDL-C			
Desirable (≤3.4 mmol/L)	7134 (95.0)	3286 (97.3)	3848 (93.2)
High (>3.4 mmol/L)	373 (5.0)	92 (2.7)	281 (6.8)
HDL-C			
Desirable (≥1.04-m, 1.3-f)	1940 (25.8)	1127 (33.4)	813 (19.7)
Undesirable (<1.04-m, 1.3-f), low	5567 (74.2)	2251 (66.6)	3316 (80.3)
HbA1-C			
Normal (≤6%)	7469 (99.7)	3359 (99.8)	4110 (99.7)
Raised (≥6.5%)	19 (0.3)	7 (0.2)	12 (0.3)

TABLE 1: Continued.

	All participants n (%)	Sex	
		Male, n (%)	Female, n (%)
Clinical characteristics			
Hypertension status			
Normal BP	6163 (82.1)	2799 (82.9)	3364 (81.5)
Normal BP on treatment	173 (2.3)	56 (1.7)	117 (2.8)
Raised on treatment	119 (1.6)	31 (0.9)	88 (2.1)
Raised BP, not on treatment	1050 (14.0)	492 (14.6)	558 (13.5)
HIV/ART status			
Negative	6821 (92.0)	3103 (93.5)	3718 (90.7)
Positive, on ART	201 (2.7)	63 (1.9)	138 (3.4)
Positive, not on ART	396 (5.3)	152 (4.6)	244 (6.0)
Atherogenic risk			
Low (<0.1)	4341 (57.8)	1878 (55.6)	2463 (59.7)
Intermediate (0.1–0.24)	1259 (16.8)	583 (17.3)	676 (16.4)
High (>0.24)	1907 (25.4)	917 (27.1)	990 (24.0)

*Riha et al. 2014 [26].
**8 missing pieces of information.

lipoprotein size [21] which may predict risk better. Participants on treatment, but with uncontrolled hypertension, were more likely to be at risk of atherosclerosis compared to those not on treatment and those with controlled hypertension. Literature shows that blood pressure control gives minimal reduction of cardiovascular risk especially among those older than 40 years [12] and in our study we found the mean age to be 49 years. This could explain why even among participants on treatment and controlled hypertension atherogenic risk was still high. Participants that were HIV infected and ART naive were more likely to have a high atherogenic risk, a finding similar to other studies done, possibly owing to their high inflammatory state [34]. The use of ART was found to be protective as ART is thought to reduce inflammatory markers and provide cardioprotection [35]. However, other studies have found the use of protease inhibitors (PI) to increase the serum levels of atherogenic lipoproteins [34]. In this population first-line therapy was non-PI based and could further explain our findings. We also observed that a high atherogenic index was less prevalent in participants aged 60 years and above and yet it is more likely that individuals in this age category are more at risk of cardiovascular events. The HIV prevalence in this cohort is higher in the younger age group and we thought this may be the main driver for the increased risk in this age group.

Abnormal HbA1c as a screen for diabetes was also found to be associated with high atherogenic risk. Diabetes affects the integrity of the vasculature and is also associated with other conditions that predispose to CHD, such as hypertension and dyslipidemia that may explain the increased risk. Previous epidemiological studies have shown cholesterol to predict risk of CHD and LDL-C to be associated with future risk [36]; however, we did not find any association between high serum cholesterol levels and atherogenic risk in this rural population. Similar to the Framingham study [36] and the INTERHEART study [32] we demonstrated that obesity and abdominal obesity were associated with increased risk of CHD in this study population. Our study showed that participants from less urbanised villages were more likely to be at high risk for CHD. However previous studies done within this same population showed that persons in less urbanised villages were more likely to indulge in physical activity and eat fruits and vegetables [26], factors thought to reduce risk for CHD. It may be possible that a different set of risk factors, yet to be explored, is responsible for the risk of CHD in this population.

Our study was limited in that we did not derive lipid parameters from fasted samples which may impact on risk estimation if there should be any variation with parameters derived after fasting. We also did not ascertain differences among the subcategories of participants with hypertension that may have accounted for differences in risk profile. The design of the study did not allow making inferences as to casualty. However this study provides insight into estimated cardiovascular risk in a widely distributed rural population taking into account environmental, infectious, and noninfectious risk factors and provides a platform for further research into possible causes of high atherogenic risk whose findings may give information on preventive strategies.

5. Conclusion

A significant proportion of persons in this rural Ugandan population are at risk of atherosclerosis. Persons with hypertension, untreated HIV infection, abnormal glycaemia, and obesity appear to be more at risk and may be considered as target groups for intervention programs. Follow-up studies are needed to further assess other risk factors including the role of genetics in cardiovascular risk in this population.

TABLE 2: Factors associated with high atherogenic risk.

Covariates	High atherogenic risk n (%)	Crude OR$^{\phi}$		Adjusted OR$^{\phi}$ b/ci95	Overall p value
Hypertension status					
Normal BP (≤140/90 mmHg) (n = 6163)	1538 (25.0)	1	**0.022**	1	**0.007**
Normal BP on treatment (n = 173)	53 (30.6)	1.34 (1.01–1.78)		1.32 (0.98–1.79)	
Raised BP (≥140/90 mmHg) on treatment (n = 119)	36 (30.3)	1.51 (1.08–2.11)		1.53 (1.07–2.18)	
Raised BP not on treatment (n = 1050)	280 (26.7)	1.04 (0.91–1.18)		1.17 (1.00–1.37)	
Sex					
Male (n = 3378)	917 (27.1)	1	**<0.001**	1	**<0.001**
Female (n = 4129)	990 (24.0)	0.85 (0.77–0.93)		0.57 (0.50–0.66)	
Age, in years					
13–29 (n = 3679)	980 (26.6)	1	**0.001**	1	**<0.001**
30–59 (n = 2978)	727 (24.4)	0.88 (0.80–0.97)		0.84 (0.75–0.94)	
60+ (n = 850)	200 (23.5)	0.84 (0.71–1.00)		0.71 (0.58–0.87)	
Urbanicity score					
Quartile 1 (least urban) (n = 1978)	488 (24.7)	1	**<0.001**	1	**0.018**
Quartile 2 (n = 1893)	535 (28.3)	1.15 (1.02–1.30)		1.16 (1.02–1.31)	
Quartile 3 (n = 1946)	473 (24.3)	0.94 (0.83–1.07)		0.96 (0.85–1.09)	
Quartile 4 (very urban) (n = 1690)	411 (24.3)	0.95 (0.83–1.10)		0.98 (0.86–1.12)	
Highest education level					
None/up to p4 (n = 2112)	596 (28.2)	1	**<0.001**	1	**<0.001**
P5–P7 (n = 3365)	880 (26.2)	0.85 (0.77–0.95)		0.81 (0.73–0.91)	
Secondary+ (n = 2030)	431 (21.2)	0.66 (0.58–0.76)		0.64 (0.55–0.74)	
Cigarette consumption					
Never smokers (n = 6747)	1718 (25.5)	1	0.992	1	0.471
Ever smokers (n = 760)	189 (24.9)	1.00 (0.86–1.16)		0.94 (0.79–1.11)	
Alcohol consumption					
Never drinkers (n = 4844)	1276 (26.3)	1	**<0.001**	1	**<0.001**
Ex-drinkers (n = 583)	155 (26.6)	1.06 (0.90–1.25)		1.00 (0.84–1.20)	
Current drinkers (n = 2080)	476 (22.9)	0.81 (0.73–0.89)		0.78 (0.69–0.88)	
HIV/ART status					
Negative (n = 6821)	1711 (25.1)	1	**<0.001**	1	**<0.001**
Positive, on ART (n = 201)	33 (16.4)	0.54 (0.39–0.73)		0.57 (0.41–0.78)	
Positive, not on ART (n = 396)	133 (33.6)	1.62 (1.34–1.96)		1.76 (1.45–2.13)	
BMI category					
Underweight (n = 1701)	459 (27.0)	1	**<0.001**	1	**<0.001**
Normal (n = 4878)	1177 (24.1)	0.85 (0.76–0.95)		0.98 (0.87–1.10)	
Overweight (n = 730)	197 (27.0)	1.07 (0.91–1.27)		1.29 (1.07–1.55)	
Obese (n = 198)	74 (37.4)	1.70 (1.29–2.24)		2.08 (1.55–2.79)	
Waist-hip ratio					
Normal, ≤0.95-m, ≤0.80-f (n = 4440)	1065 (24.0)	1	**0.001**	1	**<0.001**
Abnormal, >0.95-m, >0.80-f (n = 3067)	842 (27.5)	1.17 (1.07–1.28)		1.55 (1.36–1.77)	
Total cholesterol (mmol/L)					
Desirable (≤5.2) (n = 7084)	1814 (25.6)	1	0.291	1	0.359
High (>5.2) (n = 423)	93 (22.0)	0.90 (0.74–1.09)		0.91 (0.74–1.12)	
HbA1-C					
Normal ≤6% (n = 7469)	1891 (25.3)	1	**0.004**	1	**0.014**
Raised ≥6.5% (n = 19)	11 (57.9)	3.65 (1.49–8.93)		3.17 (1.27–7.96)	

$^{\phi}$High atherogenic risk versus intermediate and low risk.

Competing Interests

The authors do not report any potential competing interests relevant to this paper.

Authors' Contributions

Anatoli Kamali conceived and designed the experiments. Clara Wekesa and Gershim Asiki performed the experiments. Ivan Kasamba, Laban Waswa, and Rebecca N. Nsubuga analysed the data. Clara Wekesa, Gershim Asiki, Rob Newton, and Steven J. Reynolds wrote the paper.

Acknowledgments

This work was supported and funded by the UK Medical Research Council (MRC) and the UK Department for International Development (DFID) under the MRC/DFID Concordat Agreement, University of Cambridge, UK, and the Wellcome Trust Sanger. Steven J. Reynolds was supported by the Division of Intramural Research, National Institute of Allergy and Infectious Diseases, National Institutes of Health. The authors would like to acknowledge the work of the GPC team and all other MRC/UVRI staff who contributed to this study. They are grateful to all the study participants. Support for paper writing was provided by Fogarty International Center, National Institutes of Health (Grant no. D43TW009771: "HIV Coinfections in Uganda: TB, Cryptococcus, and Viral Hepatitis").

References

[1] World Health Organisation, *Cardiovascular Diseases (CVDs)*, World Health Organisation, Geneva, Switzerland, 2013.

[2] A. D. Alwan, G. Galea, and D. Stuckler, "Development at risk: addressing noncommunicable diseases at the United Nations high-level meeting," *Bulletin of the World Health Organization*, vol. 89, no. 8, pp. 546–546A, 2011.

[3] J. J. Dalal, T. N. Padmanabhan, P. Jain, S. Patil, H. Vasnawala, and A. Gulati, "Lipitension: Interplay between dyslipidemia and hypertension," *Indian Journal of Endocrinology and Metabolism*, vol. 16, no. 2, pp. 240–245, 2012.

[4] M. Twagirumukiza, D. de Bacquer, J. G. Kips, G. de Backer, R. V. Stichele, and L. M. Van Bortel, "Current and projected prevalence of arterial hypertension in sub-Saharan Africa by sex, age and habitat: an estimate from population studies," *Journal of Hypertension*, vol. 29, no. 7, pp. 1243–1252, 2011.

[5] P. Kotwani, D. Kwarisiima, T. D. Clark et al., "Epidemiology and awareness of hypertension in a rural Ugandan community: a cross-sectional study," *BMC Public Health*, vol. 13, article 1151, 2013.

[6] G. Musinguzi and F. Nuwaha, "Prevalence, awareness and control of hypertension in Uganda," *PLoS ONE*, vol. 8, no. 4, Article ID e62236, 2013.

[7] W. B. Kannel, "Fifty years of Framingham study contributions to understanding hypertension," *Journal of Human Hypertension*, vol. 14, no. 2, pp. 83–90, 2000.

[8] A. Bottger, H. A. Van Lith, V. Kren et al., "Quantitative trait loci influencing cholesterol and phospholipid phenotypes map to chromosomes that contain genes regulating blood pressure in the spontaneously hypertensive rat," *Journal of Clinical Investigation*, vol. 98, no. 3, pp. 856–862, 1996.

[9] F. Thomas, K. Bean, L. Guize, S. Quentzel, P. Argyriadis, and A. Benetos, "Combined effects of systolic blood pressure and serum cholesterol on cardiovascular mortality in young (< years) men and women," *European Heart Journal*, vol. 23, no. 7, pp. 528–535, 2002.

[10] P. Castelli and K. Anderson, "A population at risk: prevalence of high cholesterol levels in hypertensive patients in the Framingham study," *The American Journal of Medicine*, vol. 80, no. 2, pp. 33–39, 1986.

[11] P. W. F. Wilson, R. B. D'Agostino, D. Levy, A. M. Belanger, H. Silbershatz, and W. B. Kannel, "Prediction of coronary heart disease using risk factor categories," *Circulation*, vol. 97, pp. 1837–1847, 1998.

[12] M. R. Law, N. J. Wald, and S. G. Thompson, "By how much and how quickly does reduction in serum cholesterol concentration lower risk of ischaemic heart disease?" *British Medical Journal*, vol. 308, no. 6925, pp. 367–372, 1994.

[13] J. Millán, X. Pintó, A. Muñoz et al., "Lipoprotein ratios: physiological significance and clinical usefulness in cardiovascular prevention," *Vascular Health and Risk Management*, vol. 5, pp. 757–765, 2009.

[14] H. R. Superko and S. King, "Lipid management to reduce cardiovascular risk: a new strategy is required," *Circulation*, vol. 117, pp. 560–568, 2008.

[15] M. Dobiášová, "Atherogenic index of plasma [log(triglycerides/HDL-cholesterol)]: theoretical and practical implications," *Clinical Chemistry*, vol. 50, no. 7, pp. 1113–1115, 2004.

[16] V. Bittner, B. D. Johnson, I. Zineh et al., "The triglyceride/high-density lipoprotein cholesterol ratio predicts all-cause mortality in women with suspected myocardial ischemia. A Report From the Women's Ischemia Syndrome Evaluation (WISE)," *American Heart Journal*, vol. 157, no. 3, pp. 548–555, 2009.

[17] J. M. Gaziano, C. H. Hennekens, C. J. O'Donnell, J. L. Breslow, and J. E. Buring, "Fasting triglycerides, high-density lipoprotein, and risk of myocardial infarction," *Circulation*, vol. 96, no. 8, pp. 2520–2525, 1997.

[18] U. Nwagha, E. J. Ikekpeazu, F. E. Ejezie, E. E. Neboh, and I. C. Maduka, "Atherogenic index of plasma as useful predictor of cardiovascular risk among postmenopausal women in Enugu, Nigeria," *African Health Sciences*, vol. 10, no. 3, pp. 248–252, 2010.

[19] K. Wan, J. Zhao, H. Huang et al., "The association between triglyceride/high-density lipoprotein cholesterol ratio and all-cause mortality in acute coronary syndrome after coronary revascularization," *PLoS ONE*, vol. 10, no. 4, Article ID e0123521, 2015.

[20] W. P. Castelli, "Epidemiology of coronary heart disease: The Framingham Study," *The American Journal of Medicine*, vol. 76, no. 2, pp. 4–12, 1984.

[21] M. Dobiášová, "AIP—atherogenic index of plasma as a significant predictor of cardiovascular risk: from research to practice," *Vnitrni Lekarstvi*, vol. 52, no. 1, pp. 64–71, 2006.

[22] D. Guwatudde, G. Mutungi, R. Wesonga et al., "The epidemiology of hypertension in Uganda: findings from the national non-communicable diseases risk factor survey," *PLoS ONE*, vol. 10, no. 9, Article ID e0138991, 2015.

[23] G. Asiki, G. A. V. Murphy, K. Baisley et al., "Prevalence of dyslipidaemia and associated risk factors in a rural population in South-Western Uganda: a community based survey," *PLoS ONE*, vol. 10, no. 5, Article ID e0126166, 2015.

[24] G. F. Watts, "Treating patients with low HDL-cholesterol: choices, issues and opportunities," *Current Controlled Trials in Cardiovascular Medicine*, vol. 2, no. 3, pp. 118–122, 2001.

[25] G. Asiki, G. Murphy, J. Nakiyingi-Miiro et al., "The general population cohort in rural south-western Uganda: a platform for communicable and non-communicable disease studies," *International Journal of Epidemiology*, vol. 42, no. 1, pp. 129–141, 2013.

[26] J. Riha, A. Karabarinde, G. Ssenyomo et al., "Urbanicity and lifestyle risk factors for cardiometabolic diseases in rural Uganda: a cross-sectional study," *PLoS Medicine*, vol. 11, no. 7, Article ID e1001683, 2014.

[27] WHO, *Use of Glycated Haemoglobin (HbA1c) in the Diagnosis of Diabetes Mellitus*, World Health Organization, 2011.

[28] Uganda National Policy Guidelines for HIV Counselling and Testing Ministry of Health Uganda, 2003.

[29] *National Guidelines for Research Involving Humans as Research Participants*, UNCST, Kampala, Uganda, 2007.

[30] J. Idemudia, E. Ugwuja, O. Afonja, E. Idogun, and N. Ugwu, "C-Reactive proteins and cardiovascular risk indices in hypertensive Nigerians," *The Internet Journal of Cardiovascular Research*, vol. 6, no. 2, 2008.

[31] S. Niroumand, M. Khajedaluee, M. Khadem-Rezaiyan et al., "Atherogenic Index of Plasma (AIP): a marker of cardiovascular disease," *Medical Journal of The Islamic Republic of Iran (MJIRI)*, vol. 29, p. 240, 2015.

[32] S. Yusuf, S. Hawken, S. Ôunpuu et al., "Effect of potentially modifiable risk factors associated with myocardial infarction in 52 countries (the INTERHEART study): case-control study," *The Lancet*, vol. 364, no. 9438, pp. 937–952, 2004.

[33] P. L. Da Luz, D. Favarato, J. R. Faria-Neto Jr., P. Lemos, and A. C. P. Chagas, "High ratio of triglycerides to HDL-cholesterol predicts extensive coronary disease," *Clinics*, vol. 63, no. 4, pp. 427–432, 2008.

[34] D. Périard, A. Telenti, P. Sudre et al., "Atherogenic dyslipidemia in HIV-infected individuals treated with protease inhibitors," *Circulation*, vol. 100, no. 7, pp. 700–705, 1999.

[35] V. A. Triant, "HIV infection and coronary heart disease: an intersection of epidemics," *Journal of Infectious Diseases*, vol. 205, no. 3, pp. S355–S361, 2012.

[36] C. J. O'Donnell and R. Elosua, "Cardiovascular risk factors. Insights from framingham heart study," *Revista Española de Cardiología*, vol. 61, no. 3, pp. 299–310, 2008.

27

Health and Social Needs in Three Migrant Worker Communities around La Romana, Dominican Republic, and the Role of Volunteers: A Thematic Analysis and Evaluation

Aaron S. Miller,[1,2] Henry C. Lin,[2,3] Chang-Berm Kang,[2] and Lawrence C. Loh[1,2]

[1] *University of Toronto, Toronto, ON, Canada M5S 1A1*
[2] *The 53rd Week, Brooklyn, NY 11201, USA*
[3] *Perelman School of Medicine, University of Pennsylvania, Philadelphia, PA 19104, USA*

Correspondence should be addressed to Aaron S. Miller; quickdrawdoc@yahoo.com

Academic Editor: Jean P. Gonzalez

Objective. For decades, Haitian migrant workers living in bateyes around La Romana, Dominican Republic, have been the focus of short-term volunteer medical groups from North America. To assist these efforts, this study aimed to characterize various health and social needs that could be addressed by volunteer groups. *Design.* Needs were assessed using semistructured interviews of community and professional informants, using a questionnaire based on a social determinants of health framework, and responses were qualitatively analysed for common themes. *Results.* Key themes in community responses included significant access limitations to basic necessities and healthcare, including limited access to regular electricity and potable water, lack of health insurance, high out-of-pocket costs, and discrimination. Healthcare providers identified the expansion of a community health promoter program and mobile medical teams as potential solutions. English and French language training, health promotion, and medical skills development were identified as additional strategies by which teams could support community development. *Conclusion.* Visiting volunteer groups could work in partnership with community organizations to address these barriers by providing short-term access to services, while developing local capacity in education, healthcare, and health promotion in the long-term. Future work should also carefully evaluate the impacts and contributions of such volunteer efforts.

1. Introduction

Decades of economic migration from Haiti to the Dominican Republic (DR) gave rise to a sizeable minority population of Haitians that represent an inexpensive source of labour for various sectors of the Dominican economy, particularly the sugar industry [1, 2]. As a result of sociopolitical discrimination, low levels of educational attainment, and denied access to identity documents, the Haitian population in the DR is significantly marginalized [3, 4]. Those employed by the sugar industry are often housed in *bateyes*, which are rural towns characterized by endemic poverty and limited access to health and social services [2].

The marginalization of *batey* populations results in poor population health status and notable community disease burdens around HIV/AIDS, tuberculosis, and malnutrition [5–7]. Specifically, a review of medical conditions treated by mobile medical clinics in the *bateyes* found that while the most common diagnoses encountered were gastroesophageal reflux disease, hypertension, upper respiratory tract infections, otitis media, and fungal skin infections, diseases unique to an indigent tropical population were also commonly encountered, including dehydration, malnutrition, parasites, and rare infections [8].

Described barriers to healthcare experienced by this group include insufficient health insurance coverage, geographic restrictions, and limited understanding of or trust in the local healthcare system arising from reports of humiliation and discrimination [2, 9]. The issues have captured the attention of volunteer groups from the United States and Canada, which visit the DR in ever-growing numbers to provide various charitable services (e.g., primary healthcare services through mobile medical clinics) [10]. *Hospital El Buen Samaritano* (Good Samaritan Hospital or HBS), in La Romana, has hosted visiting groups since the early 1980s. As the third-largest city in the Dominican Republic and hub for the eastern Dominican sugarcane industry, La Romana presents one of the best opportunities to explore concerns around health and social status in batey communities in the Dominican Republic. Specifically, groups from HBS provide mobile medical clinics over one to two weeks throughout the year to a catchment population of 13,000 *batey* residents across an area of 160 *bateyes* (personal communication was from the Hospital El Buen Samaritano administrator Moises Sifren Juan).

Program planning and evaluation require improved evidence and data on the health status of the community, but extant literature on the subject is limited. This paper begins to address this gap by identifying key themes summarized from a community evaluation of stakeholder perceptions on the state of health determinants in the *batey* communities of La Romana. The findings of the present study represent potential areas for future exploration and service that could be targeted by visiting volunteer groups to La Romana and also will act as foundational data by which other visiting groups with efforts focused on *batey* health in the Dominican Republic might evaluate their work.

2. Methods

This community evaluation employed semistructured interview techniques to obtain insight from two key populations into the subject of local health determinants and the role of volunteer teams. Key informants from among local professionals that interact with visiting teams and members of the local community were interviewed. The initial step in developing an interview guide was to conduct a cursory literature search for relevant articles and health data on Haitian economic migrants residing in the DR. This consisted of a search of PubMed, a grey literature search, and obtaining health indicator statistics from Dominican Republic government databases and the Pan American Health Organisation. Authors identified valuable articles from abstracts by consensus. In partnership with local program collaborators, articles, along with relevant statistics and health data, were used to identify guiding questions which formed a framework for the development of an 18-item interview guide. Following translation, the guide was reviewed and revised by local partners for cultural appropriateness and nuance.

This guide was subsequently used in the conduct of semistructured interviews with the two key stakeholder populations described earlier: (1) members of the local population of migrant Haitian workers and (2) local healthcare providers and leaders. These groups were targeted to provide both professional and lay-person insight into various community needs and deficits relevant to volunteer activities. Data collection took place during a one-week field visit in December 2012 with community members from three *bateyes* of varied size and location and with staff at local partner institution. To ensure consistency in prompts, format, recording, and interpretation, all interviews were conducted by one of the investigators of this paper, with help from an interpreter who acted as a cultural interpreter and had received briefing on the overall project. Based on a sampling process developed by the local hospital partner, three bateyes were targeted as representative, and research proceeded as planned. The interpreter guided respondent selection using a systematic process in each of the *bateyes* (every fifth attendee at the community health clinic) and by a snowball method among hospital leadership and employees.

Interview responses were recorded electronically and on paper. Following data collection, these were collated and qualitatively analysed in aggregate by investigators for common themes, using an analysis framework based on the original guiding questions. For each guiding question, responses were coded by two different investigators for relevant themes. Any discrepancies between reviewers were resolved through consensus discussion and consultation with local partners. Following coding, key themes were identified based on frequency and targeted for inclusion in final results.

Institutional research ethics approval was obtained from the University of Toronto ethics review board (protocol ID 28419). Upon receiving approval from the University of Toronto REB, local community approval was granted by the leadership of HBS. As there was no local ethics review board in La Romana, HBS leadership granted approval to proceed with this study in the La Romana area provided that the researchers involved adhere to the terms of the REB approval granted by the University of Toronto.

3. Results

30 community informants were interviewed (9 male, 21 female) across three *bateyes*: *Batey* 1 ($n = 12$), *Batey* 203 ($n = 7$), and *Batey* Cacata ($n = 11$). The three *bateyes* targeted represented a collective estimated population of 3,600 inhabitants. This included *Batey* 1 which had a population of 300 inhabitants, *Batey* 203 with 300 inhabitants, and *Batey* Cacata with 3,600 inhabitants. 11 health professional informants at the local mission hospital were also interviewed and represented both administrators and direct care providers. For both groups of informants, key themes explored included community needs, health priorities, and healthcare access. Unique themes emerging among community informants centered around basic necessities, including water, electricity, food, and clothing; unique themes identified by health professional informants included specific health programs and the role of the mission hospital, as well as perceptions on disease patterns and epidemiology.

3.1. Community Informants

3.1.1. Water. Potential sources for drinking water identified by respondents included pipe, well, and bottled water. Of these, respondents uniformly reported preferring bottled water despite its cost.

Further review of responses identifying bottled water as a preferred source highlighted several common themes as rationale: respondents believed that bottled water was more palatable and safer to drink and was also inexpensive at approximately RD $40 ($1 USD) per 19-liter bottle.

Exploring the theme of price versus quality further, responses highlighted concerns about how potable municipal water delivered by pipe was, despite the fact that it was provided free of charge. Specific to potential solutions and the role of volunteers, responses occasionally referenced a water filtration and sanitation implementation initiative jointly conducted by the local mission hospital and visiting volunteers that aimed to improve access to potable water from municipal sources in all *bateyes*.

3.1.2. Electricity. While some informants reported regular and available access to electricity with reported costs in the range RD $300–$460 (approximately $7–$11 USD) per month, there were notable variations between *bateyes* that suggested infrastructure deficits. For example, respondents at *Batey* 1 reported regular access to electricity while those at *Batey* 203 reported having no access to electricity; *Batey Cacata* respondents reported partial electrification of community dwellings, with some respondents without access.

A theme arising among respondents without electric access was safety and security at night and sources of light.

Respondents identified both kerosene lamps and candles as potential lighting sources. These responses did identify slightly additional cost burden as the reported cost of kerosene and/or candles was RD $50 ($1 USD) for 3 days' use, which adds up to RD $500 monthly ($10 USD monthly).

3.1.3. Food and Clothing. Respondents noted that food was not provided by the company but was purchased out of pocket. Related to this, themes identified variations in sourcing, commonly related to finances. Small, local *batey* stores (on-*batey*) and a large supermarket in central La Romana were identified as venues, and respondents stated that the *batey* store was most commonly accessed when finances were tight.

The supermarket was more highly regarded by respondents, but many of them added the caveat that accessing this venue involved greater spending to pay both for groceries and for transport (responses estimated an average of RD $2000 or US $47 in total).

When asked about clothing supply, respondents did not identify any specific concerns. Themes in responses largely discussed the duration to which clothing remained viable, which was 6 to 24 months, and plans for replacement, which involved either attending a shop in La Romana or receiving clothing via charity.

3.1.4. Healthcare Access and Insurance. While some respondents did not attend Good Samaritan Hospital, others reported visiting up to 11 times in the previous year, with an average of two annual hospital visits. Uninsured individuals paid a range of fees for services of RD $1000–$5000 (approximately $23–$120 USD), depending on the nature of the visit. This included payments for primary care services, which were provided through the hospital. 19 respondents reported receiving medical insurance coverage through their company, which also covered their immediate family, with monthly costs in the range of RD $150–$400 (approximately $3.50–$10 USD) per month, depending on the plan. Insured respondents reported being satisfied with the cost of insurance. 11 uninsured respondents, by contrast, stated that hospital services were expensive.

The provision of care at the hospital was perceived as adequate by the vast majority of respondents. For responses that perceived care as being poor, expressed concerns around the quality of care included the nature of treatment being ineffective or a waste of time and money or the notion that competing needs prevented them from spending money on healthcare.

Alternative venues identified by respondents, considering time and financial constraints, included a community health promoter or going to a local Dominican *batey* clinic sometimes. These respondents perceived local *batey* clinics to be inferior to larger hospitals in La Romana but also saw them as more convenient.

3.1.5. Community Needs. Exploring the relationship between education and health, specific themes around further education or training were identified, with a specific focus on what would benefit the communities. Responses identified diverse content areas, including English and French language education, health promotion and nursing skills, computer skills, and improved primary education for children, particularly protected access.

Additional themes concerned social skills, sewing, and cooking.

3.2. Health Professional Interviews

3.2.1. Hospital Infrastructure and Programs. A common theme among responses was the important role that the mission hospital had played in providing care to the community for over twenty years. Growth was another commonly identified theme, with respondents highlighting that initial hospital construction efforts would reach completion in 2015 and that, over time, the hospital has emerged as a major medical hub for the estimated 20,000 Haitian workers living in the *bateyes*, as well as the wider La Romana community. Partnerships were another common theme identified by respondents, which noted that over 60 volunteering organizations visit annually, usually nonprofits, church groups, and academic institutions. Specific themes in the focus of these volunteer trips included both medical clinics and surgeries provided at no expense to the hospital or patients.

3.2.2. Batey Health Needs and Programs. As a whole, respondents viewed medical teams favorably and uniformly identified a need for more teams in the future. They cited a number of needs that could be addressed by visiting teams on locally established community work projects. These included the construction of churches and the continued development of water filtration and sanitation systems. Specifically, the impact of mobile medical clinics was positively viewed; one respondent pointed out that this outreach effort had provided service annually to nearly 13,000 *batey* residents.

Another commonly identified theme centered around the work of a local community health work (health promoter) program, which respondents identified as a potential area for collaboration with volunteer teams. Detailed descriptions provided in the responses suggested that the program recruits local *batey* community leaders into training and employment with the hospital; those recruited act as medical liaisons and first responders in their communities, providing basic medications and conducting health education. One respondent identified a deficit in the number of health promoters, however, with only 60 of 160 *bateyes* served, but this deficit was explained as arising not for lack of willing promoters but was instead due to a lack of funding to employ new promoters.

The health promoter's current scope of practice is limited to taking axillary temperatures, administering first aid, checking heart rates, administering deworming medications, and health promotion.

3.2.3. Healthcare Cost and Access. Themes matched those of community respondents in noting a difference in access, cost, and service variation for patients depending on insurance status, with insured patients paying approximately RD \$600 (approximately \$14 USD) per visit and uninsured patients paying anywhere in the range of RD \$1000–\$5000 (approximately \$23–\$120 USD) per visit, depending on the visit purpose. One respondent described other auxiliary services (such as an in-house social worker) which helped uninsured patients afford treatment. Those patients who are unable to pay are aided through establishing a payment plan or are referred to a local public hospital where the costs are generally lower.

3.2.4. Disease Patterns. Respondents suggested that the most commonly reported ailments among *batey* residents were asthma, respiratory infections, and fever. There was a concern among providers that while they were largely able to effectively meet the needs of the individual patients they see in the hospital, they felt they were not meeting the health needs of the wider community.

3.2.5. Perceptions of Visiting Teams. Respondents favorably viewed visiting groups and their mobile medical clinics and identified one potential focus area as being on local capacity development. Identified content themes included training for *batey* promoters, family planning education, sexual education (particularly around providing contraception and teaching its correct use), and nutritional counseling.

Additional responses suggested that groups could lend their perspective and advice on hospital processes, such as telemedicine, and develop an international physician-exchange program.

4. Discussion

La Romana, like many *batey* areas of the Dominican Republic, has become the focus of an ever-increasing number of short-term volunteer efforts, particularly mobile medical clinics. To interpret our findings, we applied a social determinants of health (SDOH) framework to responses in order to identify general perturbations in key determinants that might benefit from planning efforts around visiting volunteer groups in the community. The responses provided in the previous section highlight a number of key determinants that might be addressed in order to improve individual and collective community health (e.g., limited access to healthcare, education, low income and employment, and community security). This framework guides our discussion around notable trends below. The determinants for the SDOH framework were derived from the Public Health Agency of Canada website [11].

4.1. Determinant: Education and Literacy. The focus of training and programs suggested by respondents varied between both the community and health professional respondents. Themes from the former group focused on skills development, such as English and French education, and access to resources, such as added nursing care. The importance of language education reflected the extant limited level of English fluency and the preponderance of Haitian Creole and, to a lesser extent, Spanish spoken in this community.

Development of community health promoter skills represented one potential avenue to increase local capacity to address a greater range of community health needs. Successes of this nature could assist new promoter recruitment efforts while allowing for evaluation of existing health promoters and the implementation of quality improvement programs.

The favorable impression of volunteer groups by respondents in La Romana suggests community willingness to share ideas and work collaboratively with visiting groups on health education and community development. Maintaining this goodwill is essential to preventing misunderstanding and maintaining a good working relationship and can be accomplished through predeparture training that focuses on cultural sensitivity, ethics, community partnership, and responsible volunteering.

4.2. Determinant: Physical Environments. Themes around access to water, an essential necessity, highlight several areas of concern. The perception (and likely reality) that bottled water is healthier presents a notable burden in that purchasing bottled water, no matter how inexpensively it is perceived, represents an additional financial strain on the limited finances of this population. A successful water filtration project, the inception of which was identified in certain responses, would thus both meet an essential need and mitigate the financial burden associated with bottled water purchase.

Similar themes were noted in access to electricity. In particular, lack of electricity results in inconsistent access to lighting, which has implications for community safety and evening activities. There appears to be continuing work supporting ongoing electrical infrastructure installation, especially in *Batey* Cacata, where infrastructure was being extended to new growth areas in the community.

Consensus in themes favors adequate clothing supplies with continued access to new clothing. It is worth noting that neither *batey* residents nor hospital providers interviewed mentioned donation or access to clothing as being a community need.

4.3. Determinant: Health Services. Despite being established as a hospital to provide for indigent residents of *bateyes*, professional respondents seemed to indicate that many of the patients treated at HBS were patients with health insurance coverage. While this might reflect an ascertainment bias, as insured *batey* citizens might be more willing to seek care, this theme parallels a similar theme noted among community respondents who reported that local hospitals were cheaper and therefore more accessible, despite quality of care concerns.

Responses on common diseases in the community were concordant between care providers and *batey* residents. Notably, few community responses identified HIV/AIDS as a common disease on the part of *batey* residents, despite high rates of prevalence documented in the literature [12]. This concurs with published factors in Rojas et al.'s study [5] which suggest that a lack of awareness or unwillingness to address HIV/AIDS is related to social stigma, lack of knowledge as to status, and limited access to testing and care providers. The stigma that limits responses has implications for both prevention and education efforts as well as screening and treatment in this population.

It is also worth noting that the DR has specific legislation that contains publically supported provisions for various allowances, such as old age, disability, survivor coverage, sickness and maternity, and family [13]. However, Haitian migrants in the Dominican Republic are not given access to these provisions under Dominican law, which is exacerbated for Haitians who lack legal documentation of status [2].

4.4. Determinant: Gender and Culture. Perceptions of the quality of care might well determine the willingness on the part of patients to spend time and money on seeking treatment for illness. If individuals do not believe that they will receive quality care or that the provision of the care accessible to them is not in keeping with their cultural values, they may be less inclined, able, or willing to pursue it [14, 15]. Related to the responses, this raises concerns that this disenfranchised population might choose to forgo access to care to save money, especially if they feel that the care they might receive would be inadequate. This may be influenced by cultural gender roles: do men and women perceive the necessity for healthcare similarly? And whose responsibility might it be to seek treatment for children in their care? Also, to what extent might language barriers preclude or disincentivize care-seeking behaviour?

4.5. Limitations and Future Work. This preliminary work aims to provide some broad representations of barriers to health among Haitian *batey* residents in La Romana. There is a possibility that the findings from the three bateyes may not be representative of the broader 160 bateyes. However, concurrence in responses with interviewed hospital and healthcare providers mitigates this somewhat.

Additional detailed interviews and analysis could be conducted with the local general hospital in La Romana and local care providers at *batey* clinics. The development of hospital and clinic indicators based on these findings could support in-depth quantitative studies. Additionally, in interviewing *batey* residents, we did not inquire into the typical salaries of *batey* workers as well as the availability and quality of food available to residents at their local stores. This information would have been useful in drawing inferences from the illnesses reported based on the nourishment available.

5. Conclusions

Broadly reviewing the responses against a social determinant of health framework provides a descriptive summary of the environmental, cultural, educational, and systems level barriers that may diminish the health status of *batey* populations in La Romana. Limited access to potable water, adequate food, and electricity increases community susceptibility to infectious disease and injury and exacerbates safety and security concerns. These basic issues are further exacerbated by limited access to medical insurance coverage, low family wages, and access to quality healthcare services.

In addressing these determinants, respondents have indicated that volunteer teams may have a role to play in providing services and developing capacity in these communities. This study presents an initial formative assessment of barriers to health and wellbeing in the community as well as potential strategies to address them that should be explored. Additionally, given the evolving Dominican government position on migrant Haitian communities, another worthwhile line of inquiry would also be to determine whether the Dominican government might have the resources, political will, and understanding of potential benefits for costs needed to provide programs and policies that support rather than persecute this vulnerable population. Highlighting and seizing such opportunities, while being largely theoretical at this point, would provide the most lasting improvements to the health status of the migrant worker population.

Further research will also be needed to clearly identify quantitative measures on the concerns and themes identified which can be used to direct volunteer efforts more effectively. At the heart of any redirection of effort is the community goodwill that is related to the work of volunteer teams in partnership with the local hospital, which forms the basis through which collaborative work might meaningfully address these perturbations in the root causes of ill health in these *batey* communities.

Competing Interests

The authors declare that they have no competing interests.

Acknowledgments

The research team recognizes the contributions from local partners in the DR and all of the participants who took part in the conduct of the research. In particular, the authors recognize HBS leadership and numerous staff in both the approval and the implementation of this work, including interpreters who provided time and invaluable contributions to the data collection process.

References

[1] S. Alscher, "Environmental degradation and migration on Hispaniola Island," *International Migration*, vol. 49, no. 1, pp. e164–e188, 2011.

[2] J. Ferguson, *Migration in the Caribbean: Haiti, the Dominican Republic and Beyond*, Minority Rights Group International, London, UK, 2003.

[3] J. Duany, "Racializing ethnicity in the Spanish-speaking Caribbean: a comparison of Haitians in the Dominican Republic and Dominicans in Puerto Rico," *Latin American and Caribbean Ethnic Studies*, vol. 1, no. 2, pp. 231–248, 2006.

[4] J. Sidanius, Y. Peña, and M. Sawyer, "Inclusionary discrimination: pigmentocracy and patriotism in the dominican republic," *Political Psychology*, vol. 22, no. 4, pp. 827–851, 2001.

[5] P. Rojas, R. Malow, B. Ruffin, E. M. Rothe, and R. Rosenberg, "The HIV/AIDS epidemic in the Dominican Republic: key contributing factors," *Journal of the International Association of Physicians in AIDS Care*, vol. 10, no. 5, pp. 306–315, 2011.

[6] K. A. Cohn, R. Finalle, G. O'Hare, J. M. Feris, J. Fernández, and S. S. Shah, "Risk factors for intrathoracic tuberculosis in children from economic migrant populations of two dominican republic bateyes," *Pediatric Infectious Disease Journal*, vol. 28, no. 9, pp. 782–786, 2009.

[7] T. H. Brewer, J. Hasbun, C. A. Ryan et al., "Migration, ethnicity and environment: HIV risk factors for women on the sugar cane plantations of the Dominican Republic," *AIDS*, vol. 12, no. 14, pp. 1879–1887, 1998.

[8] B. J. Ferrara, E. Townsley, C. R. MacKay, H. C. Lin, and L. C. Loh, "Short-term global health education programs abroad: disease patterns observed in Haitian migrant worker communities around La Romana, Dominican Republic," *The American Journal of Tropical Medicine and Hygiene*, vol. 91, no. 5, pp. 871–875, 2014.

[9] H. M. Keys, B. N. Kaiser, J. W. Foster, R. Y. Burgos Minaya, and B. A. Kohrt, "Perceived discrimination, humiliation, and mental health: a mixed-methods study among Haitian migrants in the Dominican Republic," *Ethnicity & Health*, vol. 20, no. 3, pp. 219–240, 2014.

[10] H. L. Crouse, C. G. Macias, A. T. Cruz, K. A. Wilson, and S. B. Torrey, "Utilization of a mobile medical van for delivering pediatric care in the bateys of the Dominican Republic," *International Journal of Emergency Medicine*, vol. 3, no. 4, pp. 227–232, 2010.

[11] Public Health Agency of Canada, What makes Canadians healthy or unhealthy?, February 2014, http://www.phac-aspc.gc.ca/ph-sp/determinants/determinants-eng.php#physenviron.

[12] A. S. Bowman, L. Lerebours, S. Amesty et al., "Evaluation of patient care cascade for HIV-positive patients diagnosed in La Romana, Dominican Republic in 2011: a retrospective cohort study," *International Journal of STD & AIDS*, vol. 27, no. 5, pp. 394–401, 2016.

[13] United States Social Security Office of Retirement and Disability Policy, Social Security Programs Throughout the World: The Americas, 2011, Dominican Republic, https://www.ssa.gov/policy/docs/progdesc/ssptw/2010-2011/americas/dominican_republic.html.

[14] M. Alegría, G. Canino, R. Ríos et al., "Mental health care for Latinos: inequalities in use of specialty mental health services among Latinos, African Americans, and non-Latino Whites," *Psychiatric Services*, vol. 53, no. 12, pp. 1547–1555, 2002.

[15] A. D. Federman, E. F. Cook, R. S. Phillips et al., "Intention to discontinue care among primary care patients: influence of physician behavior and process of care," *Journal of General Internal Medicine*, vol. 16, no. 10, pp. 668–674, 2001.

28

Phlebotomines (Diptera: Psychodidae) in a Hydroelectric System Affected Area from Northern Amazonian Brazil: Further Insights into the Effects of Environmental Changes on Vector Ecology

Nercy Virginia Rabelo Furtado,[1] Allan Kardec Ribeiro Galardo,[1] Clicia Denis Galardo,[1] Viviane Caetano Firmino,[2] and Thiago Vasconcelos dos Santos[3]

[1]*Laboratório de Entomologia Médica, Instituto de Pesquisas Científicas e Tecnológicas do Estado do Amapá, Macapá, AP, Brazil*
[2]*Universidade Federal do Amapá, Campus Binacional, Oiapoque, AP, Brazil*
[3]*Instituto Evandro Chagas, Secretaria de Vigilância em Saúde, Ministério da Saúde, Ananindeua, PA, Brazil*

Correspondence should be addressed to Thiago Vasconcelos dos Santos; thiagovasconcelos@iec.pa.gov.br

Academic Editor: Aditya Prasad Dash

During 2012–2015, an entomological survey was conducted as part of a phlebotomine (Diptera: Psychodidae) monitoring program in an area influenced by the Santo Antônio do Jari hydroelectric system (Amapá State, Brazil). The purpose was to study aspects of Amazon/Guianan American cutaneous leishmaniasis (ACL) vectors subjected to stresses by anthropogenic environmental changes. For sampling, CDC light traps were positioned 0.5, 1, and 20 m above ground at five capture locations along the Jari River Basin. Fluctuations in phlebotomine numbers were analyzed to determine any correlation with rainfall, dam waterlogging, and/or ACL cases, from May 2012 to March 2015. We captured 2,800 individuals, and among 45 species identified, *Bichromomyia flaviscutellata*, *Nyssomyia umbratilis*, and *Psychodopygus squamiventris s.l.* were determined to be the main putative vectors, based on current knowledge of the Amazon/Guianan ACL scenario. Rainfall, but not complete flooding, was relatively correlated with phlebotomine fluctuation, mainly observed for *Ps. squamiventris s.l.*, as were ACL cases with *Ny. umbratilis*. Behavioral changes were observed in the unexpected high frequency of *Bi. flaviscutellata* among CDC captures and the noncanopy dominance of *Ny. umbratilis*, possibly attributable to environmental stress in the sampled ecotopes. Continuous entomological surveillance is necessary to monitor the outcomes of these findings.

1. Introduction

Insects of Phlebotominae (Diptera: Psychodidae) species are of great medical interest because of their implications in the transmission of some vector-borne diseases, in particular leishmaniasis [1–3]. American cutaneous leishmaniasis (ACL) is known to be endemic in Amazonian Brazil and is regarded as a serious risk to public health. The high biodiversity of the region induces a complex mosaic of ecological interactions among reservoirs, vectors, and parasites, and consequently a wide spectrum of ACL clinical manifestations, including disfiguring and potentially life-threatening cases [4]. Moreover, this diversity of transmission cycles becomes even more complex to understand in the context of the influence of anthropic effects on natural ecological systems. The consequences of anthropogenic environmental stress on the expansion of the geographical distribution of ACL are, therefore, difficult to predict with any certainty [5].

Over the past 30 years, one of the main causes of human influence on the environment in the Brazilian Amazon Basin is its exploitation for generating energy from hydropower. Negative effects of some of the resultant environmental changes have been observed; an example is the disturbance caused by the proliferation of *Mansonia* (Diptera: Culicidae) in the dammed lake associated with the Tucuruí hydroelectric system [6]. Vector monitoring programs, which are essential to being granted a license to operate, are included in environmental and public health planning, in order to predict and minimize the effects of vector-borne diseases in hydroelectric systems [7]. This monitoring includes spatial/temporal studies of phlebotomines and their potential implications for the transmission dynamics of leishmaniasis agents [8].

The geographically closely related Brazilian states of Pará (PA) and Amapá (AP) share a border through the Jari River and cover a region historically associated with the exploitation and processing of cellulose. Early information about leishmaniasis in the region first emerged in the 1970–1980s. In this period, studies conducted in "Monte Dourado" (Almeirim, PA) provided substantial knowledge about ACL ecoepidemiology, with particular reference to the "pian-bois," a form of cutaneous leishmaniasis caused by *Leishmania (Viannia) guyanensis* (formerly referred to as *Leishmania braziliensis guyanensis*), and its respective identity-obscured vector, *Nyssomyia umbratilis* [9–16].

Since those original studies were undertaken, the region also now hosts the Santo Antônio do Jari hydroelectric system. The present study, therefore, aimed to characterize phlebotomine fauna in the area in order to assess the potential impact of the Santo Antônio do Jari hydroelectric system and in particular the spatiotemporal implications of environmental changes on the ecology of ACL vectors in that region.

2. Materials and Methods

2.1. Study Area. The Santo Antonio do Jari hydroelectric system (0°39′02.4″S 52°30′56.9″W) is situated between the municipalities of Almeirim (PA) and Laranjal do Jari (AP), a region within the Guianan Ecoregion Complex. The hydroelectric system comprises 373.4 MW of installed potency and a reservoir area of 31.7 km^2. Its construction began in 2011, and the system was totally operative from 2014.

The Amazon Region has a "hot-humid" equatorial climate; however, only minor differences are observed in the distinct ecoregions. In this study, four Guianan Ecoregion Complex seasons were characterized as follows: a short rainy (wet) season from mid-November ("novembre humide") to late January; a short dry season between early February and mid-March; a long rainy season from late March to late July; and a long dry season from late July to mid-November [17].

2.2. Sampled Locations. Five locations, each with the following characteristics, were sampled up- and downstream of the caisson (Figure 1):

The eastern bank of the Jari River (AP), covered by alluvial dense forest:

(I) Porto Sabão (S 00°37′02.2″ W 052°30′42.1″), a forested area with only a few dwelling. A small harbor operates from the opposite side of the river.

(II) Iratapuru Village (S 00°33′50.9″ W 052°34′48.5″), a cluster of dwellings, forming a community of approximately 200 inhabitants, which primarily acts as an extractive reserve.

(III) Santo Antônio Village (S 00°38′57.4″ W 052°30′27.9″), which is the only site downstream of the caisson, comprising 27 agriculturist families inhabiting riverine wooden buildings.

The western bank of the Jari River (PA), covered by submontane (lowland) dense forest.

(IV) Traíra (S 00°37′50.7″ W 052°31′48.8″), a location with no dwellings on the Traíra river.

(V) the power Plant (S 00°39′07.7″ W 052°31′06.4″), the most affected area, close to the construction site and with very little vegetation.

2.3. Sampling. Phlebotomine captures were undertaken during 2012 to 2015 in fourteen quadrimonthly field expeditions, which aimed to sample periods in the short dry (February/March), rainy to dry (June/July), and dry to rainy (October/November) Amazon/Guianan seasons. Eight expeditions were undertaken before and six after dammed lake levels were replenished (in May 2014). In each of the above described five areas, a randomly selected horizontal transect was established in the direction of the primarily forested area, comprising a phlebotomine monitoring station (MS), sited approximately 200 m distance from the forest edge, where human settlements were present. Each MS incorporated three CDC miniature light traps (Sudia and Chamberlain model), installed between 18:00 and 06:00 for two consecutive nights. Each was placed according to the following different vertical *strata*: 0.5 m from ground level, 1 m from ground level, and at 20 m, in the tree canopy; they were placed 10 m apart from each other. Trees used for canopy placement of CDC traps were selected based on a minimum height of 20 m, regardless of species. The ground level surface was composed of humid, decomposed organic material, originating from the trees. Phlebotomines were triaged in a stereomicroscope, cleaned with neutral detergent [1% (Extran®)], washed with NaCl 0.9%, and then stored in 70% ethanol. In the laboratory, specimens were processed according to the methodology of Ryan [18], mounted in Berlese fluid (GBI Laboratories, Manchester, England), and identified according to Galati [19].

2.4. Data Analysis. Sampling effort was calculated based on number of expeditions, versus the number of installed CDC traps, versus hours of exposition. Phlebotomine frequency was analyzed for correlation with climatic data (monthly average rainfall, temperature, and air relative humidity) sourced from the Jari Meteorological Station ("Jari Energia" database) and with epidemiology (ACL monthly prevalence) obtained after interrogating the database of the "Coordenação de Vigilância em Saúde" (Coordination of Surveillance in Health) of the "Secretaria de Estado da Saúde do Amapá-SESA" (Amapá State Health Secretary). Data were tested by a single linear regression with Pearson's coefficient (r), using BioEstat 5.0, where the r-value represents a strong correlation if above 0.7, a moderate correlation if between 0.3 and 0.7, a weak correlation if between 0.1 and 0.3, and an insignificant correlation if below 0.1. The index of species abundance (ISA) and the standard index of species abundance (SISA) were calculated using Microsoft Excel for

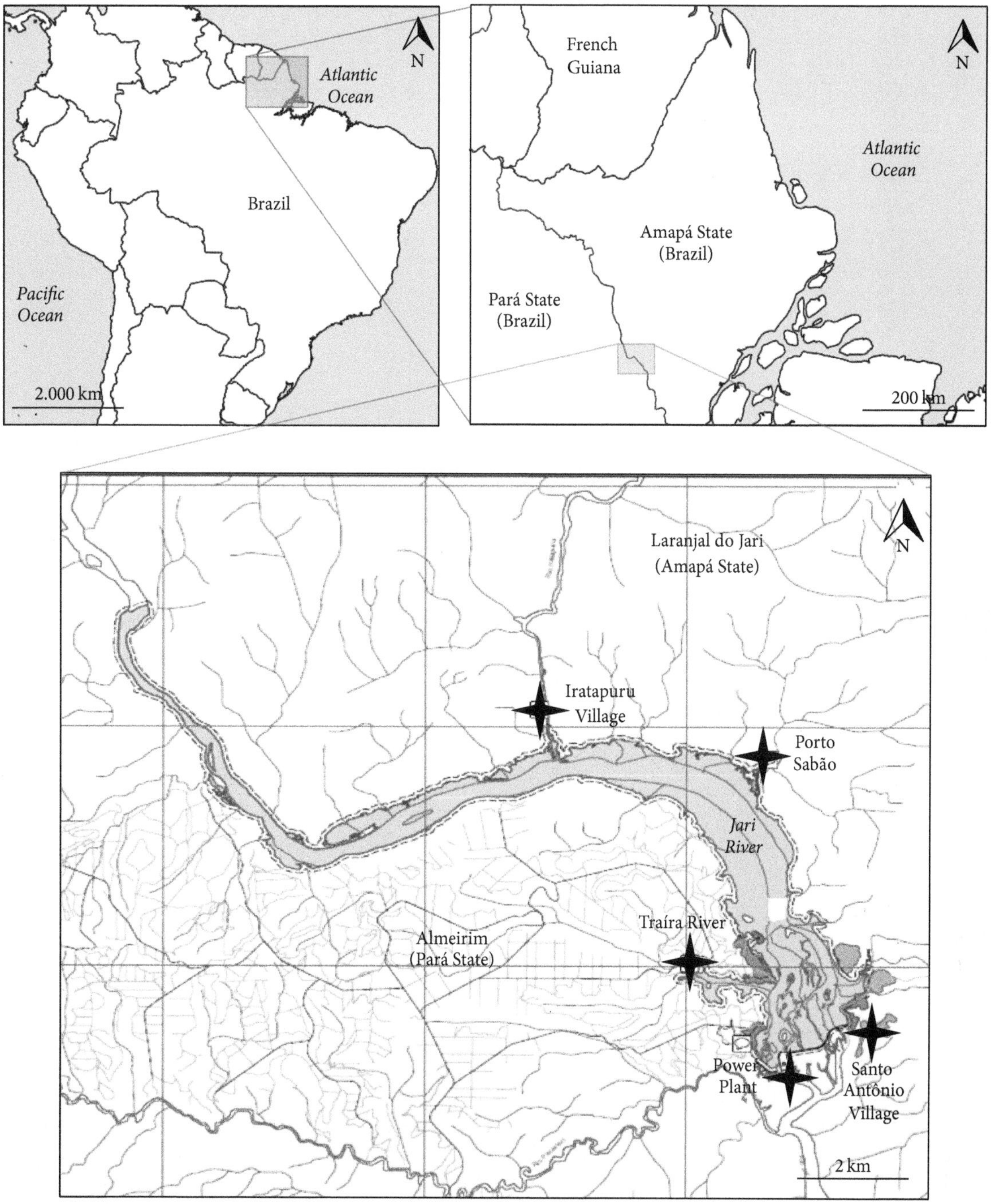

FIGURE 1: Study area. Maps showing the five surveyed locations for phlebotomine captures (2012–2015) in Santo Antônio do Jari hydroelectric system impacted area, between the states of Pará and Amapá, Brazil. ✦: locations.

the five ecotopes surveyed, as described by Roberts and Hsi [20]. Species diversity (Shannon's diversity index, H') and the coefficient of variation (S') between monthly records (climatic and epidemiological) were calculated using Past software [21]. All comparisons were performed using a t-test to determine significance level (p value ≤ 0.05).

3. Results

A total of 2,800 individuals were captured (1,894 females and 906 males), belonging to 45 species, in approximately 2,520 h of sampling effort. Females of *Trichophoromyia* (exceptionally *Th. ubiquitalis*) and *Pressatia* (not identifiable at species level), and some unidentified *Evandromyia*, *Nyssomyia*, and *Psychodopygus* species were allocated at generic level (Table 1).

New AP records included *Th. castanheirai*, *Th. eurypyga*, *Evandromyia begonae*, *Ev. bacula*, *Pressatia equatorialis*, and *Psathyromyia punctigeniculata*.

The five most frequent species captured were *Sciopemyia sordellii* (n = 316; SISA = 0.87), *Ps. davisi* (n = 314; SISA = 0.74), *Bichromomyia flaviscutellata* (n = 265; SISA = 0.95), *Ev.*

TABLE 1: Phebotomine species composition of Santo Antônio do Jari hydroelectric system impacted area (Amapá State, Amazonian Brazil) on the basis of five surveyed locations (2012–2015).

	Species	Porto Sabão		Traíra River		Iratapuru Village		Santo Antônio Village		Power Plant		ISA	SISA	Rank	Total	%
		♀	♂	♀	♂	♀	♂	♀	♂	♀	♂					
1	*Sciopemyia sordellii*	149	66	13	10	15	4	42	16	—	1	3,6	0,87	2nd	316	11,29
2	***Psychodopygus davisi***	46	37	95	56	15	10	38	17	—	—	6,4	0,74	3rd	314	11,21
—	*Trichophoromyia* spp.	177	—	34	—	40	—	17	—	—	—	—	—	—	268	9,57
3	***Bichromomyia flaviscutellata***	76	32	24	14	22	11	52	31	1	2	2	0,95	1st	265	9,46
4	*Evandromyia infraspinosa*	44	10	25	18	3	2	30	18	—	—	9,2	0,6	6th	150	5,36
5	***Nyssomyia umbratilis***	26	12	31	30	19	6	13	9	—	—	8,6	0,63	5th	146	5,21
6	*Trichophoromyia castanheirai*	—	104	—	6	—	14	—	11	—	—	11,2	0,51	9th	135	4,82
—	*Pressatia* spp.	43	—	1	—	9	—	78	—	—	—	—	—	—	131	4,68
—	*Evandromyia* spp.	52	10	4	—	39	11	12	—	—	—	—	—	—	128	4,57
7	*Viannamyia furcata*	44	4	11	5	11	1	30	5	—	—	10,4	0,55	7th	111	3,96
8	***Psychodopygus squamiventris sensu lato***	36	14	15	5	10	—	9	—	—	—	11	0,52	8th	89	3,18
9	*Trichopygomyia trichopyga*	11	16	9	8	9	—	21	12	—	—	7,2	0,7	4th	86	3,07
10	***Trichophoromyia ubiquitalis***	21	6	5	8	14	8	13	9	2	—	11,4	0,5	10th	86	3,07
11	*Evandromyia saulensis*	40	9	5	—	4	4	12	1	—	—	12,8	0,43	11th	75	2,68
12	***Psychodopygus hirsutus hirsutus***	13	—	20	4	14	4	—	—	—	—	13,6	0,4	12th	55	1,96
13	*Trichophoromyia brachypyga*	—	36	—	12	—	2	—	2	—	—	15,2	0,32	14th	52	1,86
14	*Pressatia choti*	—	17	—	3	—	5	—	25	—	—	14,2	0,37	13th	50	1,79
15	***Nyssomyia anduzei***	6	5	24	10	—	—	—	—	—	—	17	0,23	16th	45	1,61
16	***Lutzomyia gomezi***	27	11	—	—	—	—	—	—	—	—	19,4	0,12	22th	38	1,36
—	*Nyssomyia* spp.	—	—	—	1	1	—	11	25	—	—	—	—	—	38	1,36
17	***Nyssomyia antunesi***	—	2	9	—	5	2	—	—	1	—	14,2	0,37	13th	19	0,68
18	*Sciopemyia fluviatilis*	2	1	3	—	9	1	—	—	—	—	18	0,19	18th	16	0,57
19	*Micropygomyia rorotaensis*	4	—	—	—	8	—	2	1	—	—	17,8	0,2	17th	15	0,54
20	***Psychodopygus paraensis***	—	—	—	—	6	3	5	1	—	—	17,6	0,2	17th	15	0,54
21	*Psychodopygus claustrei*	7	1	—	—	—	—	2	—	3	1	15,4	0,31	15th	14	0,50
—	*Psychodopygus* spp.	4	—	2	—	6	—	2	—	—	—	—	—	—	14	0,50
22	*Trichophoromyia eurypyga*	—	8	—	—	—	3	—	1	—	—	18,2	0,18	19th	12	0,43
23	*Psathyromyia aragaoi*	—	—	5	2	—	—	4	—	—	—	18,8	0,15	20th	11	0,39
24	*Evandromyia brachyphalla*	4	3	2	1	1	—	—	—	—	—	19	0,14	21th	11	0,39
25	*Psychodopygus carrerai carrerai*	1	1	—	7	—	—	—	—	—	—	20,2	0,08	26th	9	0,32
26	*Evandromyia begonae*	2	2	—	—	4	—	—	—	—	—	19,6	0,11	23th	8	0,29
27	***Nyssomyia whitmani***	—	—	—	—	—	—	8	—	—	—	20	0,09	25th	8	0,29
28	*Psathyromyia scaffi*	3	2	—	—	2	—	—	—	—	—	19,8	0,1	24th	7	0,25
29	*Pressatia trispinosa*	—	—	—	7	—	—	—	—	—	—	20,4	0,07	27th	7	0,25
30	*Micropygomyia trinidadensis*	7	—	—	—	—	—	—	—	—	—	20,8	0,05	29th	7	0,25
31	*Viannamyia tuberculata*	6	—	—	—	—	—	—	—	—	—	21	0,04	30th	6	0,21
32	*Pintomyia damascenoi*	—	—	—	—	—	—	5	—	—	—	20	0,09	25th	5	0,18
33	*Evandromyia evandroi*	—	—	—	—	4	1	—	—	—	—	20,4	0,07	27th	5	0,18
34	*Psathyromyia lutziana*	5	—	—	—	—	—	—	—	—	—	21,2	0,03	31th	5	0,18
35	*Brumptomia travassosi*	—	—	—	—	—	—	3	1	—	—	19,6	0,11	23th	4	0,14
36	*Evandromyia bacula*	—	—	—	—	1	—	3	—	—	—	20,2	0,08	26th	4	0,14
37	*Evandromyia monstruosa*	—	—	4	—	—	—	—	—	—	—	20,6	0,06	28th	4	0,14

Table 1: Continued.

	Species	Porto Sabão		Traíra River		Iratapuru Village		Santo Antônio Village		Power Plant		ISA	SISA	Rank	Total	%
		♀	♂	♀	♂	♀	♂	♀	♂	♀	♂					
38	*Psychodopygus amazonensis*	—	—	—	—	2	2	—	—	—	—	21	0,04	30th	4	0,14
39	*Psychodopygus corossoniensis*	—	—	—	—	—	2	—	—	—	—	20,6	0,06	28th	2	0,07
40	*Pressatia equatorialis*	—	2	—	—	—	—	—	—	—	—	21	0,04	30th	2	0,07
41	*Psathyromyia inflata*	—	—	—	—	—	—	2	—	—	—	21	0,04	30th	2	0,07
42	*Micropygomyia micropyga*	—	—	—	—	—	—	1	1	—	—	21,4	0,02	32th	2	0,07
43	*Psychodopygus geniculatus*	—	—	—	2	—	—	—	—	—	—	21,8	0	33th	2	0,07
44	*Lutzomyia carvalhoi*	—	—	1	—	—	—	—	—	—	—	20,8	0,05	29th	1	0,04
45	*Psathyromyia punctigeniculata*	—	—	—	—	1	—	—	—	—	—	21,6	0,01	32th	1	0,04
	Total	*856*	*411*	*342*	*209*	*274*	*96*	*415*	*186*	*7*	*4*				*2800*	*100,0*
		1267		*551*		*370*		*601*		*11*						

Each location comprised a monitoring station (MS) sampled with 0.5, 1, and 20 m CDC traps, providing approximately 504 h/MS.
♀: female; ♂: male; ISA: index of species abundance; SISA: standard index of species abundance.
"the bold italic font" Proven and/or putative ACL vectors in the Amazon Region, based in Young and Duncan [1], Rangel and Lainson [4], Ready [2], and Lainson and Shaw [16].

Table 2: Vertical stratification of Phebotomine species composition of Santo Antônio do Jari hydroelectric system impacted area (Amapá State, Amazonian Brazil) on the basis of five surveyed locations (2012–2015).

	Species	0.5 m ground		1 m ground		20 m canopy		Total
		♀	♂	♀	♂	♀	♂	
1	*Sciopemyia sordellii*	117	71	91	23	11	3	*316*
2	*Psychodopygus davisi*	48	27	44	39	102	54	*314*
—	*Trichophoromyia* spp.	117	—	127	—	24	—	*268*
3	*Bichromomyia flaviscutellata*	85	45	79	41	11	4	*265*
4	*Evandromyia infraspinosa*	38	18	48	27	16	3	*150*
5	*Nyssomyia umbratilis*	35	23	26	13	28	21	*146*
6	*Trichophoromyia castanheirai*	—	50	—	59	—	26	*135*
—	*Pressatia* spp.	66	—	39	—	26	—	*131*
—	*Evandromyia* spp.	55	12	41	9	11	—	*128*
7	*Vianamyia furcata*	42	8	46	6	8	1	*111*
8	*Psychodopygus squamiventris s.l.*	27	11	20	1	23	7	*89*
9	*Trichopygomyia trichopyga*	18	20	10	5	22	11	*86*
10	*Trichophoromyia ubiquitalis*	28	15	16	13	9	5	*86*
—	Other species (11–45)	137	112	129	69	71	57	*575*
	Total	813	412	716	305	362	192	*2800*
	Total (♀ + ♂)	*1225*		*1021*		*554*		—

Each *stratum* was sampled with approximately 840 h of CDC trap.
♀: female; ♂: male.

infraspinosa (n = 150; SISA = 0.6), and *Ny. umbratilis* (n = 146; SISA = 0.63). Less frequently captured but nonetheless epidemiologically relevant species included *Ps. squamiventris s.l.* (n = 89; SISA = 0.52), *Th. ubiquitalis* (n = 86; SISA=0.5), *Ps. hirsutus hirsutus* (n = 55; SISA = 0.4), *Ny. anduzei* (n = 45; SISA = 0.23), *Lutzomyia gomezi* (n = 38; SISA = 0.12), *Ny. antunesi* (n = 19; SISA = 0.37), *Ps. paraensis* (n = 15; SISA = 0.2), and *Ny. whitmani* (n = 8; SISA = 0.09).

Sampling effort for each area comprised approximately 504 h of CDC trapping (14 expeditions, 3 CDC traps, and 12-hour CDC exposition). Porto Sabão was the site of the most captured specimens (1,267), followed by Santo Antônio Village (601). The highest diversity was observed in captures from Iratapuru Village (H' = 3.027). All H' value comparisons between the different environments were significant ($p \leq 0.05$), except when comparing Traíra River and the Power Plant ($p \leq 0.099$) (Figure 2).

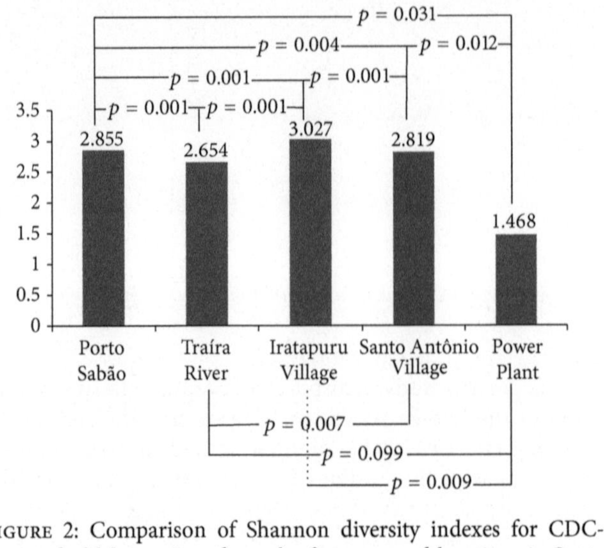

Figure 2: Comparison of Shannon diversity indexes for CDC-captured phlebotomines from the five surveyed locations in Santo Antônio do Jari hydroelectric system impacted area, between the states of Pará and Amapá, Brazil (2012–2015).

Regarding vertical distribution, sampling of the same captures described above accounted for approximately 840 h of CDC trapping by *stratum* (14 expeditions, 5 ecotopes, and 12-hour CDC exposition). CDC traps placed 0.5 m above ground level accounted for a greater number of individuals (1,225) than those placed 1 m above ground level (1,021) and 20 m above ground level in the canopy (554) (Table 2). While *Ps. davisi* was most likely to be found at canopy level (75 individuals at 0.5 m, 83 at 1 m, and 156 at 20 m) and *Bi. flaviscutellata* closer to ground level (130 at 0.5 m, 120 at 1 m, and 15 at 20 m), there was little difference in numbers of *Ny. umbratilis* individuals captured at the different levels of *strata* (58 at 0.5 m, 39 at 1 m, and 49 at 20 m).

The monthly average rainfall was the only climatic data with a representative coefficient of variance (S' = 70.81) when tested against ACL occurrence and phlebotomine frequency (S' = 65.95), in contrast to temperature (S' = 5.96), and relative air humidity (S' = 9.56). The available data enabled correlations to be determined between the periods of May 2012 to April 2015, a period within which nine of the fourteen capture efforts were undertaken. Rainfall presented a moderate correlation with overall phlebotomine frequency (r = 0.65; p = 0.00001), as also individually compared with *Ps. squamiventris s.l.* (r = 0.65; p = 0.00001), and a similarly moderate, but lower correlation with *Bi. flaviscutellata* (r = 0.48; p = 0.0021) and *Ny. umbratilis* (r = 0.48; p = 0.002).

A decrease in the overall phlebotomine population was observed after March until November 2014, coinciding with the transition between the rainy and dry periods and with flooding (Figure 3).

The number of ACL cases presented a moderate correlation with overall phlebotomine frequency ($r = 0.44$; $p = 0.0063$) and also with *Ps. squamiventris* ($r = 0.32$; $p = 0.0003$) and an insignificant negative correlation with *Bi. flaviscutellata* ($r = -0.02$; $p = 0.0001$). A similarly moderate, but higher correlation was however found with *Ny. umbratilis* ($r = 0.48$; $p = 0.002$) (Figure 4).

4. Discussion

It is important to consider current investigations of phlebotomine fauna in the Jari River Basin in the context of the historical findings from the 1970s and 1980s. These earlier studies represent comprehensive research conducted in Monte Dourado (northern PA), a region close to the area investigated in the present study and on which the present epidemiological background to ACL transmission in the associated region is based. In brief, the previous research includes a description of *Ny. umbratilis* (formerly "obscured" as *Ny. anduzei*) [13] and its incrimination as the main vector of *L.* (*V.*) *guyanensis* [9–11], confirmed by strong ecological associations [15]. Just as important, a parasite, more recently described as *L.* (*V.*) *naiffi*, was isolated from the armadillo, *Dasypus novemcinctus*, for which transmission was locally driven and attributed to *Ps. squamiventris s.l.*, and other *Psychodopygus* species [22]; this comprised a primarily enzootic ACL, occasionally infecting humans [23]. Finally, the isolation of *L.* (*L.*) *amazonensis* from rodents in an area affected by occurrence of the main vector *Bi. flaviscutellata* [11] comprised the third known Jari ACL transmission cycle. These facts described above suggest that *Ny. umbratilis*, *Ps. squamiventris s.l.*, and *Bi. flaviscutellata* are implicated in the transmission scenario of the area covered by the present study and thus merit particular attention.

The present study incorporated a representative composition of the known AP fauna. Considering the substantial sampling effort (2,520 h), the determined diversity showed agreement with the findings of other inventories from the Brazilian Amazon basin [1, 24]. Moreover, all new records for AP have already been recorded for PA [25].

Apart from *Ny. umbratilis*, *Ps. squamiventris s.l.*, and *Bi. flaviscutellata,* other species captured were noted as being epidemiologically relevant to ACL in the Brazilian Amazon Region: *Ps. paraensis*, *Ps. davisi*, and *Ps. hirsutus hirsutus*, which are putative vectors of *L.* (*V.*) *naiffi* [26, 27]; *Th. ubiquitalis*, a proven vector of *L.* (*V.*) *lainsoni* [28]; *Ny. anduzei*, a secondary vector of *L.* (*V.*) *guyanensis* [4]; *Ny. whitmani* and *Lu. gomezi*, proven and putative vectors of *L.* (*V.*) *shawi*, respectively [4, 26]; and lastly, *Ny. antunesi*, a suspected vector of *L.* (*V.*) *lindenbergi* [4].

Among the above species, *Ps. davisi* is notable as the third highest ranking according to SISA (0.74) and as having the highest presence in all vertical *strata*, in particular, at the canopy level. This species is generally anthropophilic, is widely distributed in the Amazon Basin [1, 24], and is related to *Leishmania* (*Viannia*) infections in the States of Rondônia (RO) [29] and PA [27, 30]. Interestingly, this species remains frequent in recently surveyed areas affected by hydroelectric schemes in RO [8] and PA (TVS, unpublished). These observations add weight to the need for further investigation into the putative epidemiological role of *Ps. davisi* in Jari.

The species most frequently captured, *Sc. sordellii*, would appear not to be of epidemiological concern. Firstly, the apparent abundance of a given phlebotomine species is not sufficient of itself to incriminate it as a vector [31], particularly when it does not demonstrate high levels of anthropophilic behavior. Secondly, flagellate infections isolated from this species (formerly referred to as *Lutzomyia nordestina*) are historically recognized as distinct from *Leishmania* [22] or remain undetermined, [32] and are more likely to be other trypanosomatids [22]. Furthermore, despite recent reports of molecular *Leishmania* ascribed to this fly [33, 34], currently, polymerase chain reaction-based techniques do not allow "true infection" to be distinguished from a "simple and occasionally ingested" DNA fragment [3]. Thus, there remains insufficient evidence for a potential vector role of *S. sordellii* in *Leishmania* transmission.

High frequencies of light-trapped *Bi. flaviscutellata* have been documented [8, 35], despite rodent-baited trapping being better recognized as a method for attracting the species. Additionally, the first SISA Rank (0.95) was indicative of this high presence in all five surveyed ecotopes; this has been observed in the Belém metropolitan area (PA), where *Bi. flaviscutellata* was the only omnipresent species in seven urban and ecologically isolated forest fragments surveyed [36]. Furthermore, this species has been reported as being able to adapt to plantations of introduced tree species and in other nonclimax forests in Jari [14], suggesting it is capable of responding positively to environmental change, such as the vegetal suppression and flooding caused by hydroelectric operations. Nonetheless, ecological niche model projections predict no change in spatial distribution for *Bi. flaviscutellata* in the Jari area, which is an environment that remains suitable for the species [37].

In an area in Regina, French Guiana, ecologically disturbed due to agricultural practices, flagellates infecting a *Bi. flaviscutellata* specimen have been determined to be *L.* (*V.*) *guyanensis* [38], in similar circumstances to the observed low presence of *Ny. umbratilis.* Although this possibly changing pattern in ACL transmission should be interpreted with caution, it raises an intriguing possibility about the permissiveness of *Bi. flaviscutellata* to *L.* (*V.*) *guyanensis* in the Amazon/Guianan ACL scenario.

In the present study, a higher number of *Bi. flaviscutellata* individuals was captured compared to *Ny. umbratilis* (265 versus 146, resp.). A lack of available evidence for natural infection in this unnatural vector/parasite system, however, precludes speculation about the possible involvement of *Bi. flaviscutellata*, even in the context of occasional transmission of parasites distinct from *L.* (*L.*) *amazonensis.* Nevertheless, the current high occurrence of *Bi. flaviscutellata* in the Amazon/Guianan ACL scenario may be of future concern; unnatural parasite/vector/reservoir systems, when closely related in an ecological context, can, on a century-level scale,

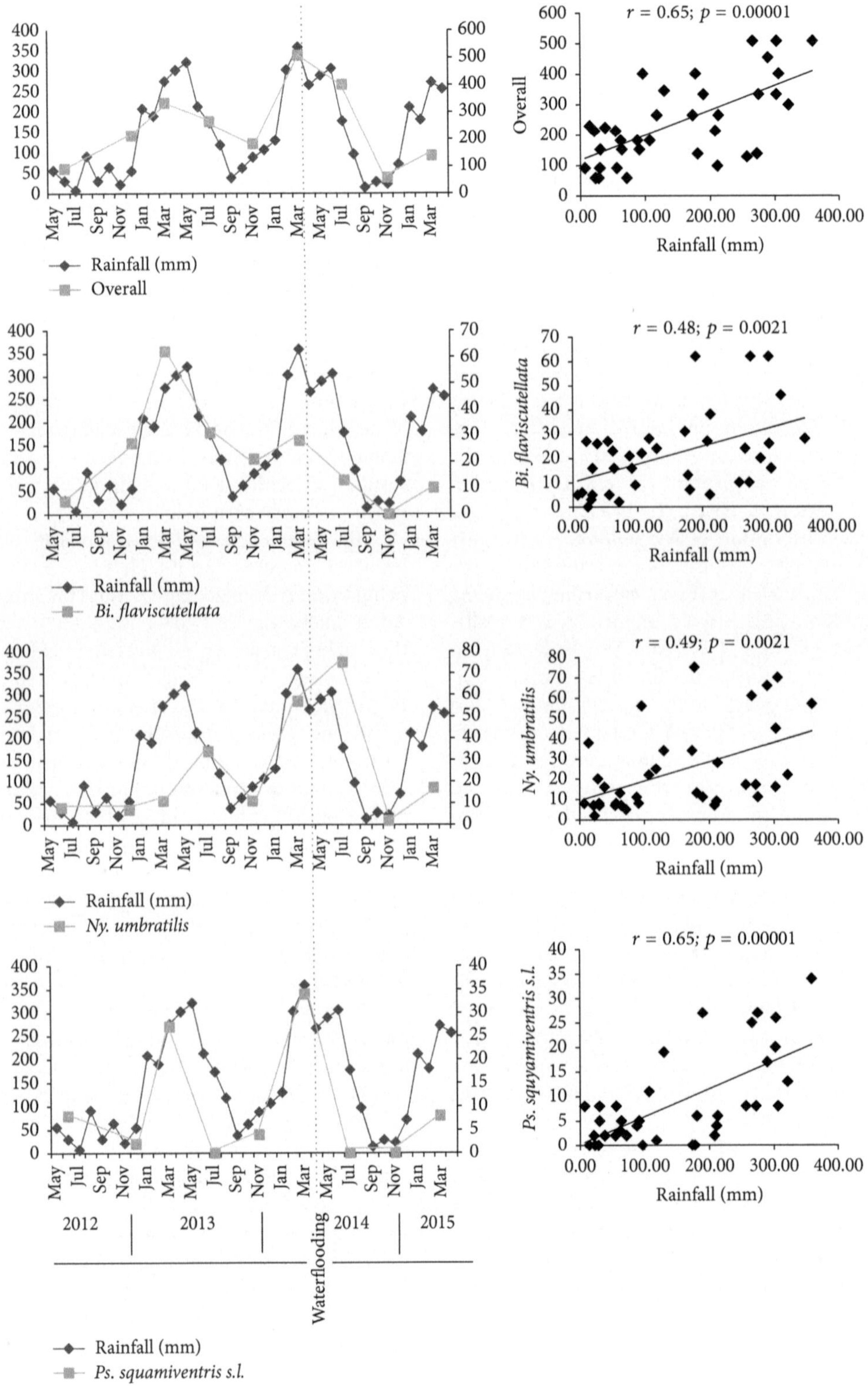

Figure 3: Correlation between rainfall and phlebotomine putative vector species captured in Santo Antônio do Jari hydroelectric system impacted area, between the states of Pará and Amapá, Brazil (2012–2015).

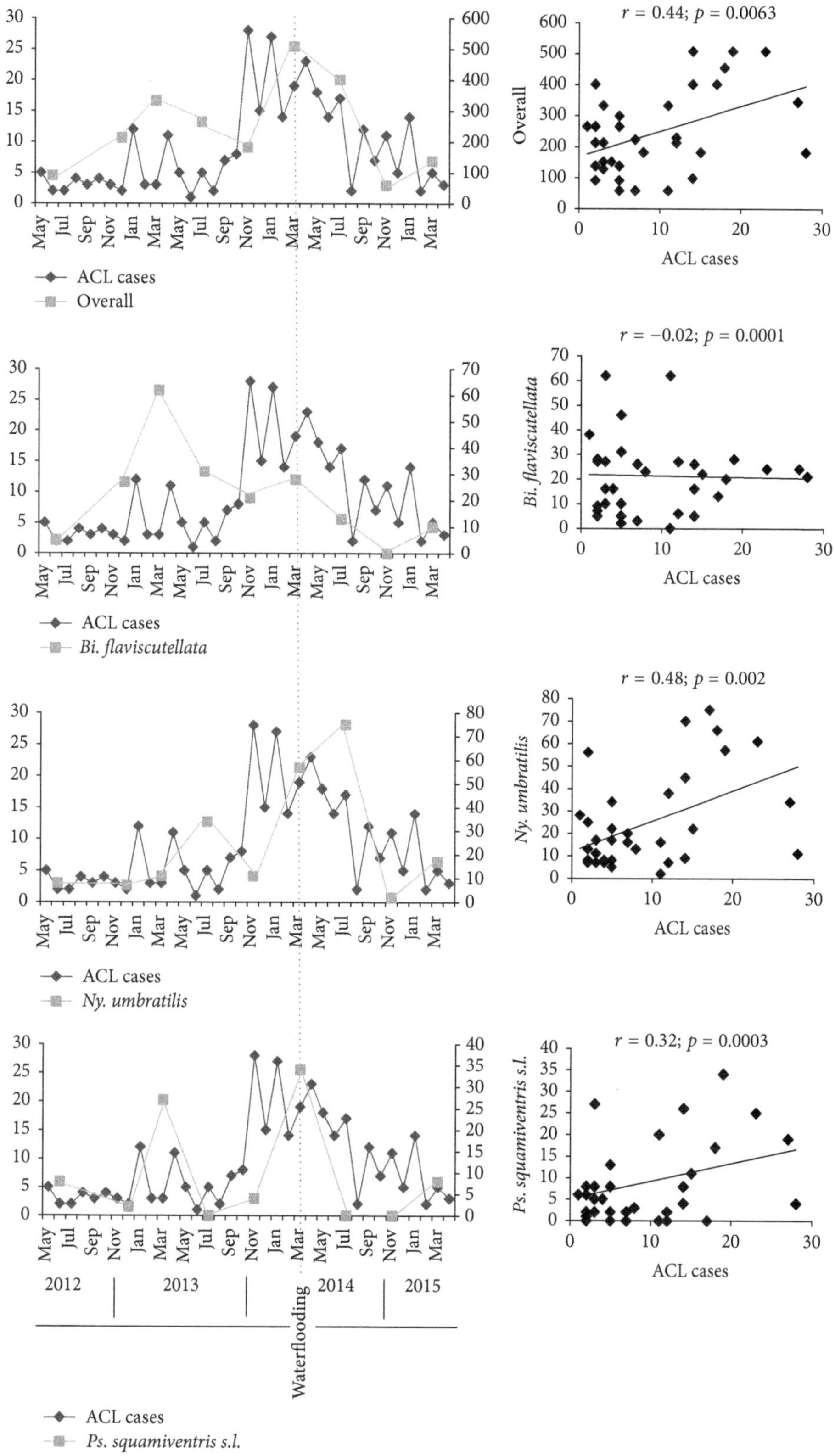

FIGURE 4: Correlation between ACL cases and phlebotomine putative vector species captured in Santo Antônio do Jari hydroelectric system impacted area, between the states of Pará and Amapá, Brazil (2012–2015).

undergo stress adaptation (evolutionary fitness) and form new ecological systems driven by coevolution [39].

There is no doubt that *Ny. umbratilis* is the main vector of ACL in the Jari River Basin [15]. Surprisingly, the well-documented tree-dwelling behavior of this species [15, 40] was not observed in CDC canopy captures in the present study; very little difference was found between the number of individuals captured in the three sampled *strata* (58 at 0.5 m, 39 at 1 m, and 49 at 20 m). Although *Ny. umbratilis* is known to climb into the canopy at night to feed on edentates (mainly sloths) [12, 41], it is possible that an alternative terrestrial source of blood, such as rodents, may be attracting females toward ground level. Sloths are very slow moving and are therefore commonly rescued for relocation during environmental monitoring operations; their resulting rareness means *Ny. umbratilis* has had to find other food sources. Conversely, blood meal analysis conducted during studies in a forest fragment of the Western Amazon has shown rodent blood to be the predominant feeding source for *Ny. umbratilis* [42]. Wild and synanthropic rodents have been shown to survive environmental disturbance in Jari and to proliferate in areas of introduced tree species [14]; this indicated a plausible reason not only for the putative adaptation of *Ny. umbratilis*, but also for the increasing population levels of the rodent blood-feeder *Bi. flaviscutellata*, as already discussed.

Given the clear importance of *Psychodopygus* of the Chagasi series (formerly referred to as the Squamiventris series) in the context of ACL transmission [22], taxonomic studies on identifying the cryptic females have been undertaken previously [43] and more recently, with interesting results (Rodrigo E. Godoy, unpublished). These techniques, however, could not be employed in the field at the time. Early consideration of the assumed geographic distribution of the complex *Ps. squamiventris s.l.* [1, 44] shows that individuals from AP are likely to be predominantly *Ps. s. maripaensis*. Determining males of the species present could clarify these taxonomic uncertainties in the area covered by the present study; however, doubts about identification of some male specimens meant they were grouped as *Ps. squamiventris s.l.*

Ryan et al. [22] did not find *Ps. squamiventris s.l.* to be naturally infected in the Jari area but proposed a link to *L. (V.) naiffi* along the same northern bank of the Amazon River through studies in Cachoeira Porteira (PA); Fouque et al. [38] came to the same conclusions in French Guiana. Interestingly, this fly species complex was found alongside *L. (V.) braziliensis* DNA in Suriname [45], an area where the known Amazonian vectors of this parasite, *Ps. complexus* and *Ps. wellcomei*, are unlikely to occur. As previously discussed in the context of *Bi. flaviscutellata*, the changing transmission patterns of unnatural vector/parasite systems must be carefully interpreted and only after strong ecological associations have been determined. Thus, the putative vector importance of *Ps. squamiventris s.l.* in Jari can only be assumed in respect of *L. (V.) naiffi*.

The five surveyed areas presented, in general, different diversity indexes, showing variations in the phlebotomine composition along the affected area. This finding can be attributed not only to the distance between capture sites, but also to forest composition, fragmentation, geographic barriers, and migration of mammal fauna between sites; this latter can occur naturally or be induced by rescue operations involved in hydroelectric planning, whereby animals are moved to suitable "dry land" environments safe from potential flooding.

A decrease in the phlebotomine population in 2014, in the period after filling the reservoir, could not be attributed exclusively either to flooding or to the transition from the rainy to the dry season. Both eventualities, although opposite in effect, are likely to lead to unsuitable conditions for phlebotomine reproduction. However, they did coincide in May 2014, when rainfall decreased and the lake was formed.

Conversely, rainfall was a valid determinant of overall phlebotomine fluctuation; *Ps. squamiventris s.l.* was the main putative vector directly correlated with this. Other variables, such as forest composition and altitudinal variation, are known to influence seasonal dynamics of species from the complex *Ps. squamiventris s.l.* For example, the dry period from October to November in Serra dos Carajás (southern PA) can be unsuitable for *Ps. wellcomei*, which is adapted to high altitudes, in contrast to *Ps. complexus*, which flourishes in lowland areas during the same months [46].

An insignificant negative to a moderate positive correlation was observed between cases of ACL and phlebotomine fluctuations. In the case of *Ny. umbratilis*, however, the apparently higher correlation when compared with other species is in agreement with its known vector importance in Amazon/Guianan ACL. A strong spatiotemporal association between a given vector and ACL cases is considered essential to maintenance of the *Leishmania* life cycle [2, 14].

In summary, the present study filled a temporal gap on phlebotomine data relating to the Jari area. It provides a meaningful update on species composition and further insights into seasonal dynamics of species under pressures caused by environmental change. The presence of ACL vectors, in particular *Ny. umbratilis*, *Bi. flaviscutellata*, and *Ps. squamiventris s.l.*, is noteworthy, due to their direct association with Amazon/Guianan-ACL transmission. For *Ny. umbratilis*, the lower frequency associated with the unpredicted lack of tree-dwelling behavior may be attributable to a reduction in numbers of canopy-dwelling mammals, due to the environmental disturbance and relocation efforts; this could consequently have led to seeking for alternative terrestrial blood sources at ground level. The possible association of *Ps. davisi* with *Leishmania* transmission cycles in other Amazon ecoregions draws attention to its high rank position in Jari. Rainfall can be partly associated with local seasonal fluctuations in fly numbers, mainly with respect to *Ps. squamiventris s.l.* Cases of ACL were also more highly correlated with *Ny. umbratilis* dynamics. Further attention was also given to results for *Bi. flaviscutellata*, which has been apparently tolerant of anthropic activity: continued phlebotomine monitoring is proposed in order to evaluate the implication for social welfare and health in the future.

Competing Interests

The authors declare that they have no competing interests.

Acknowledgments

The authors wish to thank the "Instituto de Pesquisas Científicas e Tecnológicas do Estado do Amapá, IEPA" entomology team for the technical assistance given to the field work, in particular to Aderbal Amanajás Santana, Rosalvo Dias de Castro, Noel Fernandes Santos Neto, Ósita Cleyriane Lobato do Nascimento, José Luiz dos Santos Chaves, and João do Socorro Gomes Campos. Logistical facilities were financially supported by the "Jari Energia."

References

[1] D. G. Young and M. A. Duncan, "Guide to the identification and geographic distribution of *Lutzomyia* sand flies in Mexico, the West Indies, Central and South America (Diptera: Psychodidae)," in *Memoirs of the American Entomological Institute*, pp. 1-881, Associated Publishers American Entomological Institute, Gainesville, Fla, USA, 1994.

[2] P. D. Ready, "Biology of phlebotomine sand flies as vectors of disease agents," *Annual Review of Entomology*, vol. 58, pp. 227-250, 2013.

[3] R. P. Brazil, A. A. Fuzzari, and J. D. Andrade Filho, "Sand fly vectors of *Leishmania* in the Americas—a mini review," *Entomology, Ornithology & Herpetology*, vol. 4, no. 2, Article ID 1000144, 2015.

[4] E. F. Rangel and R. Lainson, "Proven and putative vectors of American cutaneous leishmaniasis in Brazil: aspects of their biology and vectorial competence," *Memorias do Instituto Oswaldo Cruz*, vol. 104, no. 7, pp. 937–954, 2009.

[5] E. F. Rangel, S. M. Costa, and B. M. Carvalho, "Environmental changes and the geographic spreading of American cutaneous leishmaniasis in Brazil," in *Leishmaniasis-Trends in Epidemiology*, D. Claborn, Ed., Diagnosis and Treatment, InTech, Rijeka, Croatia, 2014.

[6] W. P. Taddei, "O gênero *Mansonia* (Diptera: Culicidae) e a proliferação de mosquitos na usina hidrelétrica de Tucuruí," in *Energia na Amazônia*, S. B. Magalhães, R. C. Brito, and E. R. Castro, Eds., vol. 1, pp. 311-318, MPEG/FPA/UNAMAZ, Belém, Brazil, 1996 (Portuguese).

[7] A. I. A. Oliveira, *Observações Sobre a Resolução CONAMA no. 237/97, que Dispõe Sobre o Licenciamento Ambiental*, Mimeo, Conselho Empresarial Brasileiro Para o Desenvolvimento Sustentável, Rio de Janeiro, Brazil, 1997 (Portuguese).

[8] A. K. R. Galardo, C. D. Galardo, G. A. Silveira et al., "Phlebotominae sand flies (Diptera: Psychodidae): potential vectors of American cutaneous leishmaniasis agents in the area associated with the Santo Antônio hydroelectric system in Western Amazonian, Brazil," *Revista da Sociedade Brasileira de Medicina Tropical*, vol. 48, no. 3, pp. 265–271, 2015.

[9] R. Lainson, R. D. Ward, and J. J. Shaw, "Cutaneous leishmaniasis in North Brazil: *Lutzomyia anduzei* as a major vector," *Transactions of the Royal Society of Tropical Medicine and Hygiene*, vol. 70, no. 2, pp. 171–172, 1976.

[10] R. Lainson, J. J. Shaw, R. D. Ward, P. D. Ready, and R. D. Naiff, "Leishmaniasis in Brazil: XIII. Isolation of *Leishmania* from armadillos (*Dasypus novemcinctus*), and observations on the epidemiology of cutaneous leishmaniasis in north Pará State," *Transactions of the Royal Society of Tropical Medicine and Hygiene*, vol. 73, no. 2, pp. 239–242, 1979.

[11] R. Lainson, J. J. Shaw, P. D. Ready, M. A. Miles, and M. Póvoa, "Leishmaniasis in Brazil: XVI. Isolation and identification of *Leishmania* species from sandflies, wild mammals and man in north Pará State, with particular reference to *L. braziliensis guyanensis* causative agent of "pian-bois"," *Transactions of the Royal Society of Tropical Medicine and Hygiene*, vol. 75, no. 4, pp. 530–536, 1981.

[12] R. Lainson, J. J. Shaw, and M. Póvoa, "The importance of edentates (sloths and anteaters) as primary reservoirs of *Leishmania braziliensis guyanensis*, causative agent of 'pian bois' in north Brazil," *Transactions of the Royal Society of Tropical Medicine and Hygiene*, vol. 75, no. 4, pp. 611–612, 1981.

[13] R. D. Ward and H. Fraiha, "*Lutzomyia umbratilis*, a new species of sand fly from Brazil (Diptera: Psychodidae)," *Journal of Medical Entomology*, vol. 14, no. 3, pp. 313–317, 1977.

[14] P. D. Ready, R. Lainson, and J. J. Shaw, "Leishmaniasis in Brazil: XX. Prevalence of 'enzootic rodent leishmaniasis' (*Leishmania mexicana amazonensis*), and apparent absence of 'pian bois' (*Le. braziliensis guyanensis*), in plantations of introduced tree species and in other non-climax forests in eastern Amazônia," *Transactions of the Royal Society of Tropical Medicine and Hygiene*, vol. 77, no. 6, pp. 775–785, 1983.

[15] P. D. Ready, R. Lainson, J. J. Shaw, and R. D. Ward, "The ecology of *Lutzomyia umbratilis* Ward & Fraiha (Diptera: Psychodidae), the major vector to man of *Leishmania braziliensis guyanensis* in north-eastern Amazonian Brazil," *Bulletin of Entomological Research*, vol. 76, no. 1, pp. 21–40, 1986.

[16] R. Lainson and J. J. Shaw, "*Leishmania (Viannia) naiffi* sp. n., a parasite of the armadillo, *Dasypus novemcinctus* (L.) in Amazonian Brazil," *Annales de Parasitologie Humaine et Comparee*, vol. 64, no. 1, pp. 3–9, 1989.

[17] A. Roger, M. Nacher, M. Hanf et al., "Climate and leishmaniasis in French guiana," *The American Journal of Tropical Medicine and Hygiene*, vol. 89, no. 3, pp. 564–569, 2013.

[18] L. Ryan, "Flebótomos do estado do Pará, Brasil (Diptera: Psychodidae)," Thecnical Document 1, Instituto Evandro Chagas, Belém, Brazil, 1986 (Portuguese).

[19] E. A. B. Galati, "Morfologia e Taxonomia: Morfologia, terminologia de adultos e identificação dos táxons da América," in *Flebotomíneos do Brasil*, E. F. Rangel and R. Lainson, Eds., pp. 53–75, Editora Fiocruz, Rio de Janeiro, Brazil, 2003 (Portuguese).

[20] D. R. Roberts and B. P. Hsi, "An index of species abundance for use with mosquito surveillance data," *Environmental Entomology*, vol. 8, no. 6, pp. 1007–1013, 1979.

[21] Ø. Hammer, D. A. T. Harper, and P. D. Ryan, "Past: paleontological statistics software package for education and data analysis," *Palaeontologia Electronica*, vol. 4, no. 1, pp. 1–9, 2001.

[22] L. Ryan, R. Lainson, J. J. Shaw, R. R. Braga, and E. A. Ishikawa, "Leishmaniasis in Brazil. XXV. Sandfly vectors of *Leishmania* in Pará State, Brazil," *Medical and Veterinary Entomology*, vol. 1, no. 4, pp. 383–395, 1987.

[23] R. Lainson, J. J. Shaw, F. T. Silveira, R. R. Braga, and E. A. Ishikawa, "Cutaneous leishmaniasis of man due to *Leishmania (Viannia) naiffi*," *Annales de Parasitologie Humaine et Comparee*, vol. 65, no. 5-6, pp. 282–284, 1990.

[24] E. G. C. Bermudez, *Lutzomyia Sand Flies in the Brazilian Amazon Basin (Diptera: Psychodidae)*, INPA, Manaus, Brazil, 2009.

[25] G. M. Aguiar and W. M. Medeiros, "Distribuição regional e hábitats das espécies de flebotomíneos do Brasil," in *Flebotomíneos do Brasil*, E. F. Rangel and R. Lainson, Eds., pp. 207–256, Fiocruz, Rio de Janeiro, Brazil, 2003 (Portuguese).

[26] J. R. Arias, M. A. Miles, R. D. Naiff et al., "Flagellate infections of Brazilian sand flies (Diptera: Psychodidae): isolation in vitro and biochemical identification of *Endotrypanum* and *Leishmania*," *The American Journal of Tropical Medicine and Hygiene*, vol. 34, no. 6, pp. 1098–1108, 1985.

[27] A. A. Souza, T. V. Santos, Y. L. Jennings et al., "Natural *Leishmania(Viannia)* spp. infections in phlebotomine sand flies (Diptera: Psychodidae) from the Brazilian Amazon region reveal new putative transmission cycles of American cutaneous leishmaniasis," *Parasite*, vol. 23, article 22, 2016.

[28] F. T. Silveira, A. A. Souza, R. Lainson, J. J. Shaw, R. R. Braga, and E. A. Ishikawa, "Cutaneous leishmaniasis in the Amazon Region: natural infection of the sand fly *Lutzomyia ubiquitalis* (Psychodidae: Phlebotominae) by *Leishmania (Viannia) lainsoni* in Pará state, Brazil," *Memórias do Instituto Oswaldo Cruz*, vol. 86, no. 1, pp. 127–130, 1991.

[29] L. H. S. Gil, S. A. Basano, A. A. Souza et al., "Recent observations on the sand fly (Diptera: Psychodidae) fauna of the state of Rondônia, Western Amazonia, Brazil: the importance of *Psychdopygus davisi* as a vector of zoonotic cutaneous leishmaniasis," *Memórias do Instituto Oswaldo Cruz*, vol. 98, no. 6, pp. 751–755, 2003.

[30] A. A. A. Souza, F. T. Silveira, R. Lainson et al., "The Phlebotominae fauna of Serra dos Carajás, Pará, Brazil, and its possible implication in the transmission of American tegumentary leishmaniasis," *Revista Pan-Amazônica de Saúde*, vol. 1, no. 1, pp. 45–51, 2010.

[31] R. Killick-Kendrick, "Phlebotomine vectors of the leishmaniases: a review," *Medical and Veterinary Entomology*, vol. 4, no. 1, pp. 1–24, 1990.

[32] M. E. C. Dorval, G. Cristaldo, H. C. da Rocha et al., "Phlebotomine fauna (Diptera: Psychodidae) of an American cutaneous leishmaniasis endemic area in the state of Mato Grosso do Sul, Brazil," *Memórias do Instituto Oswaldo Cruz*, vol. 104, no. 5, pp. 695–702, 2009.

[33] V. C. F. V. Guimarães, P. L. Costa, F. J. da Silva et al., "Molecular detection of *Leishmania* in phlebotomine sand flies in a cutaneous and visceral leishmaniasis endemic area in northeastern Brazil," *Revista do Instituto de Medicina Tropical de Sao Paulo*, vol. 56, no. 4, pp. 357–360, 2014.

[34] R. S. Lana, É. M. Michalsky, C. L. Fortes-Dias et al., "Phlebotomine sand fly fauna and *Leishmania* infection in the vicinity of the Serra do Cipó National Park, a natural Brazilian heritage site," *BioMed Research International*, vol. 2015, Article ID 385493, 9 pages, 2015.

[35] V. R. Alves, R. A. de Freitas, F. L. Santos, A. F. J. de Oliveira, T. V. Barrett, and P. H. F. Shimabukuro, "Sand flies (Diptera, Psychodidae, Phlebotominae) from central amazonia and four new records for the Amazonas State, Brazil," *Revista Brasileira de Entomologia*, vol. 56, no. 2, pp. 220–227, 2012.

[36] J. V. S. Ferreira, T. V. Santos, E. M. Santos, and I. S. Gorayeb, "Phlebotomine sand flies (Diptera: Psychodidae) in forest fragments of Belém metropolitan area, Pará State, Brazil, with considerations on vectors of American cutaneous leishmaniasis agents," *Revista Pan-Amazônica de Saúde*, vol. 5, no. 2, pp. 29–35, 2014.

[37] B. M. Carvalho, E. F. Rangel, P. D. Ready, and M. M. Vale, "Ecological niche modelling predicts southward expansion of *Lutzomyia (Nyssomyia) flaviscutellata* (Diptera: Psychodidae: Phlebotominae), vector of *Leishmania (Leishmania) amazonensis* in South America, under climate change," *PLoS ONE*, vol. 10, no. 11, Article ID e0143282, 2015.

[38] F. Fouque, P. Gaborit, J. Issaly et al., "Phlebotomine sand flies (Diptera: Psychodidae) associated with changing patterns in the transmission of the human cutaneous leishmaniasis in French Guiana," *Memórias do Instituto Oswaldo Cruz*, vol. 102, no. 1, pp. 35–40, 2007.

[39] R. Killick-Kendrick, "Some epidemiological consequences of the evolutionary fit between *Leishmaniae* and their phlebotomine vectors," *Bulletin de la Societe de Pathologie Exotique et de ses Filiales*, vol. 78, no. 5, pp. 747–755, 1985.

[40] F. X. Pajot, F. Le Pont, B. Gentile, and R. Besnard, "Epidemiology of leishmaniasis in French Guiana," *Transactions of the Royal Society of Tropical Medicine and Hygiene*, vol. 76, no. 1, pp. 112–113, 1982.

[41] H. A. Christensen, J. R. Arias, A. M. De Vasquez, and R. A. De Freitas, "Hosts of sandfly vectors of *Leishmania braziliensis guyanensis* in the central Amazon of Brazil," *The American Journal of Tropical Medicine and Hygiene*, vol. 31, no. 2, pp. 239–242, 1982.

[42] L. C. R. Nery, E. S. Lorosa, and A. M. R. Franco, "Feeding preference of the sand flies *Lutzomyia umbratilis* and *L. spathotrichia* (Diptera: Psychodidae, Phlebotominae) in an urban forest patch in the City of Manaus, Amazonas, Brazil," *Memórias do Instituto Oswaldo Cruz*, vol. 99, no. 6, pp. 571–574, 2004.

[43] P. D. Ready, R. Lainson, J. J. Shaw, and A. A. Souza, "DNA probes for distinguishing *Psychodopygus wellcomei* from *Psychodopygus complexus* (Diptera: Psychodidae)," *Memórias do Instituto Oswaldo Cruz*, vol. 86, no. 1, pp. 41–49, 1991.

[44] P. D. Ready, H. Fraiha, R. P. Lane, J. R. Arias, and F. X. Pajot, "On distinguishing the female of *Psychodopygus wellcomei*, a vector of mucocutaneous leishmaniasis, from other *squamiventris* series females. I. Characterization of *Ps. squamiventris squamiventris* and *Ps. s. maripaensis* stat. nov. (Diptera: Psychodidae)," *Annals of Tropical Medicine and Parasitology*, vol. 76, no. 2, pp. 201–214, 1982.

[45] A. D. Kent, T. V. dos Santos, A. Gangadin, A. Samjhawan, D. R. A. Mans, and H. D. F. H. Schallig, "Studies on the sand fly fauna (Diptera: Psychodidae) in high-transmission areas of cutaneous leishmaniasis in the Republic of Suriname," *Parasites and Vectors*, vol. 6, no. 1, article 318, 2013.

[46] P. D. Ready, R. Lainson, and J. J. Shaw, "Habitat and seasonality of *Psychodopygus wellcomei* help incriminate it as a vector of *Leishmania braziliensis* in Amazônia and Northeast Brazil," *Transactions of the Royal Society of Tropical Medicine and Hygiene*, vol. 78, no. 4, pp. 543–544, 1984.

Development and Validation of a PCR-ELISA for the Diagnosis of Symptomatic and Asymptomatic Infection by *Leishmania (Leishmania) infantum*

Fernanda Alvarenga Cardoso Medeiros,[1] Luciana Inácia Gomes,[1] Edward Oliveira,[1] Carolina Senra Alves de Souza,[1] Maria Vitória Mourão,[1] Gláucia Fernandes Cota,[1] Letícia Helena dos Santos Marques,[2] Mariângela Carneiro,[2] and Ana Rabello[1]

[1]*Centro de Pesquisas René Rachou, Oswaldo Cruz Foundation (Fiocruz), Belo Horizonte, MG, Brazil*
[2]*Departamento de Parasitologia, Instituto de Ciências Biológicas, Universidade Federal de Minas Gerais, Belo Horizonte, MG, Brazil*

Correspondence should be addressed to Edward Oliveira; edwardjo@cpqrr.fiocruz.br

Academic Editor: Sukla Biswas

A *kDNA* PCR enzyme-linked immunosorbent assay (*kDNA* PCR-ELISA) for the diagnosis of human visceral leishmaniasis (HVL) was developed. The detection limit of the reaction, precision measurements, and cut-off of the *kDNA* PCR-ELISA were defined in a proof-of-concept phase. A reference strain of *Leishmania (Leishmania) infantum* and a bank of 14 peripheral blood samples from immunocompetent patients with VL were characterized using techniques considered gold standards, and 11 blood samples obtained from healthy individuals of an endemic area were also assessed. Phase II evaluation determined the performance of the assay in peripheral blood samples from 105 patients with VL (adults and children), 25 patients with *Leishmania*/HIV coinfection, 40 healthy individuals, and 33 asymptomatic individuals living in endemic areas. The *kDNA* PCR-ELISA exhibited satisfactory precision, with a detection limit of 0.07 fg of DNA from *L. (L.) infantum* and 1 parasite/mL blood. The overall sensitivity of the assay for all groups studied was 100% (95% confidence interval [CI]: 97.1–100%), and the specificity was 95% (95% CI: 83.5–98.6%). The *kDNA* PCR-ELISA was shown to be a useful tool for VL symptomatic and asymptomatic individuals diagnosis and its use in endemic countries may help monitor control interventions.

1. Introduction

Visceral leishmaniasis (VL) is a major public health problem and has an estimated annual incidence of approximately 0.2 to 0.4 million cases and a focal distribution, with more than 90% of global cases occurring in six countries: India, Bangladesh, Sudan, South Sudan, Brazil, and Ethiopia [1]. In Brazil, the disease is an endemic anthropozoonosis caused by the parasitic protozoa *Leishmania* (*Leishmania*) *infantum*, which is an obligate intracellular protozoan belonging to the *Leishmania donovani* complex. *L. infantum* is primarily transmitted by the sand fly *Lutzomyia longipalpis*, and dogs are the main reservoir of these parasites. The number of cases has increased in large Brazilian cities despite Brazilian measures to control VL [2, 3]. A mean of 3.771 cases are detected annually in Brazil [4].

A noninvasive easily implemented high performance test for the detection of symptomatic and asymptomatic infection is lacking despite several technological advances in recent years. Parasitological examination, which is a reference technique, requires invasive sample collection from the spleen or bone marrow, which must be performed by trained professionals and often exhibits low and variable sensitivity. Antibody-based tests, such as immunofluorescence antibody test (IFAT), enzyme-linked immunosorbent assay (ELISA), and recombinant antigen-based immunochromatography test (ICT), support the clinical diagnosis of VL, but these methods have drawbacks, such as cross-reactions in the presence of other diseases and an inability to distinguish between active and past infection. Some studies demonstrated that serological tests based on antigens of a single *Leishmania* sp. exhibited low diagnostic performance in regions with circulating heterologous parasites [5, 6]. The serological tests, with the exception of the Direct Agglutination Tests (DAT) and Western blotting, exhibit low sensitivity in VL patients coinfected with HIV [7–9] because of their insufficient immune humoral response.

Molecular methods are useful for the detection of low parasitic loads and exhibit high sensitivity in the diagnosis of VL [10]. PCR-based assays are the most commonly used approaches in molecular diagnostics. One additional advantage of PCR is that it is based on the identification of conserved DNA sequences, which allows the detection of specific pathogen species in a variety of clinical samples, even archived materials [11]. PCR sensitivity is directly related to the copy number of the target and the primer and cycling protocol used [12]. The internal transcribed spacers (ITS, ITS1, and ITS2) regions, gp63 gene, HSP-70 gene, miniexon (ME), and SSU-rRNA and conserved and variable regions of kinetoplast DNA (kDNA) minicircles are used for the diagnosis and characterization of *Leishmania* strains [13]. Conventional PCR techniques targeting kDNA exhibit high sensitivity for VL diagnosis [13, 14], but this technique is not automated and is laborious, which limits its use to a small number of samples. To overcome this limitation, we developed a *kDNA* PCR-ELISA, which allows simultaneous testing of a large number of blood samples without the use of commercial kits for the detection of PCR products via measurement of absorbance readings for the laboratory diagnosis of VL.

2. Materials and Methods

This work was performed in two phases:

(i) In a proof-of-concept phase, the assay was standardized using a reference strain of *L. (L.) infantum* and a bank of peripheral blood samples from nonimmunosuppressed patients with VL that were characterized using techniques considered gold standards and from healthy individuals in an endemic area.

(ii) In a phase II evaluation, the assay was validated in clinical samples from varied groups of VL patients of different ages and in asymptomatic and noninfected individuals to certify the wide use of the assay for the diagnosis of human VL. We describe the step-by-step development and internal validation of the *kDNA* PCR-ELISA below.

2.1. Parasites. Promastigotes of *L. (L.) infantum* (MHOM/BR/2002/LPC-RPV), *L. (L.) donovani* (MHOM/ET/196/HU3), *L. (Viannia) braziliensis* (MHOM/BR/75/M2903), *L. (V.) guyanensis* (MHOM/BR/1975/M4147), and *L. (L.) amazonensis* (IFLA/BR/1967/PH-8) were cultured in Schneider medium (Sigma-Aldrich, St. Louis, MO, USA) supplemented with 10% foetal bovine serum (Invitrogen, Carlsbad, CA, USA) and counted in a Neubauer chamber. An aliquot of 1 mL of the suspension of parasites was centrifuged at $2.300g$ for 2 minutes and stored at −70°C.

2.2. Samples

2.2.1. Peripheral Blood Samples. Peripheral blood samples collected from 14 patients with VL, nonimmunosuppressed, living in endemic areas in Brazil, with typical VL symptoms and parasitological confirmation (direct exam and/or culture) with a mean age of 12.7 years (range one month to 76.8 years) were used as positive controls.

Peripheral blood samples from 11 healthy individuals from the endemic area of Belo Horizonte, MG, were used as negative controls.

2.2.2. Spiked Blood Samples. Aliquots of peripheral blood samples obtained from 11 healthy individuals were added to the reference sample *L. (L.) infantum* (MHOM/BR/2002/LPC-RPV) to obtain a concentration of 10,000 parasites/mL of blood.

2.2.3. Evaluation of kDNA PCR-ELISA Performance in the Diagnosis of VL, VL-HIV Coinfected, Asymptomatic, and Noninfected Endemic Controls. A minimum sample size of 38 VL cases was calculated with a mean sensitivity of 97.5% to assess the accuracy of the assay, which is consistent with previously published molecular tests [15, 16]. The specificity in these studies was 100%, and a minimum sample size of 38 noninfected controls was estimated with a level of confidence of 95%:

$$n = z^2 \cdot p \cdot \frac{(1-p)}{x^2}, \quad (1)$$

where p is the sensitivity or specificity and x^2 is the confidence interval (95%) [17].

The following groups were included.

Children VL Group. This group was composed of 81 children admitted to Hospital João Paulo II-FHEMIG (Fundação Hospitalar de Minas Gerais), Belo Horizonte, Minas Gerais, who presented with VL symptoms and parasitological confirmation (direct exam and/or culture) and/or serological diagnosis for VL (indirect immunofluorescence antibody test-IFAT and/or immunochromatographic rK39 antigen-test) associated with clinical improvement after treatment. Patients in this group were aged 3 months to 10 years (mean 2.5 years).

Adult VL Group. This group was constituted by 24 adult patients aged 18 to 68 years (mean of 36 years) who were admitted to Hospital Eduardo de Menezes-FHEMIG and presented VL symptoms with parasitological confirmation (direct exam and or culture) and/or serological diagnosis for

VL (indirect immunofluorescence antibody test-IFAT and/or immunochromatographic rK39 antigen-test) associated with clinical improvement after treatment.

VL/HIV Group. This group was composed of 25 HIV-infected patients who were admitted to Hospital Eduardo de Menezes-FHEMIG, aged 21 to 61 years (mean of 41 years), presenting VL symptoms and parasitological confirmation (direct exam and/or culture) and/or serological diagnosis for VL (indirect immunofluorescence antibody test-IFAT and/or immunochromatographic rK39 antigen-test) associated with clinical cure after treatment. HIV infection was diagnosed by a positive ELISA or chemiluminescence followed by a confirmatory Western blot performed in two different samples.

Asymptomatic Group. This group was composed of 33 asymptomatic children, aged 3 months to 6.8 years (mean 2.8 years), living in an endemic area of Belo Horizonte and presenting positive serology (ELISA using recombinant antigen K39 and/or DAT) or molecular (SSU-rRNA qPCR) tests for *Leishmania infection.*

Noninfected Group. This group consisted of 40 children, aged 1.1 to 6.7 years (mean 3.5 years), living in an endemic area of Belo Horizonte and presenting negative serological (ELISA using recombinant antigen K39 and/or DAT) and molecular (*SSU-rRNA* qPCR) tests for *Leishmania* spp. infection.

2.3. DNA Extraction. DNA from parasites and total DNA from peripheral blood samples and spiked blood samples were extracted using the "QIAamp DNA mini" (QIAGEN GmbH, Hilden, Germany) kit according to the manufacturer's specifications. Negative DNA extraction controls were performed for each experiment by the addition of all reagents except the sample. The yield was determined by absorbance at 260 nm in a spectrophotometer (NanoDrop ND-1000, Thermo Fisher Scientific, Wilmington, DE, USA). The A260/A280 absorbance ratio was analysed to verify the purity of the DNA obtained.

2.4. kDNA PCR-ELISA

2.4.1. kDNA PCR Amplification. The reaction was made for a final volume of 25 μL containing 2 μL of DNA sample, 2 units of Platinum Taq DNA Polymerase (Invitrogen, Carlsbad, CA, USA), 1x PCR buffer (200 mM Tris-HCl, pH 8.4, and 500 mM KCl), sense primer 150 (5′-GGGG/TAGGGGCGTTCTC-/GCGAA-3′) labelled with biotin at the 5′ end and antisense primer 152 (3′-C/GC/GC/GA/TCTATA/TTTACACCA-ACCCC-5′) [18] at 0.6 μM each, 2.0 mM $MgCl_2$, and 0.2 mM dNTPs (Promega, Madison, WI, USA). The cycling protocol consisted of one step at 95°C for 5 min followed by 34 cycles at 95°C for 30 seconds, 60°C for 30 seconds, and 72°C for 30 seconds. A final step of 72°C for 5 minutes was performed. Each PCR assay included negative (PCR mix without DNA, control for the process of DNA extraction and DNA extracted from samples of healthy volunteers) and positive (genomic DNA extracted from the reference strain of *L. (L.) infantum*, MHOM/BR/2002/LPC-RPV) controls.

2.4.2. ELISA Colorimetric Assay. For the detection of the amplified products, the 5′-GATTTCTGCACCCATTTTTC-3′ probe labelled with fluorescein at the 5′ end, designed using the Primer3 program, was used [19]. A better site for annealing of the probe was verified to be among 76 to 91 bp of 120 bp *Leishmania kDNA* fragment amplified using the PCR assay. The search of the lowest homology with genomic sequences from *Leishmania braziliensis*, *Leishmania amazonensis*, *Leishmania guyanensis*, *Trypanosoma cruzi*, *Plasmodium vivax*, and *Mycobacterium tuberculosis* for selection and design of the probe was performed in the BLAST program (National Center for Biotechnology Information website), using the database nucleotides and MegaBlast option.

ELISA followed the parameters described previously [20, 21]. Briefly, wells of MaxiSorp® polystyrene microplates (Nunc Thermo Scientific, Vernon Hills, IL, USA) were coated with 100 μL of streptavidin (5 μg/mL) (streptavidin from *Streptomyces avidinii*, Sigma-Aldrich, St. Louis, MO, USA) in PBS via incubation at 37°C for 1 hour plus overnight at 2–8°C. Coated plates were washed 4 times with PBS-Tween (PBS-T) 0.05%, followed by incubation at 37°C for 2 hours with 200 μL 3% BSA in PBS-T. The plates were washed 4 times with PBS-T and stored at −20°C until use.

PCR at a volume of 100 μL diluted 1:25 in PBS were performed in duplicate in microplates at 37°C for 30 minutes. The microplates were washed 3 times with 300 μL of PBS-T and incubated for 10 minutes at room temperature in 0.1 M NaOH 100 μL/well. The microplates were washed once with 0.1 M NaOH (300 μL/well) and 3 times with 300 μL of 0.1 M Tris-HCl. Next, 100 μL/well of a fluorescein-labelled probe at the 5′ end diluted to 0.2 pM in hybridisation solution (70% SSPE5x, 0.75 M sodium chloride, 0.05 M sodium phosphate, 0.005 M EDTA, 30% formamide, and 0.1% SDS) was added and the microplate incubated for one hour at 37°C. The microplates were washed 3 times with 6x SSC solution (0.9 M NaCl and 0.09 M sodium citrate) and twice with a 3x SSC solution (0.45 M NaCl and 0.045 M sodium citrate) containing 0.1% SDS. PBS (150 μL) containing 1% BSA solution (PBS-BSA) was added to each well, and microplates were incubated for 30 minutes at 37°C. An antifluorescein conjugate (antifluorescein/Oregon Green®-peroxidase, Invitrogen-Thermo Scientific, Wilmington, DE, USA) (150 μL) was diluted 1:9,000 in PBS-BSA solution and added to each well. The microplates were incubated for one hour at 37°C. The microplates were washed 4 times with PBS-T (300 μL/well) and 100 μL/well of a chromogenic mixture (3,3′,5,5′-tetramethylbenzidine + hydrogen peroxide, Sigma-Aldrich) was added. Plates were incubated for 10 minutes at room temperature in the dark, and the reaction was stopped by the addition of 100 μL of 3N sulfuric acid. Absorbance readings were performed in a microplate reader at 450 nm (Model 550, Bio-Rad, Hercules, CA, USA).

Each ELISA was performed with the positive and negative controls described above for the PCR, and all experiments were performed in duplicate. Data represent the mean values.

2.4.3. ACTB PCR-ELISA. As a control for the DNA extraction and amplification procedure, all samples were amplified for the human beta actin *(ACTB)* gene using an Acol (5′-ACCTCATGAAGATCCTCACC-3′) primer labelled with biotin at the 5′ end and an Aco2 primer (5′-CCATCTCTT-GCTCGAAGTCC-3′), which generated a product of 120-base pairs [22]. The PCR was performed in a final volume of 20 μL containing 2 μL of DNA sample, 2 units of Platinum *Taq* DNA Polymerase (Invitrogen), 1x PCR buffer (200 mM Tris-HCl, pH 8.4, and 500 mM KCl), 0.5 μM of each primer, 2.0 mM $MgCl_2$, and 0.2 mM dNTP (Promega). The cycling protocol consisted of an initial step of 95°C for 5 min and 35 cycles at 95°C for 20 seconds, 60°C for 30 seconds, and 72°C for 1 minute. A final step at 72°C for 6 minutes was performed. Each PCR assay included negative controls (PCR mix without DNA and control for the process of DNA extraction).

The 5′-TCTCCTTAATGCACGCACG-3′ probe labelled with fluorescein at the 5′ end was used to detect the amplified products using the ELISA colorimetric assay [21]. The assay followed the same conditions described above, except that 100 μL of the PCR diluted 1 : 10 in PBS was used, and the antifluorescein conjugate (antifluorescein/Oregon Green-peroxidase, Invitrogen) was diluted 1 : 1,000 in PBS-BSA.

2.4.4. Analytical Precision (Analytical Sensitivity and Specificity). The detection limit was measured in 6% gel polyacrylamide and kDNA PCR-ELISA for the detection of PCR products from DNA *L. infantum* in the following concentrations: 700 pg, 70 pg, 7 pg, 700 fg, 70 fg, 7 fg, 0.7 fg, 0.07 fg, and 0.007 fg/μL, which were obtained by successive 1 : 10 dilution in RNase-free water. The detection limit was measured via the detection of PCR products from DNA extracted from spiked blood samples with 1, 10, 100, 1,000, and 10,000 of *L. infantum* parasites/mL, obtained by successive 1 : 10 dilutions. The analytical specificity was determined by the analysis of PCR products from genomic DNA extracted of *L. infantum, L. donovani, L. braziliensis, L. guyanensis,* and *L. amazonensis* in 6% gel polyacrylamide and kDNA PCR-ELISA.

2.4.5. Diagnostic Precision (Repeatability and Reproducibility). The intra-assay (repeatability) was performed in four replicates in a single run to detect PCR products amplified from the DNA of the reference *L. infantum* (MHOM/BR/2002/LPC-RPV) at 700 fg, 70 fg, 0.7 fg, and 0.07 fg/μL. Four DNA samples from the peripheral blood of patients with VL and four DNA samples from the peripheral blood of noninfected individuals were assayed. Interassay precision (reproducibility) was assessed using PCR products from genomic DNA extracted from *L. infantum*, VL patients, and noninfected individuals, performed in duplicate on consecutive days.

2.5. Data Analysis. In the *kDNA* PCR-ELISA development phase, the cut-off was determined using Receiver Operating Characteristic (ROC) curve analysis in GraphPad Prism 5.0 software (San Diego, CA, USA). The detection limit and analytical specificity of the *kDNA* PCR-ELISA were also assessed. The intra-assay (repeatability) and interassay (reproducibility) precision levels were measured using the variation coefficient (VC) of the results of the retested samples using the equation VC = Standard Deviation/Mean × 100.

The sensitivity and specificity were calculated by evaluating the absorbance readings of the *kDNA* PCR-ELISA in 130 DNA samples from VL patients (Children VL Group and Adult VL Group and VL/HIV Group) and 40 samples from the Noninfected Group using ROC curve analyses.

Absorbance readings were individually assessed using the Shapiro-Wilk normality test (W test) and compared using the Kruskal-Wallis test. The groups that presented normal (Adult VL and VL/HIV Groups) or nonnormal distribution (Children VL and Asymptomatic VL Groups) were compared using the unpaired t-test and Mann–Whitney U test, respectively. All tests were performed in the software GraphPad Prism 6.0, considering a level of significance of $p < 0.05$.

The cut-off value for the *ACTB* PCR-ELISA was calculated as the mean of the absorbance readings of the negative controls plus three standard deviations and was determined in the development phase of the assay.

2.6. Ethical Considerations. Informed consent was obtained from patients, individuals, or guardians at the time of blood collection and all involved centers evaluated and approved the protocol studies (Protocol Number 14/2011).

3. Results

3.1. Analytical Sensitivity, Specificity, and Precision of the kDNA PCR-ELISA. ROC curve analysis using the absorbance readings of the control samples (14 peripheral blood samples collected from patients with VL and peripheral blood samples obtained from healthy individuals of an endemic area) defined a cut-off of 0.096, which showed better sensitivity without compromising specificity, and an area under the curve of 1.0 (95% CI: 0.86 to 1.0).

This *kDNA* PCR-ELISA presented a limit of detection of 0.07 fg, which was defined using a serial dilution of the reference *L. (L.) infantum* (MHOM/BR/2002/LPC-RPV) DNA in water. The detection limit was evaluated using DNA extracted from successive dilutions of blood samples (11 samples evaluated) spiked with an initial concentration of 10,000 parasites. The *kDNA* PCR-ELISA consistently detected the lowest concentration: 1 parasite/mL of blood in all samples evaluated. Similar results were observed for electrophoresis analyses on 6% polyacrylamide gels with products from the same PCR assay (Figures 1 and 2).

In the evaluation of analytical specificity, the *kDNA* PCR-ELISA showed positive results for species from the *L. donovani* complex (*L. (L.) donovani* and *L. (L.) infantum*) and negative results for other species (*L. (V.) braziliensis, L. (V.) guyanensis,* and *L. (L.) amazonensis*). Positive results for all species of *Leishmania* were observed when the same products of the PCR assay were analysed in 6% polyacrylamide gel electrophoresis stained with silver nitrate (Table 1).

The obtained variation coefficients (VCs) in the intra-assay tests were 6.81%, 7.78%, 3.44%, and 11.22% for DNA from the culture samples at concentrations of 700 fg, 70 fg, 0.7 fg, and 0.07 fg, respectively, and ranged from 1.36% to

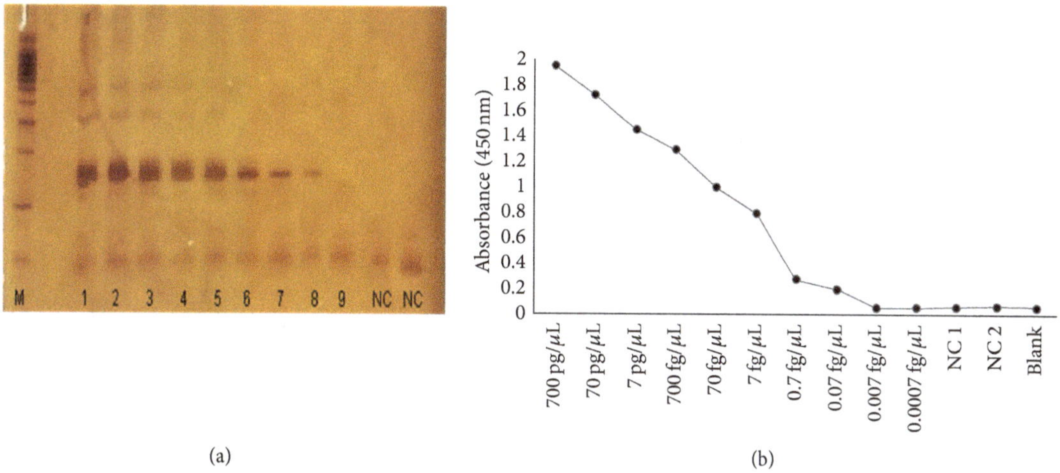

FIGURE 1: Analytical sensitivity of the conventional PCR and kDNA PCR-ELISA in *L. infantum* gDNA. (a) Analytical sensitivity of 6% polyacrylamide gel and (b) *kDNA* PCR-ELISA for the detection of PCR products from DNA extracted of *L. infantum* at concentrations of 1: 700 pg, 2: 70 pg, 3: 7 pg, 4: 700 fg, 5: 70 fg, 6: 7 fg, 7: 0.7 fg, 8: 0.07 fg, and 9: 0.007 fg/μL; NC: negative controls and M: 100 pb DNA Ladder (Promega).

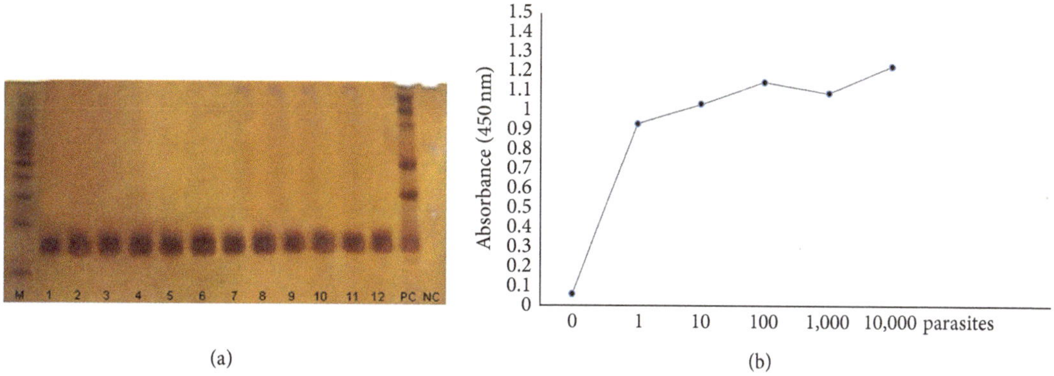

FIGURE 2: Analytical sensitivity of conventional PCR and kDNA PCR-ELISA in spiked blood samples. (a) Analytical sensitivity of 6% polyacrylamide gels and (b) *kDNA* PCR-ELISA for the detection of PCR products from DNA extracted from spiked blood samples with the addition of 1 parasite (lines 1 and 2) and 10 (lines 3 and 4), 100 (lines 5 and 6), 1,000 (lines 7, 8, and 9), and 10,000 parasites (lines 10, 11, and 12); PC: positive control, NC: negative control, and M: 100 pb DNA Ladder (Promega). The absorbance readings correspond to the mean of the duplicate for each parasite concentration.

17.55% in the positive blood samples and 2.78% to 8.81% in negative blood samples. The VC values in the reproducibility analyses (interassay precision) were calculated from the results of four different assays performed on consecutive days with the samples evaluated in duplicate. The VCs were 5.36%, 6.03%, 9.44%, and 23.13% for DNA from the culture samples at concentrations of 700 fg to 0.07 fg, respectively, and ranged from 5.44% to 12.8% for positive blood samples and 8.24% to 21.45% for negative blood samples.

3.2. Diagnostic Performance of the kDNA PCR-ELISA in Different Groups of Patients with VL, VL-HIV Coinfected, Asymptomatic, and Noninfected Endemic Controls. The *kDNA* PCR-ELISA detected infection by *L. (L.) infantum* in 100% of the VL Group (children and adult patients) and 100% of the VL/HIV group. The assay detected infection in 100% of asymptomatic individuals living in endemic areas, and only 5% of noninfected individuals (Noninfected Group) had positive results (Figure 3). Therefore, the *kDNA* PCR-ELISA produced an overall sensitivity of 100% (95% CI: 97.1 to 100%) and specificity of 95% (95% CI: 83.5 to 98.6%).

The levels of *Leishmania* DNA measured by the absorbance readings of the PCR-ELISAs were very similar in the Children VL and Adult VL and VL/HIV groups ($p = 0.18$). In contrast, the absorbance readings in the Asymptomatic Group varied from 0.115 to 1.151 (median = 0.347), which indicates lower levels of circulating *Leishmania* DNA in the children of this group (Figure 3).

All samples of the VL, VL/HIV, asymptomatic, and negative groups were assessed using the PCR-ELISA to detect the human *ACTB* gene and produced absorbance readings above the previously determined cut-off (0.099).

Table 1: Analytical specificity of the PCR detected in 6% polyacrylamide gels and the *kDNA* PCR-ELISA using DNA extracted from different *Leishmania* species.

DNA samples	Gel electrophoresis (*kDNA*)	*kDNA* ELISA	
		Absorbance readings (450 nm)	Status
L. (L.) infantum	Positive	2,237	Positive
L. (L.) donovani	Positive	1,397	Positive
L. (V.) braziliensis	Positive	0,056	Negative
L. (V.) guyanensis	Positive	0,063	Negative
L. (L.) amazonensis	Positive	0,095	Negative

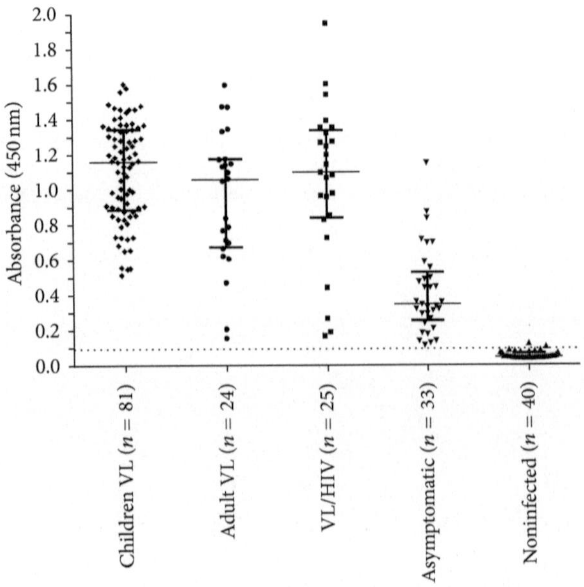

Figure 3: Circulating *L. infantum* DNA levels measured using the *kDNA* PCR-ELISA in different groups. *kDNA* PCR-ELISA absorbance results for the detection of PCR products from DNA extracted from peripheral blood samples in different groups of patients with VL, VL/HIV, asymptomatic, and noninfected endemic controls. There was no statistically difference between Adult VL and VL/HIV Groups ($p = 0.38$). In contrast, the median (0,347) in the Asymptomatic Group was lower than the Children VL Group ($p < 0.0001$). The dashed line represents the cut-off (0.096). Children VL Group: Median = 1.157, 25% Percentile = 0.886 and 75% Percentile = 1.345. Adult VL Group: Median = 1.057, 25% Percentile = 0.675 and 75% Percentile = 1.175. VL/HIV Group: Median = 1.099, 25% Percentile = 0.842 and 75% Percentile = 1.340. Asymptomatic Group: Median = 0.347, 25% Percentile = 0.255 and 75% Percentile = 0.531.

4. Discussion

Despite the technological developments of the twentieth century, VL diagnosis made little progress in recent decades, with few new or alternative tests. There are two main reasons for this lack of progress: VL is a neglected disease that provides businesses small returns on investment in research and development, and it is an infection with high biological complexity [23].

The present study improves the diagnosis of *L. infantum* in humans by presenting the development and proof-of-concept analysis and phase II evaluation of a *kDNA* PCR-ELISA. This method combines PCR and ELISA into a single analytical technique and provides an objective interpretation of the results compared to conventional PCR followed by electrophoresis because it uses a gene-specific probe to detect the amplified product. The PCR-ELISA also allows multiple sample testing and quantitative and qualitative analyses, such as quantitative real-time PCR (qRT-PCR), but using basic laboratory equipment for the processing ELISA tests that is present in most clinical laboratories [20, 21, 24]. PCR-ELISA has the additional advantage of using a whole blood sample that is obtained in a minimally invasive manner. Recently, Ruiter and colleagues [25] demonstrated that there was no statistically significant difference between the accuracy of molecular methods using whole blood samples in VL diagnosis compared with the use of more invasive bone marrow clinical samples.

The *kDNA* PCR-ELISA is based on the capture of an amplified product with a sense primer labelled with biotin at the 5′end in the polystyrene plate coated with streptavidin, followed by hybridisation with a fluorescein-labelled probe at the 5′ end and an antifluorescein-peroxidase conjugate for detection [21]. Kinetoplast DNA or *kDNA* was chosen as the DNA target for the PCR-ELISA because it is present in a large copy number in the *Leishmania* cell [26, 27]. However, it does not permit precise quantification of the DNA of *Leishmania* spp. because of the large variability in copy number of its minicircle forms (the specific *kDNA* target) in different strains, which led us to choose a qualitative type of a PCR-ELISA.

Different PCR-ELISA were developed for the diagnosis of VL, but most of these assays were evaluated in only one group of patients [28–30], which did not allow broad validation for clinical diagnosis. Other tests were not designed to specifically detect causative agents of VL [28, 29, 31], which discourages its use in surveillance and disease control programmes. Two tests were described only at the development phase [31, 32], and many others used commercial kits for the detection of PCR-amplified products that may suffer from discontinuity of production [28, 30, 33, 34].

The analytical specificity of the *kDNA* PCR-ELISA for causative VL agents was only possible because of the use of a probe designed to complement a specific nucleotide sequence for the *L. donovani* complex. Only the *L. (L.) infantum* and *L. (L.) donovani* species were detected using the assay in the proposed test (Table 1). The same result was obtained using only one platform and a probe specific to *L. (L.) infantum* compared with VL PCR-ELISA previously developed [33].

The lower detection limits of the assay (0.07 fg of purified *L. (L.) infantum* DNA and 1 parasite/mL of human blood) (Figures 1 and 2) are lower or similar to the detection of other PCR-ELISA [29, 31, 33, 35].

The *kDNA* PCR-ELISA exhibited diagnostic precision because it presented ratios of repeatability and reproducibility from 1.36 to 17.55% and 5.36 to 23.13%, respectively. The upper limit for the coefficient of variation in molecular tests is not established, but our results are similar to other reported tests based on the PCR-ELISA, which revealed intra-assay coefficients of variation (repeatability) from 1.9 to 12.0 and interassay coefficient of variation (repeatability) from 3.0 to 27.0% [21, 36–38]. The same protocol was used to develop the human beta actin *(ACTB)* PCR-ELISA for evaluations of all samples analysed. This test was developed as an internal control of DNA integrity and a control for variation in the efficiency of DNA extraction and PCR amplification primarily in peripheral blood samples that were negative in the *kDNA* PCR-ELISA test. To our knowledge, no other PCR-ELISA that was developed for the diagnosis of VL demonstrated the same type of control.

Phase II evaluation of a *kDNA* PCR-ELISA used 130 DNA samples from the peripheral blood of patients (Children VL Group and Adult VL Group and VL/HIV Group) and 40 samples from a Noninfected Group. The assay exhibited a good performance, with a sensitivity of 100% and specificity of 95%.

The equivalence of *kDNA* PCR-ELISA performance with values demonstrated by other molecular methods for the diagnosis of VL must be highlighted, including PCR assay followed by electrophoresis (sensitivity of 91 to 100% and specificity of 87 to 100%) [15, 16, 39]. The sensitivity of the *kDNA* PCR-ELISA was similar to the value of 98% for the assay developed by Costa et al. and compared with other assays that used the same methodology to diagnose VL and evaluated for test performance [28]. This study used peripheral blood and bone marrow aspirate samples for evaluations, and the DNA target was the *SSU-rRNA* coding region of *L. (L.) donovani*. The *kDNA* PCR-ELISA demonstrated superior performance compared to the assay developed by De Doncker et al. [29], which used the target *SSU-rRNA* that is conserved in *Leishmania* genus and presented a sensitivity of 83.9% (95% CI: 71.7–92.4) and specificity of 87.2% (95% CI: 72.6–95.7).

The *kDNA* PCR-ELISA was validated in this study in clinical samples from varied groups of VL patients at different ages and asymptomatic and noninfected endemic controls to ensure its widespread use as a method for the diagnosis of the disease and asymptomatic infection. Molecular tests are especially useful for VL diagnosis in immunosuppressed patients, in whom serological tests tend to be less sensitive because of impaired humoral immune response. The sensitivity of *kDNA* PCR-ELISA in VL/HIV coinfected patients was 100%. This result is superior to Piarroux et al. [40] (82%) and similar to Lachaud et al. [41] (100%) (both of these studies used bone marrow samples) and Fissore et al. [42] with serum samples (sensitivity of 97%) and PCR electrophoresis analysis on 2% agarose gel.

Two samples of noninfected individuals (negative group) that previously presented negative results in qPCR were positive in the *kDNA* PCR-ELISA, but with low absorbance readings (Figure 3). This fact may be explained by the molecular target used in the qPCR assay, the *SSU-rRNA*, and these two positive samples may be asymptomatic individuals who were not identified using the reference antibody-based methods. Lachaud et al. [14] compared various molecular targets for the detection of *Leishmania* DNA in peripheral blood samples, the ribosomal DNA target, two nuclear targets, and three kinetoplast (minicircle) targets, and the kinetoplast was generally the most sensitive. Unfortunately, the high number of kDNA copies increases the risk of carryover contamination in the handling and processing steps, mainly if not handled by trained professionals. In the development of kDNA PCR-ELISA all procedures were done by a trained researcher and physical barriers (e.g., separation of rooms and materials and the use of laminar flow hood with ultraviolet light) were utilized in the sample handling steps to minimize the risk of contamination.

Currently, one of the most important challenges in assessing *L. infantum* transmission in endemic areas is the identification of asymptomatic infection. Serological tests are the methods of choice for population studies, but our results suggest that these methods are neither adequate nor accurate for the diagnosis of the asymptomatic form. The performance of serological tests to detect *L. infantum* antibodies was evaluated primarily in patients presenting VL symptoms [43–47]. Some studies demonstrated that ELISA methods cannot be reliably used as a tool to identify asymptomatic individuals, and it may underestimate the positive rates, especially when only one antigen is used [48, 49].

The *kDNA* PCR-ELISA in this study is a potential tool to identify and follow up asymptomatic individuals, especially in population-based studies in which there are a larger number of individuals to be evaluated. The assay detected all children from the Asymptomatic VL Group as positive, with absorbance readings from 0.115 to 1.151 and a median (0,347) that was lower than the Children VL Group (Median 1.157; $p < 0.0001$), which suggests the presence of circulating DNA *L. Infantum*. These findings corroborate data published by dos Santos Marques et al. [50], who found lower circulating DNA levels in asymptomatic compared to VL children tested with qPCR targeting SSU-rRNA from *Leishmania* spp. Molecular diagnosis of asymptomatic individuals has great importance because it provides monitoring of individuals who are in contact but have not developed the disease and allows the monitoring of transmission areas to develop more effective strategies for VL control programmes.

5. Conclusions

A PCR-ELISA targeting *kDNA* from the *Leishmania donovani* complex was developed for human VL diagnosis in peripheral blood samples. The assay exhibited good performance in proof-of-concept analyses and phase II evaluation in age-variable groups of *L. infantum*-infected patients, asymptomatic individuals, and healthy endemic controls. A human beta actin *(ACTB)* PCR-ELISA was developed as an internal control for DNA extraction and PCR amplification. Therefore, the *kDNA* PCR-ELISA is safe and suitable for the diagnosis of human *L. infantum* infection in reference laboratories in endemic countries and allows the simultaneous testing of a large number of samples with broad application for disease control programmes. It is important to note that the present study is a case control evaluation which may justify the existence of bias and an exaggerated estimate of sensitivity and specificity. So, a large field trial assessing the usefulness of the PCR-ELISA as a confirmatory VL test is still necessary before the PCR-ELISA implementation, both for the evaluation of asymptomatic individuals with positive or negative serology and for the diagnosis of true VL cases among symptomatic suspected patients in an endemic region.

Competing Interests

The authors declare that they have no competing interests.

Authors' Contributions

Fernanda Alvarenga Cardoso Medeiros, Luciana Inácia Gomes, and Ana Rabello conceived and designed the study. Acquisition of the financial support for the study was by Fernanda Alvarenga Cardoso Medeiros, Luciana Inácia Gomes, and Ana Rabello. Fernanda Alvarenga Cardoso Medeiros, Carolina Senra Alves de Souza, and Letícia Helena dos Santos Marques performed the experiments. Luciana Inácia Gomes, Edward Oliveira, Ana Rabello, Gláucia Fernandes Cota, and Mariângela Carneiro analysed the data. Maria Vitória Mourão, Letícia Helena dos Santos Marques, Gláucia Fernandes Cota, and Mariângela Carneiro proved biological samples. Fernanda Alvarenga Cardoso Medeiros, Luciana Inácia Gomes, Edward Oliveira, and Ana Rabello wrote the paper. All authors contributed equally to this work.

Acknowledgments

The authors thank Eliane de Morais Teixeira for providing *Leishmania* spp.

References

[1] WHO, "Leishmaniasis in high-burden countries: an epidemiological update based on data reported in 2014," *Weekly Epidemiological Record*, vol. 22, pp. 287–296, 2016.

[2] M. O. Harhay, P. L. Olliaro, D. L. Costa, and C. H. N. Costa, "Urban parasitology: visceral leishmaniasis in Brazil," *Trends in Parasitology*, vol. 27, no. 9, pp. 403–409, 2011.

[3] V. E. M. de Araújo, L. C. Pinheiro, M. C. M. de Almeida et al., "Relative risk of visceral leishmaniasis in Brazil: a spatial analysis in urban area," *PLoS Neglected Tropical Diseases*, vol. 7, no. 11, article no. e2540, 2013.

[4] SINAN-Sistema de Informação de Agravos de Notificação, Ministério da Saúde, Brasília, 2015, http://datasus.saude.gov.br/.

[5] K. Ritmeijer, Y. Melaku, M. Mueller, S. Kipngetich, C. O'Keeffe, and R. N. Davidson, "Evaluation of a new recombinant K39 rapid diagnostic test for Sudanese visceral leishmaniasis," *American Journal of Tropical Medicine and Hygiene*, vol. 74, no. 1, pp. 76–80, 2006.

[6] E. Abass, C. Kang, F. Martinkovic et al., "Heterogeneity of Leishmania donovani parasites complicates diagnosis of visceral leishmaniasis: comparison of different serological tests in three endemic regions," *PLoS ONE*, vol. 10, no. 3, Article ID e0116408, 2015.

[7] R. Ter Horst, T. Tefera, G. Assefa, A. Z. Ebrahim, R. N. Davidson, and K. Ritmeijer, "Field evaluation of rK39 test and direct agglutination test for diagnosis of visceral leishmaniasis in a population with high prevalence of human immunodeficiency virus in Ethiopia," *The American Journal of Tropical Medicine and Hygiene*, vol. 80, no. 6, pp. 929–934, 2009.

[8] G. F. Cota, M. R. de Sousa, F. N. Demarqui, and A. Rabello, "The diagnostic accuracy of serologic and molecular methods for detecting visceral leishmaniasis in HIV infected patients: meta-analysis," *PLoS Neglected Tropical Diseases*, vol. 6, no. 5, Article ID e1665, 2012.

[9] G. F. Cota, M. R. De Sousa, B. M. De Freitas Nogueira et al., "Comparison of parasitological, serological, and molecular tests for visceral leishmaniasis in HIV-infected patients: a cross-sectional delayed-type study," *American Journal of Tropical Medicine and Hygiene*, vol. 89, no. 3, pp. 570–577, 2013.

[10] M. Andreadou, E. Liandris, I. N. Kasampalidis et al., "Evaluation of the performance of selected in-house and commercially available PCR and real-time PCR assays for the detection of *Leishmania* DNA in canine clinical samples," *Experimental Parasitology*, vol. 131, no. 4, pp. 419–424, 2012.

[11] G. Srividya, A. Kulshrestha, R. Singh, and P. Salotra, "Diagnosis of visceral leishmaniasis: developments over the last decade," *Parasitology Research*, vol. 110, no. 3, pp. 1065–1078, 2012.

[12] A. M. Montalvo, J. Fraga, I. Maes, J.-C. Dujardin, and G. Van Der Auwera, "Three new sensitive and specific heat-shock protein 70 PCRs for global Leishmania species identification," *European Journal of Clinical Microbiology & Infectious Diseases*, vol. 31, no. 7, pp. 1453–1461, 2012.

[13] I. S. Koltas, F. Eroglu, S. Uzun, and D. Alabaz, "A comparative analysis of different molecular targets using PCR for diagnosis of old world leishmaniasis," *Experimental Parasitology*, vol. 164, pp. 43–48, 2016.

[14] L. Lachaud, S. Marchergui-Hammami, E. ChabbertDereure, J. Dereure, J. P. Dedet, and P. Bastien, "Comparison of six PCR methods using peripheral blood for detection of canine visceral leishmaniasis," *Journal Clinical Microbiology*, vol. 40, no. 1, pp. 210–215, 2002.

[15] Z. Wu, Y. Bao, Y. Ding, M. Yu, L. Lu, and Y. Zhang, "An experimental study on application of PCR in detection of Kala-azar," *The Southeast Asian Journal of Tropical Medicine and Public Health*, vol. 28, no. 1, pp. 169–172, 1997.

[16] R. Maurya, R. K. Singh, B. Kumar, P. Salotra, M. Rai, and S. Sundar, "Evaluation of PCR for diagnosis of Indian kala-azar and assessment of cure," *Journal of Clinical Microbiology*, vol. 43, no. 7, pp. 3038–3041, 2005.

[17] S. Banoo, D. Bell, P. Bossuyt et al., "Evaluation of diagnostic tests for infectious diseases: general principles," *Nature Reviews Microbiology*, vol. 4, no. 9, pp. S21–S31, 2006.

[18] Â. C. Volpini, V. M. A. Passos, G. C. Oliveira, and A. J. Romanha, "PCR-RFLP to identify *Leishmania* (*Viannia*) *braziliensis* and *L.* (*Leishmania*) amazonensis causing American cutaneous leishmaniasis," *Acta Tropica*, vol. 90, no. 1, pp. 31–37, 2004.

[19] S. Rozen and H. Skaletsky, "Primer3 on the WWW for general users and for biologist programmers," *Methods in molecular biology (Clifton, N.J.)*, vol. 132, pp. 365–386, 2000.

[20] E. Luneberg, J. S. Jensen, and M. Frosch, "Detection of Mycoplasma pneumoniae by polymerase chain reaction and nonradioactive hybridization in microtiter plates," *Journal of Clinical Microbiology*, vol. 31, no. 5, pp. 1088–1094, 1993.

[21] L. I. Gomes, L. H. Dos Santos Marques, M. J. Enk, M. C. de Oliveira, P. M. Z. Coelho, and A. Rabello, "Development and evaluation of a sensitive PCR-ELISA system for detection of *Schistosoma* infection in feces," *PLoS Neglected Tropical Diseases*, vol. 4, no. 4, article e664, 2010.

[22] O. Musso, P. Sommer, E. Drouet et al., "In situ detection of human cytomegalovirus DNA in gastrointestinal biopsies from AIDS patients by means of various PCR-derived methods," *Journal of Virological Methods*, vol. 56, no. 2, pp. 125–137, 1996.

[23] S. Antinori, L. Schifanella, and M. Corbellino, "Leishmaniasis: new insights from an old and neglected disease," *European Journal of Clinical Microbiology and Infectious Diseases*, vol. 31, no. 2, pp. 109–118, 2012.

[24] M. J. Sue, S. K. Yeap, A. R. Omar, and S. W. Tan, "Application of PCR-ELISA in molecular diagnosis," *BioMed Research International*, vol. 2014, Article ID 653014, 6 pages, 2014.

[25] C. M. De Ruiter, C. Van Der Veer, M. M. G. Leeflang, S. Deborggraeve, C. Lucas, and E. R. Adams, "Molecular tools for diagnosis of visceral leishmaniasis: systematic review and meta-analysis of diagnostic test accuracy," *Journal of Clinical Microbiology*, vol. 52, no. 9, pp. 3147–3155, 2014.

[26] M. R. Rodgers, S. J. Popper, and D. F. Wirth, "Amplification of kinetoplast DNA as a tool in the detection and diagnosis of *Leishmania*," *Experimental Parasitology*, vol. 71, no. 3, pp. 267–275, 1990.

[27] W. Degrave, O. Fernandes, D. Campbell, M. Bozza, and U. Lopes, "Use of molecular probes and PCR for detection and typing of Leishmania—a mini-review," *Memorias do Instituto Oswaldo Cruz*, vol. 89, no. 3, pp. 463–469, 1994.

[28] J.-M. Costa, R. Durand, M. Deniau et al., "PCR enzyme-linked immunosorbent assay for diagnosis of leishmaniasis in human immunodeficiency virus-infected patients," *Journal of Clinical Microbiology*, vol. 34, no. 7, pp. 1831–1833, 1996.

[29] S. De Doncker, V. Hutse, S. Abdellati et al., "A new PCR-ELISA for diagnosis of visceral leishmaniasis in blood of HIV-negative subjects," *Transactions of the Royal Society of Tropical Medicine and Hygiene*, vol. 99, no. 1, pp. 25–31, 2005.

[30] A. Alborzi, B. Pourabbas, F. Shahian, J. Mardaneh, G. R. Pouladfar, and M. Ziyaeyan, "Detection of *Leishmania infantum* kinetoplast DNA in the whole blood of asymptomatic individuals by PCR-ELISA and comparison with other infection markers in endemic areas, southern Iran," *The American Journal of Tropical Medicine and Hygiene*, vol. 79, no. 6, pp. 839–842, 2008.

[31] T. Kobets, J. Badalová, I. Grekov, H. Havelková, M. Svobodová, and M. Lipoldová, "*Leishmania* parasite detection and quantification using PCR-ELISA," *Nature protocols*, vol. 5, no. 6, pp. 1074–1080, 2010.

[32] N. Rolão, S. Cortes, O. R. Rodrigues, and L. Campino, "Quantification of *Leishmania infantum* parasites in tissue biopsies by real-time polymerase chain reaction and polymerase chain reaction-enzyme-linked immunosorbent assay," *Journal of Parasitology*, vol. 90, no. 5, pp. 1150–1154, 2004.

[33] J. Martin-Sanchez, M. C. Lopez-Lopez, C. Acedo-Sanchez, J. J. Castro-Fajardo, J. A. Pineda, and F. Morillas-Marquez, "Diagnosis of infections with *Leishmania infantum* using PCR-ELISA," *Parasitology*, vol. 122, no. 6, pp. 607–615, 2001.

[34] J. Martín-Sánchez, J. A. Pineda, M. Andreu-Lopez et al., "The high sensitivity of a PCR-ELISA in the diagnosis of cutaneous and visceral leishmaniasis caused by *Leishmania infantum*," *Annals of Tropical Medicine and Parasitology*, vol. 96, no. 7, pp. 669–677, 2002.

[35] J. Martín-Sánchez and M. M. Francisco, Kit para diagnóstico específico de las leishmaniosis causadas por 'Leishmania infantum' por la técnica de PCR-ELISA, Espanha patente CI- C12Q 1/68, 01 Novmber 2003.

[36] P. Morata, M. I. Queipo-Ortuño, J. M. Reguera, M. A. García-Ordoñez, A. Ana Cárdenas, and J. D. Colmenero, "Development and evaluation of a PCR-enzyme-linked immunosorbent assay for diagnosis of human brucellosis," *Journal of Clinical Microbiology*, vol. 41, no. 1, pp. 144–148, 2003.

[37] M. I. Queipo-Ortuño, M. A. García-Ordoñez, R. Gil, J. Rojas, J. D. D. Colmenero, and P. Morata, "PCR-DIG ELISA with biotinylated primers is unsuitable for use in whole blood samples from patients with brucellosis," *Molecular and Cellular Probes*, vol. 18, no. 4, pp. 243–250, 2004.

[38] M. Musiani, G. Gallinella, S. Venturoli, and M. Zerbini, "Competitive PCR-ELISA protocols for the quantitative and the standardized detection of viral genomes," *Nature Protocols*, vol. 2, no. 10, pp. 2511–2519, 2007.

[39] J. Disch, F. C. Maciel, M. C. de Oliveira, M. Orsini, and A. Rabello, "Detection of circulating *Leishmania chagasi* DNA for the non-invasive diagnosis of human infection," *Transactions of the Royal Society of Tropical Medicine and Hygiene*, vol. 97, no. 4, pp. 391–395, 2003.

[40] R. Piarroux, F. Gambarelli, H. Dumon et al., "Comparison of PCR with direct examination of bone marrow aspiration, myeloculture, and serology for diagnosis of visceral leishmaniasis in immunocompromised patients," *Journal of Clinical Microbiology*, vol. 32, no. 3, pp. 746–749, 1994.

[41] L. Lachaud, J. Dereure, E. Chabbert et al., "Optimized PCR using patient blood samples for diagnosis and follow-up of visceral leishmaniasis, with special reference to AIDS patients," *Journal of Clinical Microbiology*, vol. 38, no. 1, pp. 236–240, 2000.

[42] C. Fissore, P. Delaunay, B. Ferrua et al., "Convenience of serum for visceral leishmaniasis diagnosis by PCR," *Journal of Clinical Microbiology*, vol. 42, no. 11, pp. 5332–5333, 2004.

[43] R. F. S. Braz, E. T. Nascimento, D. R. A. Martins et al., "The sensitivity and specificity of *Leishmania chagasi* recombinant K39 antigen in the diagnosis of American visceral leishmaniasis and in differentiating active from subclinical infection," *American Journal of Tropical Medicine and Hygiene*, vol. 67, no. 4, pp. 344–348, 2002.

[44] S. F. Guimarães Carvalho, E. Moreira Lemos, R. Corey, and R. Dietze, "Performance of recombinant K39 antigen in the diagnosis of Brazilian visceral leishmaniasis," *American Journal of Tropical Medicine and Hygiene*, vol. 68, no. 3, pp. 321–324, 2003.

[45] M. Boelaert, S. Rijal, S. Regmi et al., "A comparative study of the effectiveness of diagnostic tests for visceral leishmaniasis," *American Journal of Tropical Medicine and Hygiene*, vol. 70, no. 1, pp. 72–77, 2004.

[46] F. Chappuis, S. Rijal, A. Soto, J. Menten, and M. Boelaert, "A meta-analysis of the diagnostic performance of the direct agglutination test and rK39 dipstick for visceral leishmaniasis," *British Medical Journal*, vol. 333, no. 7571, pp. 723–726, 2006.

[47] Z. Maia, M. Lírio, S. Mistro, C. M. C. Mendes, S. R. Mehta, and R. Badaro, "Comparative study of rK39 *Leishmania* antigen for serodiagnosis of visceral leishmaniasis: systematic review with meta-analysis," *PLoS Neglected Tropical Diseases*, vol. 6, no. 1, Article ID e1484, 2012.

[48] L. de Gouvêa Viana, T. S. M. de Assis, M. Orsini et al., "Combined diagnostic methods identify a remarkable proportion of asymptomatic *Leishmania* (*Leishmania*) *chagasi* carriers who present modulated cytokine profiles," *Transactions of the Royal Society of Tropical Medicine and Hygiene*, vol. 102, no. 6, pp. 548–555, 2008.

[49] E. C. Moreno, A. V. Gonçalves, A. V. Chaves et al., "Inaccuracy of enzyme-linked immunosorbent assay using soluble and recombinant antigens to detect asymptomatic infection by Leishmania infantum," *PLoS Neglected Tropical Diseases*, vol. 3, no. 10, article no. e536, 2009.

[50] L. H. dos Santos Marques, L. I. Gomes, I. C. M. da Rocha et al., "Low parasite load estimated by qPCR in a cohort of children living in urban area endemic for visceral leishmaniasis in Brazil," *PLoS Neglected Tropical Diseases*, vol. 6, no. 12, Article ID e1955, 2012.

30

Clinical Profiles of Dengue Infection during an Outbreak in Northern India

Anish Laul,[1] Poonam Laul,[2] Vamsi Merugumala,[2] Ravi Pathak,[2] Urvashi Miglani,[2] and Pinkee Saxena[2]

[1]*Maulana Azad Medical College, No. 2, Bahadur Shah Zafar Marg, New Delhi, Delhi 110002, India*
[2]*Deen Dayal Upadhyay Hospital, Hari Nagar, Clock Tower, New Delhi, Delhi 110064, India*

Correspondence should be addressed to Poonam Laul; poonam_laul@yahoo.com

Academic Editor: Shyam Sundar

Introduction. Dengue fever is an arboviral disease, which is transmitted by mosquito vector and presents as varied clinical spectrum of dengue fever (DF), dengue hemorrhagic fever (DHF), dengue shock syndrome (DSS), and expanded dengue syndrome (EDS) with atypical presentations, thus posing a diagnostic dilemma. Unless we are aware of these presentations, diagnosis as well as early initiation of treatment becomes difficult. We studied the various clinical presentations of dengue infection during an outbreak of disease in 2015. *Materials and Methods.* A total of 115 confirmed cases of dengue infection from Department of Medicine of Deen Dayal Upadhyay Hospital, New Delhi, were enrolled in this observational study. *Results.* The common signs and symptoms of dengue infection were fever, headache, body ache, backache, retro-orbital pain, bleeding manifestations, and rash in 100%, 87%, 86%, 58%, 41%, 21%, and 21%, respectively. Nonspecific or warning signs and symptoms included vomiting, weakness, abdominal pain, breathlessness, vertigo, sweating, and syncope. Other possible signs and symptoms of coinfections, comorbidities, or complications included diarrhea, sore throat, and neurological manifestations. There were seven patients with coinfections and four with comorbidities. The final diagnosis of these patients was DF (73%), DHF (16.5%), DSS (1.7%), and EDS (4.3%). Among EDS patients, the atypical presentations included encephalopathy, lateral rectus nerve palsy, acalculous cholecystitis, and myocarditis. Four patients required ICU care and there was no death in this study. *Conclusion.* Knowledge of atypical presentations is a must for early diagnosis and timely intervention to prevent life-threatening complications.

1. Introduction

Dengue is a viral disease of tropical regions. The causative agent is one of serotypes of a single stranded RNA virus called DENV 1, 2, 3, and 4 [1]. It is a tropical disease, which is transmitted by the *Aedes aegypti* mosquito. Incubation period is 4 to 7 days (range 3–14 days) [2]. Once the symptoms start, person can remain infectious for next six to seven days. In addition to mosquito bite, dengue has been reported to be transmitted by transfusion of blood from an infected donor, injuries by infected sharps to health care workers, transplantation of organs and tissues from infected donors, and from infected pregnant mother to her fetus by vertical transmission [3–5]. This viral infection has a wide clinical spectrum ranging from asymptomatic disease to undifferentiated fever (or viral syndromes), classical dengue fever (DF), dengue hemorrhagic fever (DHF), or dengue shock syndrome (DSS) and expanded dengue syndrome (EDS) [2]. After incubation period ends, the disease is followed by three phases: febrile, critical, and recovery phase [2]. In the recent years, dengue has crossed geographic borders and has spread to many new countries. Currently, it is endemic to southeast Asia and western pacific regions [2]. So dengue fever has become a major international public concern particularly in tropical and subtropical regions affecting urban as well as rural areas. Though several measures are taken to prevent and control it, recurrent outbreaks have been reported in India. The first outbreak of dengue fever in India was in 1812 [6].

Several major outbreaks took place after this in years 1836, 1906, 1911, 1972, 2005, 2010, and 2015. An increasing number of cases of dengue are being reported with atypical presentations as frequent epidemics are occurring. As awareness of

Table 1

DF/DHF	Grade	Signs and symptoms	Laboratory
DF	With or without haemorrhagic manifestations	Fever with two of the following: (i) Headache. (ii) Retro-orbital pain. (iii) Myalgia. (iv) Arthtralgia/bone pain. (v) Rash. (vi) Haemorrhagic manifestations. (vii) No evidence of plasma leakage.	Leucopenia (wbc ≤5000 cells/mm^3). (i) Thrombocytopenia (platelet count <150 000 cells/mm^3). (ii) Rising haematocrit (5%–10%). (iii) No evidence of plasma loss.
DHF	I	Fever and haemorrhagic manifestation (positive tourniquet test) and evidence of plasma leakage.	Thrombocytopenia <100 000 cells/mm^3; HCT rise ≥20%.
DHF	II	As in Grade I plus spontaneous bleeding.	Thrombocytopenia <100 000 cells/mm^3; HCT rise ≥20%.
DHF	III	As in Grade I or II plus circulatory failure (weak pulse, narrow pulse pressure (≤20 mmHg), hypotension, restlessness).	Thrombocytopenia <100 000 cells/mm^3; HCT rise ≥20%.
DHF	IV	As in Grade III plus profound shock with undetectable BP and pulse.	Thrombocytopenia < 100 000 cells/mm^3; HCT rise ≥20%.

this disease is increasing, rare manifestations are also being reported. During an outbreak in 2015 in Northern India, the present study was conducted in tertiary care hospital in Delhi highlighting the varied clinical presentations of dengue fever.

2. Materials and Methods

This was an observational study conducted on the patients selected from indoor and outdoor Departments of Medicine of Deen Dayal Upadhyay Hospital in West Delhi, India, during the period from 1 June to 31 August 2015. 115 patients suffering from dengue fever during an outbreak of the disease were enrolled. All patients who were admitted with complaint of fever and were found positive for either NS1 antigen (Micro ELISA, J. Mitra) or dengue IgM antibodies (NIV Pune) were included in the present study. A detailed history was taken and careful clinical examination was performed. Besides routine biochemical and hematological investigations [hemoglobin, total leucocyte count (TLC) and differential leucocyte count (DLC), platelet count, hematocrit (HCT), liver function tests (LFT), blood urea, and serum creatinine], malarial antigen, Slide test for malarial parasite, IgM antibodies and Widal test for typhoid, and X-ray chest and ultrasonography (USG) of abdomen were also done in all patients. Other investigations were performed according to the clinical conditions of the patients. All subjects were classified according to WHO guidelines as shown in Table 1 [2].

2.1. Criteria for Classification of Dengue Infection. Patients having neurological, cardiac, gastrointestinal, musculoskeletal, renal, ocular, and other nonspecific manifestations were grouped in expanded dengue syndrome (EDS) category. Thrombocytopenia was taken as platelet count less than 1 lac/mm^3 and leucopenia as wbc ≤5000 cells/mm^3.

Table 2

Age groups	Frequency	%
18–20 years	23	20%
21–30 years	48	41.7%
31–40 years	22	19.1%
41–50 years	12	10.4%
>50 years	10	8.7%
Total	115	100%
Mean ± SD	31.36 ± 13.17	
Median	30	
Min–max	13–71	

3. Results

192 subjects with fever and clinical suspicion of dengue were tested for NS1 antigen and dengue IgM antibody and 115 subjects (59.8%) of confirmed dengue fever with age more than 18 years were included in the study.

4. Age-Wise Distribution of Patients

Age distribution of patients is as shown in Table 2. We had 64 (57%) males and 51 (44%) females enrolled in our study.

5. Clinical Presentations

As far as clinical spectrum was concerned, all patients had come with fever along with varied clinical manifestations as shown in Table 3. 65 patients (57%) had abdominal pain, out of which 26 had right upper quadrant pain with fever. Nine patients had positive Murphy's sign. All the 26 patients with

Table 3

Symptoms	Number of patients	Percentage%
Fever	115	100
Headache	100	87
Body ache	99	86
Backache	67	58
Retro-orbital pain	47	41
Bleed (any hemorrhagic manifestation)	24	21
Rashes	25	21
Vomiting	78	68
Weakness	79	68
Pain abdomen	65	57
Breathlessness	22	19
Vertigo	16	14
Sweating	15	13
Syncope	14	12
Diarrhoea	31	27
Sore throat	29	25
Neurological manifestations	3	2
Itching	22	19
Others	9	8

pain had edematous gall bladder without gallstones. Diagnosis of acalculous cholecystitis was made and all patients responded well to supportive therapy. 29 patients (25%) had associated hepatomegaly and six patients (5%) had ascites associated with hepatosplenomegaly. All 65 patients (57%) of pain abdomen had elevated AST and 49% had elevated ALT as shown in Table 7. There was significant difference in ALT among the four groups with elevated levels indicating the severest and atypical forms of infections in form of DHF, DSS, and EDS (p value 0.039) as shown in Table 8. All patients with raised AST and ALT were discharged once they showed falling trend and no patient reported to have any hepatic sequelae.

One patient with jaundice and enzymes in range of 200 IU also recovered completely within two weeks. All other causes of jaundice were ruled out in this. Only one patient in our study had blood urea of 42 mg% and serum creatinine 1.6 mg%; however he also recovered with supportive treatment without any complication. There was no hepatic or renal failure reported in our study.

22 patients (19%) had breathlessness, out of which 18 patients (16%) had pleural effusion on chest X-ray as shown in Table 4. Two patients were known asthmatic, one had come in respiratory failure, and another had dyspnoea due to congestive heart failure.

6. Investigations (X-Ray, Ultrasound Abdomen, Test for Coinfections)

For more details see Table 4.

7. Blood Investigations

90 patients (78%) had thrombocytopenia with platelet count less than one lac. There was significant difference in the platelet count among the four groups, with DHF and DSS having significantly low values (p value 0.003). 80 patients (70%) had leucopenia with relatively decreased lymphocyte count among the four groups, the mean value being the lowest in DSS and DHF group, respectively (p value < 0.001) (Tables 5 and 6).

Clinical categorisation of subjects was done as shown in Table 9. Nineteen patients were diagnosed with DHF and two with DSS. 24 patients (20%) had hemorrhagic manifestations in form of epistaxis, hematemesis, hemoptysis, melena, subconjunctival hemorrhage, and menorrhagia. Ten patients required both blood and platelet transfusion and five required only platelet transfusion. A total of thirty units of platelets were transfused. Intravenous fluid therapy was given according to WHO guidelines.

8. Clinical Categorisation

Four patients (3%) required ICU care because of DSS, myocarditis, and encephalopathy. One patient of DSS had come with acute respiratory distress in shock with saturation of 79% and needed intubation in casualty and was transferred to ICU and put on ventilator. He had pleural effusion as well as ascites and very low platelet count. He was monitored with central line, transfused 6 units of platelets, and required ICU care for five days. Total hospital stay was eight days and patient recovered well without any residual disease.

Another patient of DSS with BP of 60/40 and haematemesis required ICU care with platelet as well as blood transfusion. His hospital stay was of 6 days. Patient responded well to platelet, blood, and fluid therapy. Another patient of encephalopathy also required ICU care.

The fourth patient requiring ICU care was an eighteen-year-old girl. She had come with fever and breathlessness which on physical examination revealed congestive heart failure. Patient was hypoxemic and hypotensive. She had thrombocytopenia, EKG revealed sinus tachycardia, X-ray chest revealed bilateral pleural effusion, and echocardiography showed pericardial effusion, global hypokinesia, and reduced left ventricular systolic function with ejection fraction of 40%. Clinical diagnosis of myocarditis was made. She was treated in ICU with standard decongestive therapy, positive inotropic support, and platelet infusion. Patient responded well to treatment and had ejection fraction of 56% at the time of discharge with no long term sequelae on follow-up.

Five patients (4.3%) had expanded dengue syndrome (EDS) affecting nervous system (encephalopathy, facial, and lateral rectus nerve palsy) in three, cardiovascular system (myocarditis) in one, and gastrointestinal system in one (jaundice). The patient with encephalopathy was brought

Table 4

Finding	Positive cases	Total	Percentage%
Pleural effusion (PE)	18	115	15
Gall bladder edema (GBE)	26	115	22
Hepatosplenomegaly (HS)	29	115	25
Hepatosplenomegaly + ascites (HS + A)	6	115	5
Malarial antigen (R-MAT)	1	115	0.9
Slide test for malaria	2	115	1.8
Widal test	4	115	3.5

Table 5

WBC count	Mean ± SD	Median	Min–max
Total	3749.48 ± 2411	3000.00	1100–18500
N	55.58 ± 12.54	55.00	25–90
L	38.83 ± 12.58	40.00	9–64
M	2.78 ± 1.89	2.00	0–10
E	1.95 ± 1.89	1.00	0–16

Table 6

WBC count	DF		DHF		DSS		EDS		*p* value
	Mean	±SD	Mean	±SD	Mean	±SD	Mean	±SD	
Total	3398.43	±1645.59	4404.21	±2771.25	10550	±11243	4790	±3267.72	0.541
N	53.49	±11.93	63.53	±11.25	64.5	±28.99	59	±11.18	0.011
L	41.49	±12.07	29.42	±9.49	27	±24.04	31.8	±6.8	<0.001
M	2.75	±1.93	3.11	±1.91	3	±1.41	1.75	±0.96	0.499
E	1.99	±2.07	1.74	±1.24	3.5	±0.71	1.5	±0.58	0.265

Table 7

	Mean ± SD	Median	Min–max
PL count (K)	52.70 ± 38.54	41.00	10–204
HCT	38.86 ± 5.91	39.00	18.10–67.30
UREA	18.97 ± 5.21	18.00	10–42
Creatine	1.16 ± 1.69	1.00	0.20–17
Serum bilirubin	1.13 ± 0.63	1.10	0.20–6.30
AST	69.50 ± 51.52	50.00	24–346
ALT	60.10 ± 38.55	45.00	20–234

Table 8

	DF		DHF		DSS		EDS		*p* value
	Mean	±SD	Mean	±SD	Mean	±SD	Mean	±SD	
Hb	12.74	±9.81	12.36	±4.16	15.25	±0.35	12.14	±2.14	0.074
PL count (K)	58.24	±41.31	41.11	±15.68	27.5	±17.68	14.4	±3.78	0.003
HCT	38.48	±4.39	39.82	±10.21	43.5	±9.19	40.06	±7.64	0.706
Urea	18.5	±4.75	20.75	±6.22	25	±14.14	19.38	±4.89	0.696
Creatine	1.24	±1.88	0.83	±0.23	0.7	±0.42	0.85	±0.45	0.142
Serum bilirubin	1.18	±0.67	0.89	±0.23	0.7	±0.42	1.08	±0.58	0.042
ALT	62.85	±47.07	89.6	±63.61	128	±11.31	92.2	±65.74	0.039
AST	56.18	±32.61	71.6	±54.61	79	±62.23	80.8	±59.91	0.758

Table 9

Categorisation	Frequency	%
DF	84	73%
DF with Hg	5	4.3%
DHF	19	16.5%
DSS	2	1.70%
EDS	5	4.3%
Total	115	100%

to casualty with history of fever and altered sensorium. On examination he was found to be responding only to painful stimuli with normally reacting pupils and fundus examination. His all investigations were normal except low platelet, mildly raised ALT and AST, and positive NS1 antigen. MRI brain was inconclusive. CSF was sterile on culture with lymphocytosis and normal glucose values. Diagnosis of dengue encephalopathy was made. Patient was given supportive care in ICU with strict monitoring of electrolyte and fluid balance. He started to recover after 6 days. Recovery was prolonged with slight slurring of speech which recovered fully within next two months.

One patient reported drooping of saliva and slurred speech and another acute onset of diplopia with squint. MRI was done to exclude intracranial space occupying lesion or bleed. Provisional diagnosis of facial and lateral rectus nerve palsy was made in consultation with ophthalmologist. Both patients responded well to conservative treatment and recovered without any sequelae within eight weeks.

Out of 115 patients, seven had coinfections with malaria in three (confirmed by Slide test positive for *Plasmodium vivax* malarial parasite and malarial antigen) and typhoid in four confirmed with Widal test as shown in Table 3. Four patients had comorbidities with diabetes and asthma (two subjects each). Diabetic patients had their blood glucose monitored regularly. There was no death or long term disability in our study patients.

9. Discussion

The present study highlighted the varied spectrum of dengue fever ranging from some known clinical presentations of fever, rash, headache to some atypical presentations like acalculous cholecystitis, encephalopathy, myocarditis, and facial and lateral rectus nerve palsy. The atypical manifestations of dengue fever are increasing in recent outbreaks as evidenced by various studies.

Headache and retro-orbital pain are well-known features of dengue fever. In present study we found that 87% of patients had headache as chief complaint and 41% had typical retro-orbital pain. In study by Mandal et al. [6], 62.16% patients presented with headache. In some studies like Itoda et al. [7], 90% of patients presented with headache. On the other hand, Awasthi et al. [8] conducted a study in north India and reported that only 9% of cases had headache as their chief symptom.

With technological advancements like ultrasonography, more and more cases of dengue fever are being reported with ascites and pleural effusion but it is to be done at right time. We have detected third space collection in form of ascites in 6% and pleural effusion in 16% of patients. In a study by Mandal et al., [6] ascites was present in 8.1% and pleural effusion in 18.9% of cases. In Bangladesh based study by Mia et al. [9], 42% had pleural effusion and 41% of patients developed ascites. In ultrasound based study by Kalayanarooj et al. [10], pleural effusion was diagnosed in 18%, which corroborated with the findings of the present study.

Hemorrhagic manifestations are a well-known complication of dengue fever due to decreased platelet count and leakage from blood vessels. Thrombocytopenia may be because of spontaneous aggregation of platelets to virus-infected endothelium, bone marrow suppression, or immune mediated clearance. In our study we found that 20% of patients had hemorrhagic manifestations in the form of epistaxis, hematemesis, hemoptysis, melena, subconjunctival hemorrhage, hematomas, and menorrhagia. Hemorrhagic manifestations were present in 40% of patients in a study by Karoli et al. [11].

In the present study, 78% of patients had platelet count <1 lakh. Singh et al. [12] observed thrombocytopenia in 61.39% of cases. In a study by Mandal et al. [6], 37.8% had platelet count below 50,000 per cubic mm and 13.51% had hemorrhagic manifestations in the form of melena and gum bleeding. In a study by Tripathi et al. [13], only 12.8% had platelet count <70,000 but 28% cases had hematemesis, 26% had melena, and 14.28% had epistaxis. In a Hyderabad based study by Khan et al. [14], only 5% of patients had bleeding while 40% had thrombocytopenia.

Low leucocyte count may be due to virus-induced inhibition of myeloid progenitor cells or due to destruction. We found that 70% had leucocyte count <5000 almost similar to a study by Itoda et al. [7] in which leucopenia was observed in 71% of cases. Ageep et al. [15] detected leucopenia in 90% of cases while Mandal et al. [6] found leucopenia in 29.73% of cases. Elevated transaminases are found to be raised in a large percentage of our study. Dengue fever can cause hepatic injury and elevation of transaminases. 57% of patients had elevated ALT and 49% had raised AST.

57% of patients presented with pain abdomen along with fever. 22% had acalculous cholecystitis with right upper quadrant abdominal pain, positive Murphy's sign, abnormal liver function tests, and thickened gall bladder wall without stones on ultrasonography. The exact mechanism of acalculous cholecystitis in dengue is not known. It could be due to viral invasion of gall bladder wall causing microangiopathic injury and increased vascular permeability leading to protein rich plasma leakage. This could be the cause of thickening of gall bladder wall [1]. Severity as well as progression of dengue fevers has been found to be significantly associated with thickening of gall bladder wall in some studies. The course of disease is usually self-limiting but, in a few patients, acalculous cholecystitis progresses rapidly to ischemic gangrene and perforation. Cholecystectomy is reserved for such patients who progress to peritonitis.

We had five cases of EDS with neurological, cardiovascular, and gastrointestinal involvement. The unusual atypical manifestations, in this study, were of neurological involvement in 3 (2.6%) patients. Neurological involvement in dengue may occur because of neurotropism of the virus, immunological mechanisms, cerebral anoxia, intracranial hemorrhage, hyponatremia, cerebral edema, hepatic failure, renal failure, or release of toxic products. Peter et al. [16] reported isolated facial nerve palsy in dengue fever and Shivanthan et al. [17] have also reported isolated 6th nerve palsy. Donnio et al. [18] reported dengue with a rare presentation of oculomotor nerve palsy. Sanjay et al. [19] reported a case of optic neuropathy associated with dengue fever.

One patient was categorised as EDS due to myocarditis. This patient had benign though prolonged self-limiting course. Bhasin et al. [20] also reported a case of DHF with myocarditis mimicking DSS with hypotension and pulmonary edema.

One patient reported acute respiratory distress syndrome and needed ICU care. ARDS in dengue is due to increased permeability of alveolar capillary membrane, which results in alveolar edema leading to pulmonary dysfunction [21]. Anam et al. [22] had an unusual EDS case presenting as pancreatitis and haemothorax with respiratory distress. This complication requires early recognition and prompt management for favorable outcome.

10. Conclusion

Dengue is a challenging disease with multisystemic, varied, atypical, and sometimes life-threatening presentations. Awareness of these rare manifestations goes a long way in early recognition, correct diagnosis, prompt intervention, and appropriate treatment. Every aspect of dengue viral infection remains a clinical challenge. A continuous seroepidemiological surveillance, timely interventions, vaccines research, and vector control measures are needed to identify the cases so that outbreaks, complications, and mortality can be minimized.

Competing Interests

The authors declare that there is no conflict of interests regarding publication of this paper.

References

[1] S. Gulati and A. Maheshwari, "Atypical manifestations of dengue," *Tropical Medicine and International Health*, vol. 12, no. 9, pp. 1087–1095, 2007.

[2] WHO, "Comprehensive guidelines for prevention and control of dengue and dengue hemorrhagic fever," World Health Organization, Regional Office for South-East Asia, http://apps.searo.who.int/pds_docs/B4751.pdf?ua=1.

[3] B. Pozzetto, M. Memmi, and O. Garraud, "Is transfusion-transmitted dengue fever a potential public health threat?" *World Journal of Virology*, vol. 4, no. 2, pp. 113–123, 2015.

[4] F. L. Tan, D. L. Loh, K. Prabhakaran, P. A. Tambyah, and H. K. Yap, "Dengue haemorrhagic fever after living donor renal transplantation," *Nephrology Dialysis Transplantation*, vol. 20, no. 2, pp. 447–448, 2005.

[5] S. H. Pouliot, X. Xiong, E. Harville et al., "Maternal dengue and pregnancy outcomes: a systematic review," *Obstetrical and Gynecological Survey*, vol. 65, no. 2, pp. 107–118, 2010.

[6] S. K. Mandal, J. Ganguly, K. Sil et al., "Clinical profiles of dengue fever in a teaching hospital of eastern India," *National Journal of Medical Research*, vol. 3, no. 2, pp. 173–176, 2013.

[7] I. Itoda, G. Masuda, A. Suganuma et al., "Clinical features of 62 imported cases of dengue fever in Japan," *American Journal of Tropical Medicine and Hygiene*, vol. 75, no. 3, pp. 470–474, 2006.

[8] S. Awasthi, V. K. Singh, S. Kumar, A. Kumar, and S. Dutta, "The changing clinical spectrum of Dengue fever in the 2009 epidemic in north India: a tertiary teaching hospital based study," *Journal of Clinical and Diagnostic Research*, vol. 6, no. 6, pp. 999–1002, 2012.

[9] M. W. Mia, A. M. Nurullah, A. Hossain, and M. M. Haque, "Clinical and sonographic evaluation of dengue fever in Bangladesh: a study of 100 cases," *Dinajpur Medical College Journal*, vol. 3, pp. 29–34, 2010.

[10] S. Kalayanarooj, D. W. Vaughn, S. Nimmannitya et al., "Early clinical and laboratory indicators of acute dengue illness," *The Journal of Infectious Diseases*, vol. 176, no. 2, pp. 313–321, 1997.

[11] R. Karoli, J. Fatima, Z. Siddiqi, K. I. Kazmi, and A. R. Sultania, "Clinical profile of dengue infection at a teaching hospital in North India," *Journal of Infection in Developing Countries*, vol. 6, no. 7, pp. 551–554, 2012.

[12] N. P. Singh, R. Jhamb, S. K. Agarwal et al., "The 2003 outbreak of dengue fever in Delhi, India," *Southeast Asian Journal of Tropical Medicine and Public Health*, vol. 36, no. 5, pp. 1174–1178, 2005.

[13] B. K. Tripathi, B. Gupta, R. S. K. Sinha, S. Prasad, and D. K. Sharma, "Experience in adult population in dengue outbreak in Delhi," *Journal of Association of Physicians of India*, vol. 46, no. 3, pp. 273–276, 1998.

[14] A. H. Khan, A. S. Hayat, N. Masood, N. M. Solangi, and T. Z. Shaikh, "Frequency and clinical presentation of dengue fever at tertiary care hospital of Hyderabad/Jamshoro," *Journal of the Liaquat University of Medical and Health Sciences*, vol. 9, no. 2, pp. 88–94, 2010.

[15] A. K. Ageep, A. A. Malik, and M. S. Elkarsani, "Clinical presentations and laboratory findings in suspected cases of dengue virus," *Saudi Medical Journal*, vol. 27, no. 11, pp. 1711–1713, 2006.

[16] S. Peter, N. Malhotra, P. Peter, and R. Sood, "Isolated Bell's palsy—an unusual presentation of dengue infection," *Asian Pacific Journal of Tropical Medicine*, vol. 6, no. 1, pp. 82–84, 2013.

[17] M. C. Shivanthan, E. C. Ratnayake, B. C. Wijesiriwardena, K. C. Somaratna, and L. K. G. K. Gamagedara, "Paralytic squint due to abducens nerve palsy: a rare consequence of dengue fever," *BMC Infectious Diseases*, vol. 12, article 156, 2012.

[18] A. Donnio, L. Béral, S. Olindo, A. Cabie, and H. Merle, "Dengue, a new etiology of oculomotor paralysis," *Canadian Journal of Ophthalmology*, vol. 45, no. 2, pp. 183–184, 2010.

[19] S. Sanjay, A. M. Wagle, and K. G. Au Eong, "Optic neuropathy associated with dengue fever," *Eye*, vol. 22, no. 5, pp. 722–724, 2008.

[20] A. Bhasin, R. Kumar, K. Chandra, and R. K. Singal, "Dengue fever with myocarditis," *Journal, Indian Academy of Clinical Medicine*, vol. 14, no. 2, pp. 187–189, 2013.

[21] L. C. S. Lum, M. K. Thong, Y. K. Cheah, and S. K. Lam, "Dengue-associated adult respiratory distress syndrome," *Annals of Tropical Paediatrics*, vol. 15, no. 4, pp. 335–339, 1995.

[22] A. M. Anam, R. Rabbani, F. Shumy, and M. M. I. Polash, "Subsequent pancreatitis and haemothorax in a patient of expanded dengue syndrome," *Tropical Doctor*, vol. 46, no. 1, pp. 40–42, 2016.

Permissions

All chapters in this book were first published in JTM, by Hindawi Publishing Corporation; hereby published with permission under the Creative Commons Attribution License or equivalent. Every chapter published in this book has been scrutinized by our experts. Their significance has been extensively debated. The topics covered herein carry significant findings which will fuel the growth of the discipline. They may even be implemented as practical applications or may be referred to as a beginning point for another development.

The contributors of this book come from diverse backgrounds, making this book a truly international effort. This book will bring forth new frontiers with its revolutionizing research information and detailed analysis of the nascent developments around the world.

We would like to thank all the contributing authors for lending their expertise to make the book truly unique. They have played a crucial role in the development of this book. Without their invaluable contributions this book wouldn't have been possible. They have made vital efforts to compile up to date information on the varied aspects of this subject to make this book a valuable addition to the collection of many professionals and students.

This book was conceptualized with the vision of imparting up-to-date information and advanced data in this field. To ensure the same, a matchless editorial board was set up. Every individual on the board went through rigorous rounds of assessment to prove their worth. After which they invested a large part of their time researching and compiling the most relevant data for our readers.

The editorial board has been involved in producing this book since its inception. They have spent rigorous hours researching and exploring the diverse topics which have resulted in the successful publishing of this book. They have passed on their knowledge of decades through this book. To expedite this challenging task, the publisher supported the team at every step. A small team of assistant editors was also appointed to further simplify the editing procedure and attain best results for the readers.

Apart from the editorial board, the designing team has also invested a significant amount of their time in understanding the subject and creating the most relevant covers. They scrutinized every image to scout for the most suitable representation of the subject and create an appropriate cover for the book.

The publishing team has been an ardent support to the editorial, designing and production team. Their endless efforts to recruit the best for this project, has resulted in the accomplishment of this book. They are a veteran in the field of academics and their pool of knowledge is as vast as their experience in printing. Their expertise and guidance has proved useful at every step. Their uncompromising quality standards have made this book an exceptional effort. Their encouragement from time to time has been an inspiration for everyone.

The publisher and the editorial board hope that this book will prove to be a valuable piece of knowledge for researchers, students, practitioners and scholars across the globe.

List of Contributors

Maria Gabriela Silva Guimarães, Athos Muniz Braña, Humberto Oliart-Guzmán, Fernando Luiz Cunha Castelo Branco, Breno Matos Delfino, Thasciany Moraes Pereira, Saulo Augusto Silva Mantovani, Antonio CamargoMartins, Ana Paula Santos, José Alcântara Filgueira-Júnior, Alanderson Alves Ramalho, Andreia da Silva Guimarães, Cristieli Sérgio de Menezes Oliveira, Thiago Santos de Araújo and Mônica da Silva-Nunes
Centro de Ciências da Saúde e do Desporto, Universidade Federal do Acre, Campus Universitário, BR 364, km 04, Bairro Distrito Industrial, 69920-900 Rio Branco, AC, Brazil

Carlos Hermógenes Manrique de Lara Estrada
Dirección Regional de Salud de Madre de Dios, Avenida Ernesto Rivero N□ 475, Puerto Maldonado, Peru

Nancy Arróspide
Instituto Nacional de Salud, Cápac Yupanqui 1400, Jesus María, 15072 Lima 11, Peru

Syed Raza Shah,Muhammad Shahzeb Khan, Muhammad Tanveer Alam, Adnan Salim,Mehwish Hussain and Areeba Altaf
Dow University of Health Sciences (DUHS), Baba e Urdu Road, Karachi 75500, Pakistan

Keneuoe Hycianth Thinyane and Keanole Mofona Motsemme
Department of Pharmacy, National University of Lesotho, Roma 180, Lesotho

Varsay Jim Lahai Cooper
Department of Internal Medicine, Queen Mamohato Memorial Hospital, Maseru 100, Lesotho

Antonio Ortega-Pacheco, Juan F. J. Torres-Acosta, Alejandro Alzina-López, Eduardo Gutiérrez-Blanco, Manuel E. Bolio-González, Armando J. Aguilar-Caballero, Roger I. Rodríguez-Vivas, Edwin Gutiérrez-Ruiz and Alberto Rosado-Aguilar
Departamento Salud Animal y Medicina Preventiva, Cuerpo Académico en Salud Animal, Facultad de Medicina Veterinaria y Zootecnia, Universidad Autónoma de Yucatán, Km 15.5 Carr. Mérida Xmatkuil, AP 4-116, Mérida, YUC, Mexico

Karla Y. Acosta-Viana, Eugenia Guzmán-Marín and Matilde Jiménez-Coello
Laboratorio de Biología Celular, CA Biomedicina de Enfermedades Infecciosas y Parasitarias. C.I.R. "Dr. Hideyo Noguchi", Universidad Autónoma de Yucatán, Avenida Itzaes, No. 490 x C. 59, 97000Mérida, YUC, Mexico

Alberto Tobón-Castaño, EstebanMesa-Echeverry and Andrés Felipe Miranda-Arboleda
Grupo Malaria, Facultad de Medicina, Universidad de Antioquia, Calle 70, No. 52-21, Medellín, Colombia

Muhammad Redzwan S. Rashid Ali
Department of Respiratory Medicine, Queen Elizabeth Hospital, 88000 Kota Kinabalu, Sabah, Malaysia

Uma Parameswaran
Infectious Diseases Unit, Clinical Research Centre, Queen Elizabeth Hospital, 88000 Kota Kinabalu, Sabah, Malaysia

Elspeth Bird and Christopher S. Wilkes
3Infectious Diseases Society Sabah-Menzies School of Health Research Clinical Research Unit, 88000 Kota Kinabalu, Sabah, Malaysia

Timothy William
Infectious Diseases Unit, Clinical Research Centre, Queen Elizabeth Hospital, 88000 Kota Kinabalu, Sabah, Malaysia
Infectious Diseases Society Sabah-Menzies School of Health Research Clinical Research Unit, 88000 Kota Kinabalu, Sabah, Malaysia
Sabah Department of Health, 88000 Kota Kinabalu, Sabah, Malaysia

Wai Khew Lee
Luyang Outpatient Clinic, 88000 Kota Kinabalu, Sabah, Malaysia

Tsin Wen Yeo
Infectious Diseases Society Sabah-Menzies School of Health Research Clinical Research Unit, 88000 Kota Kinabalu, Sabah,Malaysia
Global and Tropical Health Division, Menzies School of Health Research, Darwin, NT 0811, Australia

Nicholas M. Anstey and Anna P. Ralph
Infectious Diseases Society Sabah-Menzies School of Health Research Clinical Research Unit, 88000 Kota Kinabalu, Sabah,Malaysia
Global and Tropical Health Division, Menzies School of Health Research, Darwin, NT 0811, Australia
Department of Medicine, Royal Darwin Hospital, Darwin, NT 0811, Australia

Iraj Khodadadi, Heidar Tavilani and Ebrahim Abbasi Oshaghi
Department of Clinical Biochemistry, Medical School, Hamadan University of Medical Sciences, Hamadan, Iran

Mohammad Taghi Goodarzi
Research Center for Molecular Medicine, Hamadan University of Medical Sciences, Hamadan, Iran

Reza Taherkhani, Fatemeh Farshadpour, Behrouz Naeimi and Saeed Tajbakhsh
Department ofMicrobiology and Parasitology, School ofMedicine, Bushehr University ofMedical Sciences, Bushehr 7514633341, Iran
Persian Gulf Tropical Medicine Research Centre, Bushehr University of Medical Sciences, Bushehr 7514633341, Iran

Samad Akbarzadeh
Persian Gulf Tropical Medicine Research Centre, Bushehr University of Medical Sciences, Bushehr 7514633341, Iran

Manoochehr Makvandi and Ali Reza Samarbafzadeh
Health Research Institute, Infectious and Tropical Disease Research Centre, Ahvaz Jundishapur University of Medical Sciences, Ahvaz 6135715794, Iran

Hamid Rajabi Memari
Department of Agronomy and Plant Breeding, Faculty of Agriculture, Ahvaz Shahid Chamran University, Ahvaz 6135715794, Iran

Nasrin Sharifi
Department of Nutrition, School of Medicine, Kashan University of Medical Sciences, Kashan 8715988141, Iran

Aristide S. Hien, Sanata Coulibaly, Abdoulaye Diabaté and Roch K. Dabiré
IRSS/Centre Muraz, Bobo-Dioulasso, Burkina Faso

Ibrahim Sangaré, Moussa Namountougou, Léa Paré-Toé and Anicet Georges Ouédraogo
Université Polytechnique de Bobo-Dioulasso, Bobo-Dioulasso, Burkina Faso

Brian D. Foy
Colorado State University, Fort Collins, CO, USA

Samuel Anu Olowookere, Emmanuel Akintunde Abioye-Kuteyi, Olusegun Kayode Adepoju, Oluwaseun Taiwo Esan, TemitopeMichael Adeolu, Tolulope Kola Adeoye, Adesola Adebayo Adepoju and Adedayo Titilayo Aderogba
Department of Community Health, College of Health Sciences, Obafemi Awolowo University, Ile-Ife, Nigeria

Ibrahim Shady
Community Medicine Department, Faculty of Medicine, Mansoura University, Mansoura 35516, Egypt

Muhammad Azharuddin Azali
School of Agriculture Science and Biotechnology, Faculty of Bioresources and Food Industry, Universiti Sultan Zainal Abidin, Tembila Campus, 22200 Besut, Terengganu, Malaysia

Chan Yean Yean, Azian Harun, Nurul Najian Aminuddin Baki and Nabilah Ismail
Department of Medical Microbiology and Parasitology, School of Medical Sciences, Health Campus, Universiti Sains Malaysia, 16150 Kubang Kerian, Kelantan, Malaysia

Umar Muhammad Lawan
Department of Community Medicine, Bayero University and Aminu Kano Teaching Hospital, Kano 700001, Nigeria

Idris Usman Takai
Department of Obstetrics and Gynaecology, Bayero University and Aminu Kano Teaching Hospital, Kano 700001, Nigeria

Hamza Ishaq
College of Health Sciences, Bayero University, Kano 700001, Nigeria

Ramachandran Sudarshan
Department ofOralMedicine and Radiology, Best Dental Science College andHospital, Madurai 625104, India

G. Sree Vijayabala
Department of Dentistry, ESIC Medical College and PGIMSR, Ashok Pillar Road, KK Nagar, Chennai 600078, India

Y. Samata and A. Ravikiran
Department of Oral Medicine and Radiology, SIBAR Institute of Dental Sciences, Guntur 522509, India

Gerardo Alvarez-Uria, ManoranjanMidde, Raghavakalyan Pakam, Pradeep Sukumar Yalla and Praveen Kumar Naik
Department of Infectious Diseases, RDT Bathalapalli Hospital, Kadiri Road, Bathalapalli 515661, India

Raghuprakash Reddy
Department of Microbiology, RDT Bathalapalli Hospital, Kadiri Road, Bathalapalli 515661, India

Mida Kautako-Kiambi and Smith Kama-Lemba
Centre de Santée de Référence et Maternité de la Cité de Mbanza-Ngungu, Mbanza-Ngungu, Bas-Congo, Democratic Republic of the Congo

Mathilde B. Ekila
Division of Infectious Diseases, Department of Internal Medicine, University Hospital of Kinshasa, School of Medicine, University of Kinshasa, Kinshasa, Democratic Republic of the Congo

Roger Wumba
Department of Tropical Medicine, University Hospital of Kinshasa, Faculty of Medicine, University of Kinshasa, Kinshasa, Democratic Republic of the Congo

Michel N. Aloni
Division of Hemato-Oncology and Nephrology, Department of Pediatrics, University Hospital of Kinshasa, School of Medicine, University of Kinshasa, Kinshasa, Democratic Republic of the Congo

Sin-Yeang Teow
Sunway Institute for Healthcare Development (SIHD), Sunway University, 47500 Bandar Sunway, Selangor Darul Ehsan, Malaysia

Kitson Liew
Molecular Pathology Unit, Cancer Research Centre (CaRC), Institute for Medical Research (IMR), 50588 Jalan Pahang, Kuala Lumpur, Malaysia

Syed A. Ali
Advanced Medical and Dental Institute (AMDI), Universiti Sains Malaysia (USM), 13200 Kepala Batas, Pulau Pinang, Malaysia

Alan Soo-Beng Khoo
Molecular Pathology Unit, Cancer Research Centre (CaRC), Institute for Medical Research (IMR), 50588 Jalan Pahang, Kuala Lumpur, Malaysia
Institute for Research, Development and Innovation, International Medical University (IMU), 57000 Bukit Jalil, Kuala Lumpur, Malaysia

Suat-Cheng Peh
Sunway Institute for Healthcare Development (SIHD), Sunway University, 47500 Bandar Sunway, Selangor Darul Ehsan, Malaysia
Anatomical Pathology Department, Sunway Medical Centre, 47500 Bandar Sunway, Selangor Darul Ehsan, Malaysia

Chai Lee Tan, Evelyn Li Min Tai, Julieana Muhammed, Liza Sharmini Ahmad Tajudin and Wan-Hazabbah Wan Hitam
Department of Ophthalmology, School of Medical Sciences, Universiti Sains Malaysia, Health Campus, 16150 Kubang Kerian, Kelantan, Malaysia

Lai Chan Fhun
Department of Ophthalmology, School of Medical Sciences, Universiti Sains Malaysia, Health Campus, 16150 Kubang Kerian, Kelantan, Malaysia
2Department of Ophthalmology, Hospital Raja Permaisuri Bainun, 30990 Ipoh, Perak, Malaysia

Nor Hasnida Abdul Gani and Tengku Norina Tuan Jaafar
Department of Ophthalmology, Hospital Raja Perempuan Zainab 2, 15586 Kota Bharu, Kelantan, Malaysia

Jasem Saki and Reza Asadpouri
Health Research Institute, Infectious and Tropical Diseases Research Center, Ahvaz Jundishapur University of Medical Science, Ahvaz, Iran
Department of Medical Parasitology, Faculty of Medicine, Ahvaz Jundishapur University of Medical Sciences, Ahvaz, Iran

Masoud Foroutan-Rad
Department of Parasitology, Faculty of Medical Sciences, Tarbiat Modares University, Tehran, Iran

Williams H.Makunde
National Institute for Medical Research, Tanga Research Centre, P.O. Box 5004, Tanga, Tanzania

Happyness J. Mshana
National Institute for Medical Research, Tanga Research Centre, P.O. Box 5004, Tanga, Tanzania
Sokoine University of Agriculture, Morogoro, Tanzania

Vito Baraka
National Institute for Medical Research, Tanga Research Centre, P.O. Box 5004, Tanga, Tanzania
Global Health Institute, University of Antwerp, Antwerp, Belgium

Gerald Misinzo
National Institute for Medical Research, Tanga Research Centre, P.O. Box 5004, Tanga, Tanzania

Samarendra Mahapatro, Amit Kumar Satapathy and Rashmi Ranjan Das
Department of Pediatrics, All India Institute of Medical Sciences, Bhubaneswar, India

Nijwm Mahilary
Department of Pediatrics, Hi-Tech Medical College and Hospital, Bhubaneswar, India

Aniekan Jumbo Etokidem
Department of Community Medicine, University of Calabar, Calabar 540001, Cross River State, Nigeria

Ofonime Johnson
Department of Community Medicine, University of Uyo, Uyo 520101, Akwa Ibom State, Nigeria

Voravuth Somsak, Preeyanuch Borkaew, Chokdee Klubsri, Kittiyaporn Dondee, Panatda Bootprom and Butsarat Saiphet
Department of Clinical Chemistry, Faculty of Medical Technology,Western University, Kanchanaburi 71170,Thailand

Muhammad Faruk Bashir
Department of Paediatrics, Abubakar Tafawa Balewa University Teaching Hospital, Bauchi 740222, Nigeria

Hassan Abdullahi Elechi, Mohammed Garba Ashir, Adamu Ibrahim Rabasa, Modu Gofama Mustapha and Mohammad Arab Alhaji
Department of Paediatrics, University of Maiduguri, Maiduguri 600243, Nigeria

David Nadeba Bukbuk
Department of Microbiology, University of Maiduguri, Maiduguri 600243, Nigeria

Ahmadu Baba Usman
Department of Paediatrics, Federal Medical Centre Yola, Yola 640101, Nigeria

Gitonga N. Mburugu
School of Health Sciences, Meru University of Science and Technology, P.O. Box 972-60200, Meru, Kenya

Zablon K. Njiru
School of Health Sciences, Meru University of Science and Technology, P.O. Box 972-60200, Meru, Kenya
School of Health Professions, Murdoch University, Mandurah Campus, Education Drive, Mandurah,WA 6210, Australia

Cecilia K. Mbae
Kenya Medical Research Institute, Centre for Microbiology Research, P.O. Box 19464-00202, Nairobi, Kenya

Clara Wekesa, Gershim Asiki, Ivan Kasamba, LabanWaswa, Rebecca N. Nsubuga, Rob Newton and Anatoli Kamali
Medical Research Council/Uganda Virus Research Institute Uganda Research Unit on AIDS, Entebbe, Uganda

Steven J. Reynolds
Division of Intramural Research, National Institute of Allergy and Infectious Diseases, National Institutes of Health, Bethesda, MD 20892, USA
Johns Hopkins School of Medicine, Baltimore, MD 21205, USA

Aaron S.Miller and Lawrence C. Loh
University of Toronto, Toronto, ON, Canada M5S 1A1
The 53rdWeek, Brooklyn, NY 11201, USA

Chang-Berm Kang
The 53rdWeek, Brooklyn, NY 11201, USA

Henry C. Lin
The 53rdWeek, Brooklyn, NY 11201, USA
Perelman School of Medicine, University of Pennsylvania, Philadelphia, PA 19104, USA

Nercy Virginia Rabelo Furtado, Allan Kardec Ribeiro Galardo and Clicia Denis Galardo
Laboratório de Entomologia Médica, Instituto de Pesquisas Científicas e Tecnológicas do Estado do Amapá, Macapá, AP, Brazil

Viviane Caetano Firmino
Universidade Federal do Amapá, Campus Binacional, Oiapoque, AP, Brazil

Thiago Vasconcelos dos Santos
Instituto Evandro Chagas, Secretaria de Vigilância em Saúde, Minist´erio da Saúde, Ananindeua, PA, Brazil

Fernanda Alvarenga CardosoMedeiros, Luciana Inácia Gomes, Edward Oliveira, Carolina Senra Alves de Souza, Maria Vitória Mourão, Gláucia Fernandes Cota and Ana Rabello
Centro de Pesquisas René Rachou, Oswaldo Cruz Foundation (Fiocruz), Belo Horizonte, MG, Brazil

Letícia Helena dos Santos Marques and Mariângela Carneiro
Departamento de Parasitologia, Instituto de Ciências Biológicas, Universidade Federal de Minas Gerais, Belo Horizonte, MG, Brazil

Anish Laul
Maulana Azad Medical College, No. 2, Bahadur Shah Zafar Marg, New Delhi, Delhi 110002, India

Poonam Laul, Vamsi Merugumala, Ravi Pathak, Urvashi Miglani and Pinkee Saxena
Deen Dayal Upadhyay Hospital, Hari Nagar, Clock Tower, New Delhi, Delhi 110064, India

Index